HANDBOOK OF
PALLIATIVE CARE

E00924

Handbook of Palliative Care

EDITED BY

CHRISTINA FAULL
MB BS, BMed Sci, MD, MRCP
Medical Director and Consultant in Palliative Care
St Mary's Hospice, Raddlebarn Road
Selly Park, Birmingham

YVONNE CARTER
MB BS, MD, FRCGP
Professor of General Practice and Primary Care
Department of General Practice and Primary Care
St Bartholomew's and
The Royal London School of Medicine and Dentistry
Queen Mary and Westfield College, University of London

RICHARD WOOF
MB BS, MRCGP
Clinical Lecturer
Department of General Practice
The Medical School, University of Birmingham
Edgbaston, Birmingham

Blackwell
Science

© 1998 by
Blackwell Science Ltd
Editorial Offices:
Osney Mead, Oxford OX2 OEL
25 John Street, London WC1N 2BL
23 Ainslie Place, Edinburgh EH3 6AJ
350 Main Street, Malden
    MA 02148 5018, USA
54 University Street, Carlton
    Victoria 3053, Australia
10, rue Casimir Delavigne
    75006 Paris, France

Other Editorial Offices:

Blackwell Wissenschafts-Verlag GmbH
Kurfürstendamm 57
10707 Berlin, Germany

Blackwell Science KK
MG Kodenmacho Building
7-10 Kodenmacho Nihombashi
Chuo-ku, Tokyo 104, Japan

The right of the Authors to be
identified as the Authors of this
Work has been asserted in accordance
with the Copyright, Designs and
Patents Act 1988.

First published 1998
Reprinted 1999, 2000

Set by Setrite Typesetters, Hong Kong
Printed and bound in the United Kingdom
at the University Press, Cambridge

The Blackwell Science logo is a
trade mark of Blackwell Science Ltd,
registered at the United Kingdom
Trade Marks Registry

DISTRIBUTORS

Marston Book Services Ltd
PO Box 269
Abingdon Oxon OX14 4YN
(*Orders*: Tel: 01235 465500
        Fax: 01235 465555)

USA
Blackwell Science, Inc.
Commerce Place
350 Main Street
Malden, MA 02148 5018
(*Orders*: Tel: 800 759 6102
                781 388 8250
        Fax: 781 388 8255)

Canada
Login Brothers Book Company
324 Saulteaux Crescent
Winnipeg, Manitoba R3J 3T2
(*Orders*: Tel: 204 837 2987)

Australia
Blackwell Science Pty Ltd
54 University Street
Carlton, Victoria 3053
(*Orders*: Tel: 03 9347 0300
        Fax: 03 9347 5001)

A catalogue record for this title
is available from the British Library

ISBN 0-632-04779-8

Library of Congress
Cataloging-in-Publication Data

Handbook of palliative care / edited by
    Christina Faull, Yvonne Carter and
    Richard Woof.
        p.   cm.
    Includes bibliographical references
    and index.
    ISBN 0-632-04779-8
    1. Palliative treatment—Handbooks,
manuals, etc. I. Faull, Christina. II. Carter,
Yvonne, 1959-. III. Woof, Richard.
    [DNLM: 1. Palliative Care handbooks.
WB 39 H23653 1998]
R726.8.H355 1998
362.1′75—dc21
DNLM/DLC   98-9866
for Library of Congress   CIP

For further information on
Blackwell Science, visit our website:
www.blackwell-science.com

Contents

List of Contributors

RACHAEL BARTON *Clinical Research Fellow in Oncology, Institute for Cancer Studies, University of Birmingham, The Medical School, Edgbaston, Birmingham, B15 2TT*

CAROLE ANN BLACKSHAW *Lecturer and Clinical Course Manager, Department of Medicines Management, University of Keele, Keele, Staffordshire, ST5 5BG*

YVONNE CARTER *Professor of General Practice and Primary Care, Department of General Practice and Primary Care, St Bartholomew's and The Royal London School of Medicine and Dentistry, Queen Mary and Westfield College, University of London, London, E1 4NS*

MARIE FALLON *Senior Lecturer in Palliative Medicine, Department of Palliative Medicine, Western Infirmary, West Glasgow University Hospital NHS Trust, Dunbarton Road, Glasgow, G11 6NT*

CHRISTINA FAULL *Medical Director and Consultant in Palliative Care, St Mary's Hospice, Raddlebarn Road, Selly Park, Birmingham, B29 7DA; Honorary Senior Lecturer, Institute for Cancer Studies, University of Birmingham, Edgbaston, Birmingham, B15 2TT*

KAREN FORBES *Senior Lecturer in Palliative Medicine, Department of Palliative Medicine, Oncology Centre, Horfield Road, Bristol, BS2 8ED*

ANN GOLDMAN *Senior Lecturer in Palliative Care and Consultant Paediatrician, Haematology and Oncology Unit, Hospital for Sick Children, Great Ormond Street, London, WC1N 3JH*

DENISE HARDY *Clinical Nurse Specialist in Lymphoedema, Saint Giles' Hospice, Fisherwick Road, Whittington, Lichfield, WS14 9LH*

BOB HARRISON *Clinical Nurse Specialist in Palliative Care, Home Care Team Leader, Saint Mary's Hospice, 176 Raddlebarn Road, Selly Park, Birmingham, B29 7DA*

FIONA HICKS *Consultant in Palliative Medicine, K Block, Saint James' University Hospital, Beckett Street, Leeds, LS9 7TF*

IRENE HIGGINSON *Professor of Palliative Care, King's College London and St Christopher's Hospice, 51–59 Lawrire Park Road, Sydenham, SE26 6DZ*

DAVID JEFFREY *Consultant in Palliative Care, Three Counties Cancer Centre, Sandford Road, Cheltenham, Gloucester, GL53 7AN*

JEREMY JOHNSON *Medical Director and Consultant in Palliative Care, Shropshire and Mid Wales Hospice, Bicton Health, Shrewsbury, SY3 8HS*

GWYNETH JONES *Infectious Diseases Specialist, Dumfries and Galloway Royal Infirmary, Bankend Road, Dumfries, DG1 4AP*

BRIAN NYATANGA *Lecturer in Palliative Care, Saint Richard's Hospice, Rose Hill House, Rose Hill, Worcester, WR5 1EY*

NICKY RUDD *Consultant in Palliative Medicine, LOROS, Groby Road, Leicester, LE3 9QE*

ELIZABETH THOMPSON *Senior Registrar, Glasgow Homoeopathic Hospital, 1000 Great Western Road, Glasgow, G12 0NR*

MARY WALDING *Ward Sister, Sir Michael Sobell House, Churchill Hospital, Headington, Oxford, OX3 7DU*

JOHN WELSH *Macmillan Professor in the Olav Kerr Chair of Palliative Medicine, Department of Palliative Medicine, Beatson Oncology Centre, Western Infirmary, Glasgow, G11 6NT*

ANDREW WILCOCK *Macmillan Senior Lecturer in Palliative Medicine and Medical Oncology, Hayward House Specialist Palliative Care Unit, City Hospital, Hucknall Road, Nottingham, NG5 1PB*

PATRICIA WILKIE *Lay Chairman of Patient's Liaison Group, Dennington, Ridgeway, Horsell, Woking, Surrey, GU21 4QR*

RICHARD WOOF *Clinical Lecturer, Department of General Practice, The Medical School, University of Birmingham, Edgbaston, Birmingham, B15 2TT; Corbett Medical Practice, 36 Corbett Ave, Droitwich Spa, Worcestershire, WR9 7BE; Clinical Assistant, St Richard's Hospice, Worcester*

JANE WORLDING *Registrar, Department of Clinical Oncology, Leicester Royal Infirmary, Infirmary Square, Leicester LE1 5WW*

CATHERINE ZOLLMAN *Director Medical Education Services, Research Council for Complementary Therapies, 60 Great Ormond St, London WC1N 3JF*

Foreword

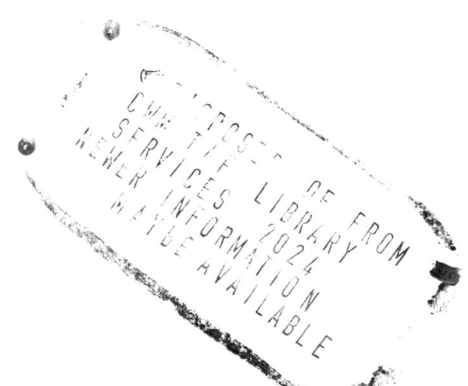

Most people if given a choice and a supportive home, would choose to die at home and the care of the dying is a traditional part of good general practice. It is a different and rather special form of medical practice and it can be both very demanding and rewarding. In recent years two organizational developments have greatly strengthened the potential for good care: the expanding primary health care team, and especially the practice-attached district nurses, and support from outside the practice through Marie Curie or hospice staff.

A third important development has been the advent of new drugs and techniques and research clarifying how best to manage the many symptoms which can occur. Medicine has more to offer than ever before, but only at the price of systematic study and learning. Despite the growing number of courses and electronic information on offer, most doctors and nurses learn mainly from reading. They therefore need a book with a broad comprehensive approach and which covers the entire spectrum of common symptoms and problems experienced by patients. This book provides a logical and ordered way of responding in the light of advancing medical practice. It often introduces its topics from an epidemiological perspective and it meets all reasonable needs. In addition, it offers thoughtful contributions on some wider aspects of palliative care, including HIV infections, teamwork, and audit. Unlike many other texts it includes a chapter on complementary medicine. It is an attractive feature that the chapters are well referenced and it is easy to check and follow sources used.

This is a relatively big book and it is packed with information. It brings together in one text the information now needed by primary healthcare teams as they care for what is likely to be an increasing number of patients who will choose in future to die at home. It can be confidently recommended as a useful addition both to practice and hospital libraries.

Denis Pereira Gray OBE
*President of the Royal College
of General Practitioners*

Preface

The aim of this book is to outline the principles, and to serve as a reference point, for both the everyday and unusual practical issues of palliative care. The handbook provides a solid basis for the management of patients whilst also introducing the range of skills in palliative care relevant to health care professionals in community and hospital settings. Its contents are aimed towards readers from medicine, nursing, pharmacy and other health professions; it should also prove invaluable to undergraduates.

The care of patients with an advanced disease at their home is a common part of the work of family doctors and the primary health care team. Within a hospital environment this care, including the breaking of bad news, is frequently the role of junior doctors. Although palliative care can be extremely rewarding, many tend to shy away from this work. We are not always confident in our skills in symptom control and communication, and can be reluctant to use powerful analgesics in effective doses. Often we can fail to anticipate the problems that disease progression and the side effects of treatments can bring and the work is carried out using underdeveloped teams. *The Handbook of Palliative Care* deals with all of these difficult areas in some detail. For example, when discussing therapeutic interventions we have used the most up-to-date information possible to help professionals with recent developments and have shown no intentional favouritism between drugs or preparations of drugs unless there is a clear basis of evidence to do so. Where possible, we have looked to the future, particularly when discussing challenges to the provision of services for patients and new therapeutic potentials.

Some health care workers worry about the demands good palliative care requires of their time; others are afraid to expose themselves to painful and often unresolved emotions. Many find care of the dying a stressful and draining experience. These are recognized issues in this handbook. We will discuss the ethical dilemmas that are faced and the potential emotional cost to ourselves in caring for patients with advanced disease.

All patients with advanced disease need a holistic approach to their care, focusing on the quality of their life. Patients should have access to comprehensive community based services, including specialist palliative care services such as hospices. Their care should be *patient centred* and as such the views of patients and their carers have been included in this handbook.

It is difficult to define the scope of palliative care. This book does not set out to encompass all of the subject nor does it deal solely with patients who have cancer. Each chapter considers the needs of patients with advanced disease. In addition chapters specifically on motor neurone disease and AIDS are included since good palliative care is vital in these particularly complex disorders. Those stimulated to further exploration of any topic will find suggestions for further reading at the end of each chapter.

In order to continue to improve services and develop confidence in the delivery of palliative care GPs, primary health care teams, and hospital doctors need to monitor the care that they provide and audit their experience and practice against standards and examples of good practice. We hope that the inclusion of a chapter on audit and outcomes will facilitate this.

To provide good palliative care for all, effort is required. The skills of symptom control must be applied holistically by a multidisciplinary team. Good interdisciplinary working depends on mutual respect for the training, knowledge, skills, experience and inexperience of each other. It demands a level of communication that often requires training and active team building.

In background, the three editors of this book are all experienced teachers of both undergraduates and postgraduates. Perhaps more importantly we are experienced in day-to-day clinical care in both community- and secondary-care settings. We recognize that as doctors we also are prone to default to a medical model of illness, need and care. This book has gathered together what we consider to be an impressive array of contributors, with a wide variety of experience. *The Handbook of Palliative Care* conveys the excitement and enthusiasm each contributor feels for their subject, and will, we hope, provide practical guidance for those delivering care for patients and their carers.

The editors would like to acknowledge their thanks to the co-authors and to the commissioning editor, Marcela Holmes for her patience and professional guidance in the preparation and development of this book.

Christina Faull, Yvonne Carter, Richard Woof

Abbreviations List

5HT	5-hydroxytryptophan (serotonin)
ACh(m)	acetylcholine (muscarinic)
ACT	Association for Children with life-threatening or Terminal conditions and their families
AIDS	acquired immune deficiency syndrome
b.d.	*bis die* (Latin) 'twice a day'
BMA	British Medical Association
CM	complementary medicine
CNS	central nervous system
COPD	chronic obstructive pulmonary disease
CT	chemotherapy
D	dopamine
GABA	gamma-amino-butyric acid
GI	gastrointestinal
GP	general practitioner
H	histamine
h	hour
HIV	human immunodeficiency virus
i.d.	intradermal
i.m.	intramuscular
i.p.	intraperitoneal
i.v.	intravenous
kPa	kilopascal
l	litre
mg	milligram
ml	millilitre
mmol	millimole
MND	motor neurone disease
MRI	magnetic resonance imaging
NHS	National Health Service
NSAID	non-steroidal anti-inflammatory drug
o.d.	*omni die* (once daily)
PCP	*Pneumocystis carinii* pneumonia

PEG	percutaneous endoscopic gastrostomy
PHCT	primary health care team
p.o.	*per os* (Latin); oral administration
p.r.	*per rectum* (Latin); rectal administration
p.r.n.	*pro re nata* (Latin) 'as required'
q.d.s.	'four times a day'
RCGP	Royal College of General Practitioners
RPSGB	Royal Pharmaceutical Society of Great Britain
RT	radiotherapy
s.c.	subcutaneous
SSRI	selective serotonin reuptake inhibitor
stat.	*statim* (Latin) 'immediately'
SVCO	superior vena cava obstruction
TCA	tricyclic antidepressant
t.d.s.	'three times a day'
TENS	transcutaneous electrical nerve stimulation
t.i.d.	*ter in die* (Latin) 'three times a day'
μg	microgram

1: The History and Principles of Palliative Care

CHRISTINA FAULL

Introduction

Palliative care is an important part of the work of most health care professionals, whatever their particular setting. All should feel confident in the core skills and knowledge of basic physical and non-physical symptom control. Moreover, it is necessary to have a grasp of the communication skills surrounding issues in incurable and advanced illness, and to be able to identify the need for referral to specialist and other services.

Palliative care is not an alternative to other care but is a complementary and vital part of total patient management.

> *I need my doctor to explain to me, to be cheerful, to share his experience and guide me, not only in the treatment but with my feelings as well. I need my doctor to discuss the possibility of death, and to find options that are unknown to me, because without him, I don't even know where to look for them. I would also like to feel free to talk to him about trying alternative treatments, without fear of his resentment or contempt, that would destroy my hope and enthusiasm, or spoil the relationship [1].*

Much of our understanding and knowledge of the philosophy, science, and art of palliative care has developed and grown through the work of the hospice movement. The word 'hospice' originates from the Latin *hospes* meaning host; *hospitalis*, a further derivative, means friendly, a welcome to the stranger. The word *hospitium* perhaps begins to convey the vital philosophy of the hospice movement: it means the warm feeling between host and guest. Hence a hospice denotes a place where this feeling is experienced, a place of welcome and care for those in need.

The word 'palliative' derives from the Latin *pallium*, a cloak. Palliation means cloaking over, not addressing the underlying cause but ameliorating the effects. The bedrock of the hospice philosophy, in Western society at least, is that of patient-centred holistic care focusing on quality of life and extending support to significant family and carers. This is encompassed in the following adapted quotations:

*You matter because you are you, and you matter until the last
moment of your life. We will do all that we can to help you not
only to die peacefully, but to live until you die.*

*What links the many professionals and volunteers who work in
hospice or palliative care is an awareness of the many needs of a
person and his/her family and carers as they grapple with all the
demands and challenges introduced by the inexorable progress of
a disease that has outstripped the possibilities of cure [2].*

Hospice has perhaps become thought of as solely a *place* of care. It is,
however, much more than this and in essence is synonymous with palliative
care. Both have a philosophy of care not dependent on a place or buildings
but on attitudes, expertise, and understanding. More recently the term
specialist palliative care has been used to represent those professionals
and services that concentrate on this area of health care as their main role
and expertise, recognizing that almost all health care professionals provide
elements of palliative care for patients as part of their practice.

The focus of modern palliative care came with the founding of Saint
Christopher's Hospice in London in 1967 by Dame Cecily Saunders. This
institution advocated an approach to care which ensured:
- quality of care for patients and relatives;
- a range of services to help provide optimum care whether the patient
was at home, in hospital, or required specialist in-patient care;
- education, advice, and support to other professionals;
- evidence-based practice;
- research and evaluation.

The growth of specialist palliative care services for patients has been
mostly unplanned and uncoordinated by health authorities. Development
has been largely in response to local pressure, enthusiasm, and fund-raising
activity, and remained mostly within the charitable, independent sector.
Some development, mostly in the hospital setting, has been prompted by
and within the National Health Service (NHS). This has led to a wide
variety in models of service provision, distribution, and funding across
the country, with some areas, and therefore patients, being better served
than others. As workloads increase, and specialist knowledge and the use
of new interventions and drugs develops, the sources and methods of
funding will undoubtedly need consideration and debate [3,4].

Recent developments of palliative care services are based on the recommendations of three national reports: the Wilkes report, *Terminal Care*,
published in 1980 [5]; the SMAC and SNMAC report, *The Principles and
Provision of Palliative Care*, published in 1992 [6]; and the Calman–Hine

report, *A Policy Framework for Commissioning Cancer Services*, published in 1995 [7].

Each report builds on the former, with the Calman–Hine report focusing solely on cancer care. In essence these reports suggest that:
• Palliative care is an important part of the work of most health care professionals, and that all should have knowledge in this area and feel confident in the core skills required.
• Palliative care should be regarded as a vital and integral part of health care for many patients and should complement other health care in a parallel, not sequential model of care.
• The primary health care team (PHCT) has a central role in, and responsibility for, the provision of palliative care and accessing and developing specialist palliative care services.
• Specialist palliative care should be seen as complementing, not replacing the care provided by other health care professionals.

The reports also stress that specialist palliative care services should be available to all patients in need wherever they are and whatever their disease. Furthermore, such services should be planned, integrated, and co-ordinated, and bear responsibility for education, training, and research.

Definitions

Palliative care

Palliative care is the active, total (holistic) care of patients and their families by a multiprofessional team when the patient's disease is no longer responsive to curative treatment [8].

The goals of palliative care are:
• achievement of the best possible quality of life for patients and their families;
• good control of symptoms;
• to facilitate adjustment to the many 'losses' of advanced and terminal illness;
• to facilitate and guide completion of unfinished 'business';
• a dignified death, with minimum distress, in the patient's place of choice;
• prevention of problems in bereavement.

To this end palliative care is a partnership between the patient, carers, and various professionals. It affirms life and regards dying as a normal process, neither hastening nor postponing death. It integrates the psychological, physical, social, and spiritual aspects of a patient's care.

The palliative care approach

Palliative care overlaps with, but should not be confused with the palliative care approach, which aims to promote both physical and psychosocial well-being in all patients. It is a vital and integral part of *all* clinical practice, whatever the illness or its stage, and is informed by a knowledge and practice of palliative care principles [9].

Specialist palliative care services

Specialist palliative care services are those with palliative care as their core speciality [10]. Effective palliative care requires an experienced, multiprofessional team. No individual or individual profession can provide the breadth of expertise and services that patients require.

Specialist palliative care has various roles. It is a resource of specialist expertise, services, and equipment for the PHCT and hospital staff. It takes a lead role in the provision of education for those working in other areas of health and social care who provide the bulk of non-specialist palliative care for patients.

Specialist palliative care provides a range of services for patients and their carers with complex needs, and takes a lead role in training specialist practitioners of medical, nursing, occupational therapy, and other disciplines. It also undertakes research, and suggests and implements, where appropriate, innovations in palliative care and palliative care services.

Terminal care

Terminal care is one important part of palliative care and usually refers to the management of patients during their last few days or weeks, or even months of life from a point at which it is clear that the patient is in a progressive state of decline.

Issues facing palliative care worldwide and the UK hospice movement

Fifty-two million people die across the world each year. Of these deaths 80% occur in the developing countries of the world, and 1 in 10 deaths is due to cancer. Tens of millions die in unrelieved suffering. The Barcelona declaration on palliative care in 1996 [11], like the World Health Organization in 1990 [8], called for palliative care to be included as part of every governmental health policy. Every individual has the right to pain relief. Inexpensive, effective methods exist to relieve pain and other symptoms. Cost need not be an impediment.

The challenges for palliative care in developing countries

A multiplicity of challenges face the development of palliative care globally, but the issues are more pronounced in the developing world for several reasons, principally: poverty; the ageing population; and the increase in cancer-related deaths. Cancer caused 10% of deaths in 1985 and this figure is estimated to rise to 15% by 2015 [12,13]. By the year 2015 it is estimated that two-thirds of all new cancer cases will occur in the developing world [13]. The problems are compounded by late presentation of cancer and the limited treatment resources available for cancer. The developing world has only 5% of the world's total resources for cancer control although it must cope with almost two-thirds of the world's new cancer patients. The developing world is currently suffering from an epidemic of lung cancer. The annual number of tobacco-related deaths is expected to rise from 3 million to 10 million by the year 2025 [14]. In India, for example, the years 1970–80 witnessed a 400% increase in smokers.

There is also an AIDS epidemic. It is projected that the cumulative total of adults with AIDS will be 10 million by the year 2000 (for HIV positivity, the figure is 30–40 million), of whom 90% will be in developing countries [15]. The sociological effect of AIDS deaths in the developing world is catastrophic. It affects those most likely to be breadwinners for the extended three-generation family, and leaves many children orphaned. The situation for patients is exacerbated in many regions by war, settlement of refugees, or natural disasters.

Availability of opioids

Under the international treaty, *Single Convention on Narcotic Drugs* [16], governments are responsible to ensure that opioids are available for pain management. The 1996 report from the International Narcotics Control Board (INCB) showed that opioids are still widely unavailable for medical needs [17].

The main impediments to opioid availability are: government concern about addiction; insufficient training of health care professionals; and restrictive laws over the manufacture, distribution, prescription, and dispensing of opioids. There is also considerable reluctance on the part of the health care profession concerning their use, due to concerns about legal sanctions. This is made worse by the burden of regulatory requirements, the often insufficient import or manufacture of opioids, and the potential for diversion of opioids for non-legitimate use.

Unmet need and continued suffering in the developed world

The hospice movement and palliative care has come a long way in the past 30 years. There is a considerable body of knowledge and expertise, and services have grown enormously in number and character. There is, however, still a major unmet need. The majority of people are not living and dying with the comfort and the dignity that it is possible to achieve for most patients. Identified areas for improvement include:
- management of pain in advanced cancer [18–20];
- management of other symptoms;
- information and support for patients and carers;
- attention to comfort and basic care for those dying in hospitals [21];
- the needs of patients dying from non-malignant illness [22,23].

One of the major challenges for those who seek to improve the care for patients with advanced disease is to ensure that all health care professionals consider palliative care an important part of their role, and have adequate skills, knowledge, and specialist support to undertake it effectively. This will require more formal consideration of palliative care and specialist palliative care services within strategic planning and commissioning of health care [24], with incentives for a stronger response in primary and secondary care. An essential step along this path may be the formation of new alliances [25].

Ethnicity and palliative care: the gaps in the UK

Recent studies have shown that the minority ethnic groups are underusers of palliative care services, in the UK at least, and that the services may be insensitive and inappropriate to the needs of these groups [26]. It may also be that GPs under-refer to specialist services for a variety of reasons. Almost 6% of the total population of England and Wales is from a minority ethnic group. In 1991 this fraction numbered almost 3 million individuals, the largest number belonging to the Indian and Pakistani groups. Black and ethnic minority patients face the potential obstacles of language and communication difficulties; attitudes that are culture-specific; cultural insensitivity; and ignorance and racism (overt and covert).

The principles of palliative care

What do patients and their carers need?

The uniqueness of each individual's situation must be acknowledged and the manner of care adapted accordingly. The essence of what patients and their carers may need is outlined in Box 1.1.

It should be clear from this that communication skills (see Chapter 8) play a fundamental role in achieving good palliative care and quality of life for the patient.

> *Almost invariably, the act of communication is an important part of the therapy; occasionally it is the only constituent. It usually requires greater thought and planning than a drug prescription, and unfortunately it is commonly administered in subtherapeutic doses [27].*

The principles of good symptom management

Twycross amongst others has done much to ensure an evidence-based, scientific rigour in palliative care [28]. The management of any problem should be approached by:
* anticipation;
* evaluation and assessment;
* explanation and information;
* individualized treatment;
* re-evaluation and supervision;
* attention to detail.

ANTICIPATION

Many physical and non-physical problems can often be anticipated and in some instances prevented. Failure to anticipate problems is a common source of dissatisfaction for patients [29]. Understanding the natural history of the disease with specific reference to an individual patient, awareness of the patient's psychosocial circumstances, and identification of 'risk factors' allows planning of care by the team. For example, in a 45-year-old woman, recently found to have spinal metastases from her breast cancer, several potential issues may be anticipated.
* Pain—may need NSAID, opioids, and radiotherapy.
* Spinal cord compression—examine neurology if unsteady or 'numb'.
* Young children—may need help, practically and in telling the children.

Box 1.1 The needs of patients and their carers

The patient's need for autonomy and choice includes the right to deny the illness, to confidentiality, and, wherever possible, to choose the setting of death and the degree of carer involvement.

Information
The patient has a need for sensitive, clear explanations of:
- the diagnosis and its implications
- the likely effects of treatments on activities of daily living and well-being
- the type and extent of family/carer support that may be required and how it may be addressed
- expected symptoms and what may be done about them.

Quality of life
The patient has a need to lead a life that is as normal, congenial, and dignified as possible. An individual's quality of life will depend on minimizing the gap between their expectations and aspirations and their actual experiences. This may be achieved by:
- general respect, as a person as well as a patient, from properly motivated, trained and experienced staff, who see themselves as partners in living
- effective relief from pain and other distressing symptoms
- an appropriate and satisfying diet
- comfort and consolation, especially from those who share the patient's religious beliefs and/or belong to the same ethnic, cultural community
- companionship from family and friends, and from members of the care team
- continuity of care within the primary health care team and from different parts of a specialist service
- consistent and effective response to changes in physical and psychosocial discomfort
- information about support and self-help and other groups and services.

Support for Carers
The patient's family or other carers have a need for support at times of crises in the illness and in their bereavement. These needs include:
- practical support with financial, legal, or welfare problems
- information about the illness (with the patient's consent) and the available support
- planned respite from the stress of caring in the home situation

Continued

> **Box 1.1** *Continued*
> • suitable involvement of carers in the moment of death and in other aspects of care
> • bereavement support
> • special support where the patient's death may directly affect young children, or where the patient is a child or adolescent.

• Work—may need financial and benefit advice.
• Hypercalcaemia—check blood if nauseated or confused.

EVALUATION AND ASSESSMENT

An understanding of the pathophysiology and likely cause(s) of any particular problem is vital in selecting and directing appropriate investigations and treatment. This is illustrated by the following specific examples.
• Sedation for an agitated patient with urinary retention is not as helpful as catheterization.
• Antiemetics for the nausea of hypercalcaemia are important but so too is lowering the serum calcium (if appropriate).
• A patient who is fearful of dying may be more helped by discussing and addressing specific fears rather than taking benzodiazepines.
• Pain in a vertebral metastasis may be helped by analgesics, radiotherapy, orthopaedic surgery, TENS, and acupuncture. A decision as to which to prescribe is made only by careful assessment.

Co-morbidity is common and should *always* be considered. For example, it is easy (and unfortunately common) to assume that pain in a patient with cancer is caused by the cancer. In one series almost a quarter of pains in patients with cancer were unrelated to the cancer or the cancer treatment [30].

EXPLANATION AND INFORMATION

Management of a problem should always begin with explanation of the findings and diagnostic conclusions. This usually reduces the patient's anxieties even if it confirms their worst suspicions—a monster in the light is usually better faced than a monster unseen in the shadows. Further information may be useful to some patients. A clear explanation of the suggested treatments and follow-up plan is important for the patient to gain a sense of control and security.

INDIVIDUALIZED TREATMENT

The physical, social, and psychological circumstances of the patient and their views and wishes should be considered in planning care. For example, lymphoedema compression bandages may be unused unless there is someone available to help the patient fit them daily.

RE-EVALUATION AND SUPERVISION

The symptoms of frail patients with advanced disease can change frequently. New problems can occur and established ones worsen requiring proactive follow-up. Interventions may be complex (many patients take >20 tablets a day) and close supervision is vital to ensure optimum efficacy and tailoring to the patient.

ATTENTION TO DETAIL

The quality of palliative care is in the detail of care. For example, it is vital to ensure that the patient not only has a prescription for the correct drug but also that they can obtain it from the pharmacy, have adequate supplies to cover a weekend, and understand how to adjust it if the problem worsens.

Limits of symptom control

There is always something more that can be done to help a patient but it is not always possible to completely relieve symptoms. Specialist advice should usually have been sought for help in the management of intractable symptoms. This extra support is in itself an important way of helping the patient.

In such situations an acceptable solution must be found to provide adequate relief of distress for the patient. For management of a physical symptom and sometimes of psychological distress this may be a compromise between the presence of the symptom and sedation from medications. It is hard for a team to accept suboptimum relief of symptoms, and discussions with the patient and the family may be very difficult. It is important for the team to remember the great value of their continuing involvement to the patient and their carers; to acknowledge how difficult the situation is and not to abandon the patient because it is painful and distressing for the professionals.

Slowly, I learn about the importance of powerlessness.
I experience it in my own life and I live with it in my work.
The secret is not to be afraid of it—not to run away.
The dying know we are not God.
All they ask is that we do not desert them [31].

References

1 Kfir N, Slevin M. *Challenging Cancer: From Chaos to Control*. London: Tavistock/Routledge, 1991.

2 Saunders C. Foreword. In: Doyle D, Hanks GWC, Macdonald N, eds. *Oxford Textbook of Palliative Medicine*. Oxford: Oxford University Press, 1993: v–viii.

3 Clark D. Whither the hospices? In: Clark D, ed. *The Future for Palliative Care: Issues of Policy and Practice*. Buckingham: Open University Press, 1993: 167–177.

4 Working Party on Clinical Guidelines in Palliative Care. *Direction and Dilemma: the Development of Palliative Care*. London: National Council for Hospices and Specialist Palliative Care Services, 1996.

5 Wilkes E. *Terminal Care: Report of a Working Party*. London: Standing Medical Advisory Committee/HMSO, 1980.

6 Joint Report of the Standing Medical Advisory Committee and the Standing Nursing and Midwifery Advisory Committee. *The Principles and Provision of Palliative Care*. London: Department of Health, 1992.

7 Report by the Expert Advisory Group on Cancer to the Chief Medical Officers of England and Wales. *A Policy Framework for Commissioning Cancer Services*. London: Department of Health, 1995.

8 *Cancer Pain Relief and Palliative Care*. Technical Report Series: 804. Geneva: World Health Organization, 1990.

9 National Council for Hospices and Specialist Palliative Care Services. *Specialist Palliative Care: A Statement of Definitions*. London: National Council for Hospices and Specialist Palliative Care Services, 1995.

10 Working Party on Clinical Guidelines in Palliative Care. *Information for Purchasers: Background to Available Specialist Palliative Care Services*. London: National Council for Hospices and Specialist Palliative Care Services, 1995.

11 The Barcelona Declaration on Palliative Care. *Prog Palliat Care* 1996; 4: 113.

12 Lopez AD. Causes of death: an assessment of global patterns of mortality around 1985. *World Health Statistics Quarterly* 1990; 43: 91–104.

13 Bulato RA, Stephens PW. Estimates and projections of mortality by cause: a global overview 1970–2015. In: Jamison DT, Mosley HW, eds. *The World Bank Health Sector Priorities Review*. Washington DC: World Bank, 1991.

14 World Health Organization. Tobacco—attributable mortality: global estimates and projections. In: *Tobacco Alert*, January 1991. Geneva: WHO.

15 World Health Organization. Current and future dimension of the HIV/AIDS pandemic: a capsule summary. In: *Global Programme on AIDS*, April 1991. Geneva: WHO.

16 United Nations. *Single Convention on Narcotic Drugs, 1961*. United Nations sales No. E62.XI.1, New York: UN 1962.
17 International Narcotics Control Board. *Availability of Opiates for Medical Needs*. New York: United Nations, 1996.
18 Larue F, Collequ SM, Brasser L, Cleeland CS. Multicentre study of cancer pain and its treatment in France. *BMJ* 1995; 310: 1034–1037.
19 Cleeland CS, Gonin R, Hatfield AK *et al*. Pain and its treatment in outpatients with metastatic cancer. *N Engl J Med* 1994; 330: 592–596.
20 Addington-Hall J, McCarthy M. Dying from cancer: results of a national population-based investigation. *Palliat Med* 1995; 9: 295–305.
21 Mills M, Davies HTO, Macrae WA. Care of dying patients in hospital. *BMJ* 1994; 309: 583–586.
22 Jones RVH. *A Parkinson's Disease Study in Devon and Cornwall*. London: Parkinson's Disease Society, 1993.
23 Addington-Hall JM, Lay M, Altmann D, McCarthy M. Symptom control, communication with health professionals and hospital care of stroke patients in the last year of life, as reported by surviving family, friends and carers. *Stroke* 1995; 26: 2242–2248.
24 Department of Health. A Policy Framework for Commissioning Cancer Services: Palliative Care Services. EL (96) 85. Leeds: Department of Health, 1996.
25 Bosanquet N. New challenge for palliative care. *BMJ* 1997; 314: 1294.
26 Hill D, Penso D. *Opening Doors: Improving Access to Hospice and Specialist Palliative Care Services by Members of Black and Ethnic Minority Communities*. London: National Council for Hospices and Specialist Palliative Care Services, 1995.
27 Buckman R. Communication in palliative care: a practical guide. In: Doyle D, Hanks GWC, Macdonald N, eds. *Oxford Textbook of Palliative Medicine*. Oxford: Oxford University Press, 1993: 47–61.
28 Twycross R. *Symptom Management in Advanced Cancer*, 2nd edn. Oxford: Radcliffe Medical Press, 1997.
29 Blyth A. An audit of terminal care in general practice. *BMJ* 1987; 294: 871–874.
30 Twycross RG, Fairfield S. Pain in far advanced cancer. *Pain* 1982; 14: 303–310.
31 Cassidy S. *Sharing the Darkness*. London: Darton, Longman and Todd, 1988.

2: Palliative Care: the Team, the Services, and the Need for Care

RICHARD WOOF, YVONNE CARTER AND
CHRISTINA FAULL

This chapter will outline the principles of multidisciplinary teamwork, the roles of different team members in the community, and the function and structure of the specialist palliative care services.

Teamworking

A team is a group of individuals with a common purpose working together.

The benefits from working in teams are various. In order to answer the diverse needs of patients, it is necessary to employ a range of services. The combined effect of individuals with specialist skills working together in a team, is greater than the sum of the parts. What is more, teams provide patients with a selection of personalities with which to interact. Consequently patients have a greater opportunity to find a particular individual with whom they have the most beneficial therapeutic relationship.

On a professional level, teamworking can provide mutual support in what can be very emotionally draining work. This activity should not be underestimated as it ensures personal and team survival. Collaboration can also raise clinical standards by facilitating the educational exchange of knowledge, ideas, and experience.

Although the aim of the team may be consistent (e.g. good palliative care), the precise strategy to achieve this aim requires foresight, flexibility, and co-ordination. This is no easy task and requires efficient organization combined with a cohesive effort from the team. Care is further complicated by continued role change in line with professional development and a constantly evolving team membership. It must also be recognized that effective collaboration is expensive in terms of time and money. In spite of these challenges, the collective and personal satisfaction gained from good team care can be rewarding.

Different people make different teams

There is no single description that adequately illustrates the typical team in community palliative care. Not least because team membership has few limits and there is no standardized structure. Also, people vary. For instance, the potential role of individuals within the team is a product of their values, capabilities, and behaviour, which is a combination of personal attributes and training. Consequently, although individuals may share an educational background and vocation, they are not professional clones. Vive la différence! This varied membership will give teams their own characteristics, with particular strengths and weaknesses. However, with training, care can be co-ordinated effectively, as long as there is a mutually held belief in the philosophy of palliative care (see Chapter 1). For instance, all team members should recognize that quality of life should be defined by the patient, and that professional intervention should be directed in that light.

The diversity of professional behaviour has other consequences for patient care. Professionals can interact with patients in different ways. Generally speaking, activity within the team will be in the best interest of the patient and the team. However, occasionally individuals can act in a way that is detrimental to patient care and counterproductive to teamworking.

HOW TO PROMOTE GOOD TEAMWORK

Good teamwork needs active development, and various techniques have been devised to facilitate effective teamwork. It is beyond the scope of this book to give a detailed account of these activities; interested readers should consult the quoted references. However, some of the approaches to team-building are listed below.

- Quality assurance:
  audit (see Chapter 4) [1];
  clinical guideline development [2];
  significant event analysis [3].
- Education:
  interdisciplinary education in any form [4].
- Team development:
  team manager (e.g. practice manager);
  team planning meetings [5,6];
  external facilitator;
  team-building 'away days';
  workbooks;
  formal professional appraisal.
- Interdisciplinary communication [7]:

patient-held records;
clinical team meetings;
key worker/liaison officer;
structured models of interprofessional communication [8].

Community palliative care services: who does what?

Patient/family/friends as team members

An important theme of palliative medicine is that the patient is the focus of care. This cannot be overstated as every professional is capable of making decisions that ease their working day, but ignore the patient's wishes. Patients should therefore be given repeated opportunities to actively participate in team decision-making. Failure to do so can result in care plans that are inappropriate and less likely to answer patient need. Consequently the patient's role in the team is pivotal. Equally the patient's family and friends often perform vital roles in caring for their loved ones. In encouraging this activity, the professional sustains a caring environment that is personal, empowering, and gives carers the opportunity to express affection. This concept is supported by the assertion that the patient/family/ friends be the unit of care.

The level of input from family and friends cannot be predicted or assumed. This support can range from heroic acts of selfless care to an inability to provide any assistance. The professional has to skilfully assess patient and carer needs and aim to achieve a balance between a perceived vulnerability and the imposition of the care. This requires repeated review and accomplished communication skills.

Professional roles

The variety of potential professional contact with a terminally ill patient is illustrated in Table 2.1. In practice only a few individuals will be regularly involved in any one case: commonly the district nurse, general practitioner (GP), and specialist palliative home care nurse. Yet there are additional specialist skills that can be called upon as required.

Although teamwork is valued by the primary health care team (PHCT), the structure, distribution of responsibilities, traditions, and workload combine to make it function in a more hierarchical way. In contrast the specialist palliative care team is typically more egalitarian.

Table 2.1 Professional carers.

Background	Primary health care team	Palliative care team	Other contributors (secondary care, private, voluntary organizations)
Medical	GP GP registrar	Palliative medicine specialist	Medical specialist (domiciliary opinions)
Nursing	District nurse Practice nurse Health visitor	Palliative home care nurse Marie Curie nurse Lymphoedema sister	Community psychiatric nurse Nursing home nurse Private nursing agency staff Stoma nurse Breast care nurse Oncology nurse Incontinence advisor
Other health care professionals	Physiotherapist Occupational therapist Chiropodist Social worker Practice counsellor Care assistants	Social worker Physiotherapist Occupational therapist	Pharmacist Dentist Clinical psychologist Speech therapist Dietician
Others	Meals on wheels Home help	Complementary therapist Volunteers Spiritual advisor Bereavement advisor	Spiritual advisor Voluntary organizations Private carers Complementary therapist Residential home carer
Administrative	Practice receptionist Practice secretary	Hospice secretary	

MEDICAL ROLES

General practitioner (GP)

This individual is a medical generalist who will be responsible for the ongoing care of approximately 2000 patients in the community. He/she is commonly in partnership with other GPs and is based within practice premises that are shared with other PHCT members.

The principal roles of the GP are to: prevent disease and anticipate care requirements; to diagnose disease (e.g. by arranging appropriate investigations); and to manage disease (e.g. by having sole responsibility for prescribing). The GP also provides undifferentiated, first-contact care, is responsible for 24-hour cover, and acts as gatekeeper to many other services (e.g. hospital referrals).

Hence, the GP co-ordinates many aspects of care and is often perceived as the team leader. He or she holds overall responsibility for patients and for staff employed by the practice, and is charged with the continuing care of those who are registered. This often involves caring for the family of a terminally ill patient, as well as the patient.

Palliative care physician

A consultant in palliative medicine has gained appropriate postgraduate qualifications and completed a period of specialist training. They are usually accessed by another doctor directly or via any member of the palliative care team.

The consultant's principal roles in a community context are to support the specialist palliative care nurse and the PHCT in their care of patients. This involves providing telephone advice, domiciliary visits, and out-patient facilities, in order to advise the PHCT on all aspects of palliative care (particularly symptom control).

Although a member of a less hierarchical specialist palliative care team, the consultant is often required to perform a leadership role within this team. He or she thus plays a key role in promoting education and research for specialists and primary health care teams, and the development of services for patients within a health authority district.

Domiciliary specialist opinion

Hospital consultants from any speciality (e.g. anaesthetist, geriatrician) can also be accessed to perform a home visit and supply an opinion to the rest of the team.

NURSING ROLES

District nurse

District nurses play an important part in domiciliary palliative care (malignant and non-malignant disease), having considerable contact with many patients. They are contacted either via the GP's surgery or their central base.

The district nurse has several key roles in the care team. Paramount among these are: assessment of need; general nursing care (e.g. dressings, pressure area care, bowel care, etc.); providing emotional support to patients and their family; and giving health education and advice to patients and family. Indeed, she or he is often the key worker for patients and family in the community. For example, they supply basic dietary advice, and organize equipment (e.g. mattresses, commodes, syringe drivers, etc.). Another valuable role is in co-ordinating and accessing other services (e.g. GP, Marie Curie nurses, hospital nurses).

The experience, knowledge of the community, and skills of the district nurse make her or him a vital team member. District nurses provide essential input in guideline development, and in the training of pre- and post-registration nursing students. Increasingly they are receiving additional training at diploma and degree level in palliative care. However, heavy workloads can pressurize this service.

Specialist palliative care nurse

These nurses have added to their basic and post-registration education, a period of specific palliative care training. Some will be termed 'Macmillan nurses' in recognition of the charity that supported their specialist training. They may be part of the specialist palliative care team based in a hospice or hospital, but practise within the community (home care team). Some specialist palliative care nurses can work in the community in isolation from other specialist professionals.

Specialist palliative care nurses fulfil several roles. They are equipped to assess the palliative care needs of patients referred by the PHCT or hospital, and can bring specialist knowledge in their support of the PHCT (e.g. symptom control, nursing care, etc.).

They may also access hospice-based services (e.g. day care, additional aids, volunteers), and in difficult cases may refer problems back to the specialist palliative care team for additional advice. Nurses provide emotional support to patient, carers, and staff, and some will provide bereavement follow-up. They may also be involved in the education of other community workers.

Some home care teams will work 9 a.m. to 5 p.m. Monday through Friday; other teams will provide a 24-hour service seven days a week.

Marie Curie nurses

These are nurses who are organised and funded by the nationwide charity, Marie Curie Cancer Care, in partnership with the NHS. They provide nursing care and support to patients and carers in their own homes. Typically this means staying with the family for a period of time, usually overnight, but occasionally through the day as well. This enables patients to be cared for at home, especially during a period of crisis and provides terminal care for patients and respite to carers.

The nurse's experience is matched to the needs of the patient. Many Marie Curie Nurses have considerable experience and can become actively involved in treatment.

Practice nurses

These are employed by the practice and their numbers are rapidly increasing. Although there is no standardized training, they often have considerable experience.

Practice nurses are based in the practice premises and have working roles (e.g. health promotion, health education, prevention) that will not immediately bring them in contact with terminally ill patients. However, they will share with the GP an intimate knowledge of the practice population and can occasionally be involved in palliative care. This is often in the early stages of investigation and treatment, with less input as the care becomes more home based.

Their main role is one of general practice-based nursing (e.g. dressings, venepuncture, administration of drugs), as well as providing emotional support and education for patients and carers. They may be able to give advice concerning locally based services.

Other nursing specialities

In response to some particularly difficult areas of care, specialist fields of nursing have arisen. These are new services and as yet no uniform pattern of care has been established nationally. Clinical nurse specialists have usually completed relevant post-registration experience and training, which allows them to confidently hold some clinical autonomy and advise other professionals.

Lymphoedema nurse. This specialist nurse is often based in a hospice, oncology unit, or breast unit, and is trained to relieve lymphoedema with massaging and bandaging techniques (see Chapter 19).

Breast care nurse. These hospital-based nurses support patients who are diagnosed as having breast cancer. They can provide explanation and emotional support to patients and their families. In particular they give advice on prostheses and clothing.

Oncology nurse. These nurses are part of the oncology services and are hospital based. However, they also make themselves available to patients at home for information and support, particularly during oncological treatment. They have a key role in liaison between hospital and community teams. They may advise the PHCT on aspects of chemotherapy and radiotherapy, and may become increasingly involved in the delivery of chemotherapy at home.

OTHER HEALTH CARE PROFESSIONALS

Pharmacist

Hospital pharmacy departments and community pharmacies are a source of a great deal of information and support for patients, carers, and prescribers. In addition hospital and community pharmacists are now encouraged by the Royal Pharmaceutical Society of Great Britain (RPSGB) to liaise with each other in order to provide seamless care for patients transferred from hospital to home or to hospice (see Chapter 3) [9].

Physiotherapist

Basic training for physiotherapists is now at degree level. They are increasingly being employed in the community. Although regional variations exist as regards service content and referral mechanisms, all PHCT teams will have access to a community physiotherapist. The GP is often required to sanction the service. Private physiotherapists can also provide domiciliary input and are often more accessible.

The main roles of physiotherapists in palliative care are symptom control (e.g. lymphoedema, neuropathic pain, chest drainage) and improving patient mobility, including providing walking aids (working closely with occupational therapists). They also give advice to carers and patients on lifting and transferring. In palliative care, holistic physiotherapy includes the setting of achievable treatment goals that foster hope, quality of life, control, and independence. There is a developing interest in specialist palliative care physiotherapy.

Occupational therapist

Occupational therapy has a role in maximizing patients' potential for safe independent living. Traditionally this therapy has concentrated on the transition between hospital and home. Changes in the delivery of the health service have resulted in greater community-based work. Referrals can be made by any individual, although the GP is often asked to provide additional information and authorize the service. Some services are organized by local authorities, and are accessed though social services.

The occupational therapist's main role in palliative care is assessing the patient's capabilities for independent living, and making practical suggestions for improvements (e.g. equipment, splints, seating, bath aids, housing adaptations, lifting equipment, coping skills). They also provide practical advice and support to carers.

Many hospices employ occupational therapists with particular expertise in meeting the needs of patients. The traditional role of providing activities for patients is being developed within hospices by diversional therapists, whose training may be outside the health service.

Social worker

Social workers are employed by local authorities and work closely with the PHCT. They often come from a variety of backgrounds, but will all need to be qualified with a Diploma in Social Work (a modular diploma, equipping the holder with different skills). They can be contacted through the GP's surgery or local social services office. They will accept referrals from any source.

They fulfil several roles in palliative care. Among these are giving advice on government financial benefits (special rules apply for terminally ill patients to receive benefits promptly—form DS 1500; see p. 22). They also assess the patient's social and continuing health care needs, and can, for example: provide access to particular forms of social care (e.g. meals on wheels, home help, emergency alarm systems); liaise with occupational therapists about housing adaptations; or advise on child care issues. They also work with both patients and carers in arranging residential and nursing home placements.

Social workers also frequently provide a counselling service for patients and families in adverse circumstances. However, in community palliative care, they are less involved in this work, leaving it to other professionals (e.g. specialist palliative care nurse). (See the Appendix (p. 31) for summary of common benefits.)

Practice counsellor

Recent changes in the delivery of services by general practitioners have resulted in an expansion of practice-based counselling. Practices vary in whether they provide this service, and in the experience/training of the counsellor employed [10]. However, practice counsellors can give emotional support to patients and their family. This will often occur in practice-based clinics and may be helpful in cases where support needs to be more focused than the general help given by the rest of the team. Counsellors can be accessed through the GP's surgery.

Clinical psychologists

This group of specialists use techniques helpful in complex psychological maladjustment to a terminal illness (e.g. cognitive, behavioural, marital therapies). Patients with past psychiatric history are particularly at risk of adverse responses. Although infrequently needed, clinical psychologists can be contacted through the psychiatric team.

Dietician

The dietician's specialist knowledge and experience can make useful contributions to the team. Their basic training is at degree level and they can be hospital or community based. A community-based dietetic service, including home assessment, is available to the PHCT. In particular they give advice to patients and staff on diet and nutritional supplements, and work closely with the speech therapists in patients with swallowing difficulties.

OTHER CARERS

Home care

Home care workers ('home helps') have a role in such things as housework, shopping, laundry, and collecting prescriptions. They are employed on the strength of their experience and attitude, and have recently taken on some basic nursing duties with patients, such as getting them in and out of bed, dressing, washing, and toileting. They can be contacted through the local social services office (home care manager). For some patients this sort of care is vital for successful palliative care at home.

Meals

Social services can arrange the home delivery of midday meals for housebound patients—'meals on wheels'. Alternatively, bulk delivery of precooked frozen meals can be organized. There is a fixed charge for this service but at low cost. Special diets can be catered for.

Residential staff

Vulnerable patients (especially the elderly) can be housed in a variety of accommodation staffed to provide additional cover and security. These include state services (e.g. Part III accommodation, i.e. 'old people's home'), voluntary organizations (e.g. alms houses), and private schemes (e.g. private residential homes, sheltered accommodation). The accommodation is usually adapted according to need and is staffed to provide various degrees of support. The staff can provide the team with considerable insight into the patient's predicament and can be crucial in liaison work. They cannot be expected to perform nursing duties.

Voluntary organizations

The role of the voluntary organizations is variable according to clinical need and the availability of services.

Private carers

Private agencies can provide registered or auxiliary nurse input at home. They can be employed privately by individuals or to cover shortfalls in statutory services. Agencies need to hold a Certificate of Licence issued by the local authority. This confirms basic standards in staff recruitment and personnel management. These agencies can also organize staff to provide social care (e.g. domestic duties, companionship).

Hospice volunteers

Volunteers can come from all walks of life and provide a wide array of services. They are organized through the hospice. Their specific roles in the community are varied (e.g. befriending, sitting, acting as driver).

Spiritual advisor

This team member can come in many forms, but typically is a recognized religious figure or layperson who can facilitate a patient's spiritual health (see Chapter 7). Their influence on patient well-being can be great, particularly if one considers suffering in a holistic sense. This role can be filled by health care workers, a religious leader assigned to a health institution (e.g. hospice/hospital chaplain), or the more traditional religious figure from the community (e.g. priest, rabbi, mullah).

Complementary therapist (see Chapter 21)

Many patients receive benefits from complementary therapists, and consequently this help is often encouraged by traditional health professionals. However, one should be mindful of unregulated services, involving people who may be practising unethically (e.g. raising hope of cure inappropriately, advising against traditional treatment of proven benefit). With close liaison, however, professional behaviour can be assured and patients helped by complementary therapy. Indeed many hospices and some GP practices offer an 'in-house' service.

Bereavement visitor

Bereavement visitors are volunteers organized and supervised through hospices (usually by a social worker) to provide support following a bereavement. Standards of recruitment and training are the responsibility of the hospice. Other organizations, such as CRUSE, also support bereaved people.

Other community-based services

The cost for these services is met by a combination of personal money and state support. Decisions on finance depend on complex calculations and involved documentation, which often require the assistance of a social worker.

Nursing homes

These are homes registered with the health authority to provide residential nursing care. They can be charitable or private organizations and need to achieve certain basic standards of care. Patients are often admitted when ongoing home care is impossible, or for periods of respite. The quality of this care can be variable, given that patients can be highly dependent and resources sometimes stretched.

Residential homes

Residential homes come under local authority administration. They can be government funded (Part III accommodation), run by voluntary organizations, or established privately. They need to provide 'the type of care which might be provided by a caring relative at home' (dressing, washing, toileting, etc.). Standards of care are heavily resource dependent. Both long-term placements and respite admissions are possible in residential homes.

Day care

Patients can visit various units for day care. These typically allow patients to get out of the house once or twice a week and receive the stimulation of group activities. Carers have some respite from their ongoing responsibility to the patient, while the patient can benefit from time away from a carer. Certain units have been developed to provide specialist input and are hospital- or hospice-based. The following is a list of possible day care units:

- hospice day care (see p. 28);
- geriatric day hospital;
- psychogeriatric day hospital;
- psychiatric day hospital;
- local authority-run day centre;
- residential home;
- nursing home;
- voluntary organized centre.

Specialist palliative care services

As can be seen from the above descriptions, community palliative care in the UK is supported by an array of specialist services. Hospital practice also benefits from specialist input.

Specialist palliative care has various functions. Firstly, it is a resource of specialist expertise, services, and equipment to the PHCT and hospital staff. Secondly, it takes a lead role in the provision of education for those working in other health-related environments, because it is the latter who provide the bulk of non-specialist palliative care for patients. It is also at the forefront of training specialist practitioners of medical, nursing, occupational therapy, and other disciplines.

Thirdly, it provides a range of services to cater for the complex needs of patients and their carers. Finally, it is charged with undertaking research, and suggesting and, where appropriate, implementing innovations in palliative care and palliative care services.

The focus of palliative care services for patients is often a hospice or specialist unit, department, or directorate. These services should aim to have a team of professionals, made up as follows [11].
- One or more doctors holding a recognized appointment in palliative medicine equivalent to consultant in palliative medicine, with supporting junior, career grade staff and trainees.
- Nursing staff who have had at least introductory training in hospice and palliative care philosophy and practices. Nurses above grade E should hold a recognized post-registration qualification, diploma, or higher award in palliative care.
- Access to physiotherapists and occupational therapists.
- Access to a recognized minister of religion (or equivalent spiritual practitioner) with training in the care of dying people and their carers.
- Access to the services of social workers, psychologists, or counsellors with demonstrable skills in palliative care.
- Access to some appropriate complementary therapeutic techniques.

Components of a specialist palliative care service

Because of the historically unplanned provision of palliative care services, the precise model of specialist palliative care services will differ between districts. In particular, the provision of services is more comprehensive in some districts than in others. All districts should, however, provide the necessary components of specialist care to fulfil the roles discussed above. Since it is more likely that a comprehensive service is provided by a number of different teams with different remits and organization; the co-ordination of patient care is potentially very complex.

HOME CARE

For many patients, a specialist nurse working in the community alongside the PHCT is the only component of specialist palliative care they will need. The role of the specialist home care nurse is outlined above (see pp. 18–19). If the specialist home care nurse works from a hospice or specialist palliative care unit he or she will provide the contact point for the other components of the specialist service (e.g. medical advice, access to in-patient services).

HOSPICE-AT-HOME

Hospice-at-home teams are a relatively new development and are not available in all health districts. Their aim is to provide 24-hour specialist care in the patient's own home in order to avoid unwanted admission to a hospital or palliative care in-patient unit in the last days of a patient's life. They may sometimes be called 'respite-at-home teams' or 'rapid-response teams'.

The core team comprises a skill mix of nurses with training in palliative care. There is formal access to specialist medical and other professional advice. The team works with the district nursing and Marie Curie nursing services providing practical, hands-on nursing care. The PHCT retains the key worker role and responsibility for care.

IN-PATIENT CARE

In-patient care may be provided in designated palliative care beds, staffed by a specialist multiprofessional team, in several different settings; these include: specialist palliative care units of hospices; palliative care beds in acute hospitals; community hospitals; and nursing homes. However, it is the team of professionals, their knowledge, skills, and philosophy of care, not the actual place of care, that is the essence of specialist in-patient care.

Patients may need admission to a specialist unit for various reasons. One is terminal care when continued care at home is not possible and hospital or nursing-home care is inappropriate because of the patient's and/or the carer's specific needs. Patients may also be admitted for short stays for complex symptom control, or for respite care in order to allow continued care in the community through adequate support of the carer. Furthermore, such units can provide rehabilitation for patients with a late-stage disease who require particular skills from staff, working together rapidly for realistic, achievable objectives outlined by the patient and the carer.

Environmental considerations

It is vital for the successful delivery of palliative care in institutional settings to establish the right physical environment. The accommodation needs to satisfy the following criteria:
- a safe, non-threatening, welcoming environment;
- an atmosphere of calm;
- responsive to individual needs and wishes;
- a comfortable atmosphere of individuality expressed through furnishings, decor, personal possessions, etc.;
- a pleasant outlook;
- privacy for the patients and their families.

DAY CARE

The day-care unit can provide support not only for patients at home but also those in in-patient units. It normally offers an environment of security, understanding, and mutual support aiming to normalize life and gain control and choices in living with an advancing illness. The unit also promotes rehabilitation and helps the patient towards independence in certain aspects of daily living. Patients also obtain support and therapy in the form of social activities, the relief from isolation and depression, and the general enhancement of well-being through, for example, chiropody, hair care, aromatherapy, and massage.

Some nursing is carried out, including changing of dressings and help with stoma care, and there can be assessment, monitoring, advice, and intervention in symptom control. The patient has access to medical advice, with the chance to discuss their diagnosis and prognosis. Such units also give valuable respite for carers.

OUT-PATIENT CLINICS

Out-patient clinics may be held in specialist units/hospices or community health clinics. Referral is made doctor to doctor. Most such clinics provide general assessment, advice, intervention and monitoring of physical and non-physical symptoms. Specific clinics may be provided by doctors and other health care professionals for the management of lymphoedema and dyspnoea, access to complementary therapies, psychological support in early disease, and administration of nerve blocks and other interventional pain management techniques.

HOSPITAL SUPPORT TEAMS

The hospital support team works mainly in an advisory capacity alongside other hospital professionals, for instance in oncology, surgery, or general medicine. The team requires a multiprofessional membership, similar to teams working in the community.

The team can have several roles, including assessing patient needs (e.g. symptom control, counselling, quality of life), giving specialist advice on symptom control and other needs, and monitoring palliative care management. It also provides support, information, and advice to patients, families, and informal carers, as well as to professional carers in hospital and other professionals. The support team acts to promote palliative care to professional groups within hospital, and encourages continuity of care upon discharge of the patient. It also participates in research.

Hospital palliative care teams are essentially the catalyst to the provision of good palliative care, enabling all hospital staff to respond consistently and appropriately to the needs of patients and carers.

BEREAVEMENT SUPPORT

The role of this service is to assess the need for support for carers and to offer this support in a carefully monitored and supervised way. Ideally this work should begin before bereavement to prevent problems, particularly with those at risk of an abnormal or difficult bereavement (see Chapter 7). The service offered may comprise telephone contact, bereavement visiting, attendance at a bereavement group, bereavement counselling to individuals and families, and referral on to other agencies. Some units may offer specific services for bereaved children.

EDUCATION

All members of the specialist multidisciplinary team have a commitment to education and training as part of the ongoing development of palliative care. This has been recognized as a vital function of specialist teams. Most teams will be involved in teaching skills and competencies to a variety of staff where palliation is a significant element of care. Some will be involved in the training of specialist practitioners in medical, nursing, and other disciplines.

The primary care: specialist care interface

This chapter has illustrated the complexities of multidisciplinary teamwork. It is important to remember that the overall responsibility for the patient in the community remains with the PHCT. Good palliative care for patients depends on the PHCT. It is this team that will provide the majority of care. They also co-ordinate care from other services and professionals. This may be difficult for many GPs [12].

As with the optimum provision of any other secondary service there needs to be close dialogue between the PHCT and specialist palliative care services to ensure:
- excellent palliative care for individual patients and their families;
- adequate provision and development of services;
- exchange of knowledge;
- audit and evaluation of care;
- mutual support and understanding.

Summary

Good quality palliative care in the community can be achieved with effective collaboration between different professionals. Many services exist to assist in this process and it is important that they are employed promptly and appropriately. The dynamics that influence teamworking are complex, but with effort can result in considerable patient benefit and professional satisfaction.

Appendix

Summary of commonly used benefits

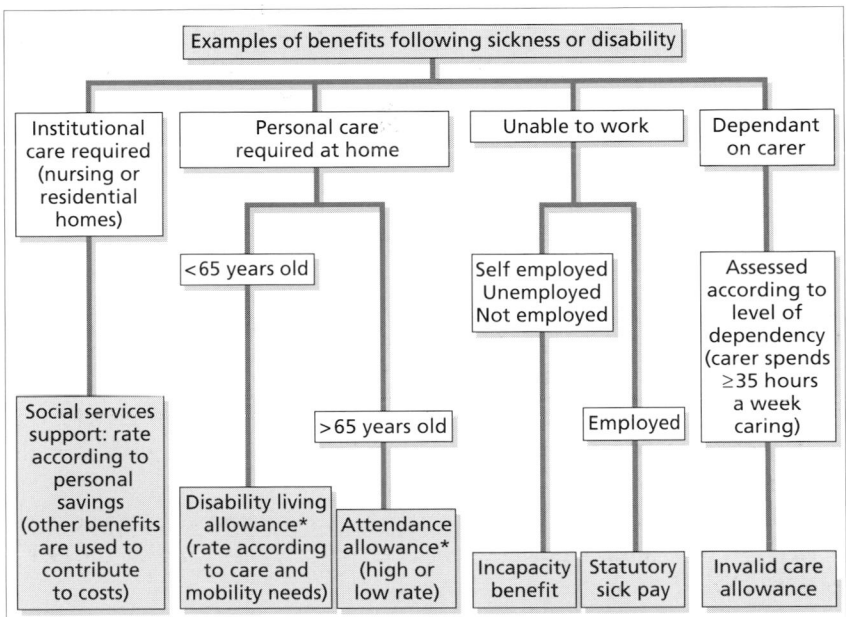

* Special rules apply in terminal illness for patients to receive these benefits promptly. Other benefits which may be appropriate include: income support, widows benefits, war pension. The rules of eligibility are complex and likely to undergo change with different governments.

References

1 Blyth AC. Audit of terminal care in a general practice. *BMJ* 1990; 300: 983–986.
2 Robinson L, Stacy R. Palliative care in the community: setting practice guidelines for primary care. *Br J Gen Pract* 1994; 44: 461–464.
3 Bennet I, Danczak AF. Terminal care: improving teamwork using significant event analysis. *Euro J Cancer Care* 1994; 3: 55–57.
4 Nash A, Hoy A. Terminal care in the community—an evaluation of residential workshops for general practitioners/district nurse teams. *Palliat Med* 1993; 7: 5–17.
5 Hobbs FDR, Drury M. Meeting and chairmanship. *BMJ* 1992; 304: 1616–1618.
6 Adelaide Medical Centre Primary Health Care Team. A primary care manifesto. *Br J Gen Pract* 1991; 41: 31–33.
7 Hampson JP, Roberts RI, Morgan DA. Shared care: a review of the literature. *Family Pract* 1996; 13: 264–279.
8 Smith S, Robinson J, Holleyer J. Combining specialist and primary health care

teams for HIV positive patients: retrospective and prospective studies. *BMJ* 1996; 312: 416–426.

9 Royal Pharmaceutical Society. *Medicines Ethics and Practice, A Guide for Pharmacists*, No. 17. London: Pharmaceutical Press, 1996.

10 Sibbald B, Addington Hall J, Brenneman D *et al.* Counsellors in English and Welsh general practices: their number and distribution. *BMJ* 1993; 306: 29–33.

11 Working Party on Clinical Guidelines in Palliative Care. *Information for Purchasers: Background to Available Specialist Palliative Care Services.* London: National Council for Hospices and Specialist Palliative Care Services, 1995.

12 Cartwright A. *The Role of the General Practitioner in Caring for People in the Last Year of their Lives.* London: King's Fund, 1990.

3: Medicines Management in Palliative Care

CAROLE ANN BLACKSHAW AND
CHRISTINA FAULL

Introduction

The complex mix of problems that arise in advanced illness may often require the patient to take a large number of medicines, which need frequent modification and change to achieve optimum symptom management. This raises many practical and pharmacological problems for the patient, their carer, and the health care team. To deal with these problems and achieve quality care requires close teamwork and efficient organization.

This chapter will describe how pharmacists can make a valuable contribution to the care of patients with advanced illness, through the application of their expertise in medicines management. The chapter will also highlight some of the unusual prescribing issues in advanced illness, particularly problems of access to drugs in the community and the prescribing of controlled drugs.

The pharmacist in palliative care: a key team member

As most prescribed medication nowadays requires no formulation by the pharmacist, and with the increasing use of prepackaged medicines, the nature of the pharmacist's professional role has changed and continues to develop. The services offered by pharmacists additional to their dispensing activities have become known as the 'extended role'.

In essence the pharmacist can play several vital roles: helping to maintain a high standard of prescribing; making doctors and nurses aware of new and alternative drugs and drug preparations; and checking for drug interactions. By ensuring that patients and their carers clearly understand the purpose of each medicine, how to take their medicines, and how to recognize side-effects and the action to be taken, the pharmacist helps to achieve optimum compliance. He or she also plays an important role in helping to manage an efficient service so that patients obtain the medicines they need promptly, in an appropriate formulation, and with helpful compliance aids.

There is enormous potential for the community pharmacists to work with other members of the primary health care team (PHCT) and specialist home care teams to strengthen the support offered to patients in the community. The extended and specific role of the pharmacist in the PHCT is being developed and appears to be a successful way forward in health care [1,2]. Community and hospital pharmacists are also key members of the specialist palliative care teams, providing services and expertise to hospices and specialist units [3].

Pharmaceutical care

The responsible provision of drug therapy for the purpose of achieving definite outcomes that improve a patient's quality of life [4,5].

This quotation clearly describes the pharmacist's role as a patient-focused health care provider, not just a dispenser of medicines. The use of pharmaceutical care plans is particularly valuable in achieving these objectives for patients with advanced illness whether in hospital, hospice, or in the community. A typical plan might include the information shown in Box 3.1.

Domiciliary services

Many pharmacists deliver medicines to their patients. Some have close links with GP surgeries to pick up prescriptions or have them delivered

---

Box 3.1 Outline of a typical hospital pharmaceutical care plan

• Consider all the symptoms and their potential origins and ensure optimum choice and use of drugs
• Identify and monitor possible adverse drug reactions and interactions
• Ensure that the patient can manage the prescribed medicine regimen (e.g. appropriate dosage forms; patient can physically and mentally manage the medicine regimen). Consider the use of compliance aids
• Talk to the patient and carers about the medicines, to enhance understanding and help to allay fears or anxieties about the medicines
• Monitor any relevant laboratory tests which may be available
• Ensure that the drugs prescribed are easily available in the community and if they are not arrange for their supply
• Review the regimen regularly to ensure that all drugs and doses are relevant to the current problems

direct to the pharmacy. Both these services are vital for frail, unwell people, particularly those without carers.

In addition health authorities may be involved in providing domiciliary pharmaceutical services to patients who would otherwise be denied access to a pharmacy service. Local arrangements are established between health commissioning authorities, social services departments, and local community pharmacists. Patients needing such a service can be identified by their GP, community nurse, community pharmacists, or social services department. The local health authority pharmaceutical adviser can be contacted to check if such arrangements are available in any particular area.

Helping patients to understand their medicines

A traditional role of the pharmacist has been to advise patients about their medicines. Pharmacists can expand on and reinforce the instructions given by the prescribing doctor and explain and provide further information about: why and how medicines should be taken; the dosage regimen for effective pain or other symptom management, and specific drugs, symptoms and other aspects of care.

Unwanted medicines

A patient, or his or her representative, may return unwanted medicines, including controlled drugs, to any pharmacist for destruction.

The provision of and access to medicines for terminally ill patients in the community

Patients with advanced disease, particularly those that are dying, commonly need rapid access to new and unusual medications. For example a GP called to the house of a terminally ill restless patient who is vomiting may wish to prescribe a subcutaneous infusion of methotrimeprazine, a drug seldom stocked by pharmacists. Difficulty in accessing medicines promptly, for a variety of reasons, is unfortunately a common issue for patients and their carers and requires careful thought and attention to detail by the primary health care team (PHCT), pharmacists, and hospital and specialist services.

Seamless care and discharge planning

The complexity of medicines used in the care of terminally ill patients in

---

Box 3.2 Examples of prescription medicines which may not be routinely stocked by community pharmacists

- Large quantities or high dosages of morphine-containing analgesics
- New morphine preparations
- Other strong opioids
- Diazepam suppositories or rectal liquid
- Midazolam injection
- Methotrimeprazine
- Ondansetron
- Dexamethasone tablets in high doses
- Enteral feeds
- Hyoscine hydrobromide or butylbromide injection

---

the community serves to highlight the importance of careful planning of the discharge of a patient from secondary to primary care, or from hospice to home. The patient and their carers may need assistance in organization of supplies so that essential equipment and medications are always available. For example, they may be advised to obtain their prescriptions well before their current stock of medicines runs out. This is extremely important as many community pharmacists will need to order unusual, or large quantities of medicines. Examples of prescription medicines which may not be routinely stocked by community pharmacists are shown in Box 3.2.

Forms for the transfer of information about patients and their medicines between pharmacists have been produced by the Royal Pharmaceutical Society of Great Britain (RPSGB) [6]. These forms are usually copied to general practitioners, community pharmacists, and appropriate community or specialist nurses. The form may also be given to the patient if it is appropriate to do so. There are similar forms to aid the smooth admission of patients to hospital or hospice [7].

Pharmacy networks

With the necessary organization and funding, community pharmacists may be prepared to keep stocks of drugs used in terminal care. In some areas, for example Islington in London, a formal network has been set up to ensure easy access to these drugs by patients and home care nurses [8,9]. These arrangements are usually administered and funded by the local health authority.

'Unlicensed' or 'special' medicines

Rarely used or new drugs may be available only as unlicensed 'specials', or on a named patient basis from the pharmaceutical industry. Community pharmacists may have to call on the local hospital pharmacy department, or pharmaceutical manufacturing specialist, to obtain these medicines. Time and advanced warning are particularly important in these situations.

The prescribing and dispensing of controlled drugs

Controlled drugs are subject to the requirements of the Misuse of Drugs Regulations 1985 [10]. The legislation is split into five Schedules. Schedule 1 lists drugs such as LSD which have no recognized place in the treatment of disease and have the strictest control imposed on them. Schedule 2 drugs included the principal opioids and cocaine, while buprenorphine and most barbiturates fall into Schedule 3. Schedule 4 drugs consist mainly of the benzodiazepines. Schedule 5 covers the low dose and dilute preparations of some of the Schedule 2 drugs and has the lowest level of control. Controlled Drugs are distinguished in the *British National Formulary* by the symbol CD (Controlled Drugs). The status of compounds can be checked in the *Medicines, Ethics and Practice Guide* obtained from the RSPGB [6].

The prescription

It is an offence for a doctor to issue an incomplete prescription and it is illegal for a pharmacist to dispense a controlled drug unless all the information required by law is given on the prescription. Failure to comply with the handwriting regulations (see below) will result in inconvenience to the patient and delay in supplying the necessary medicines.

The Misuse of Drugs Regulations 1985 requires that prescriptions for Schedule 2 and 3 drugs (all strong opioids, barbiturates and temazepam) must be completed in the following manner:
• prescriptions ordering controlled drugs must be signed and dated by the prescriber and specify the prescriber's address;
• the prescription must always be written in the prescriber's own handwriting in ink or be otherwise indelible and include the details shown in Box 3.3. Examples of prescriptions are given in Fig. 3.1. The use of computer-generated forms for repeat prescriptions of controlled drugs is thus generally inappropriate.

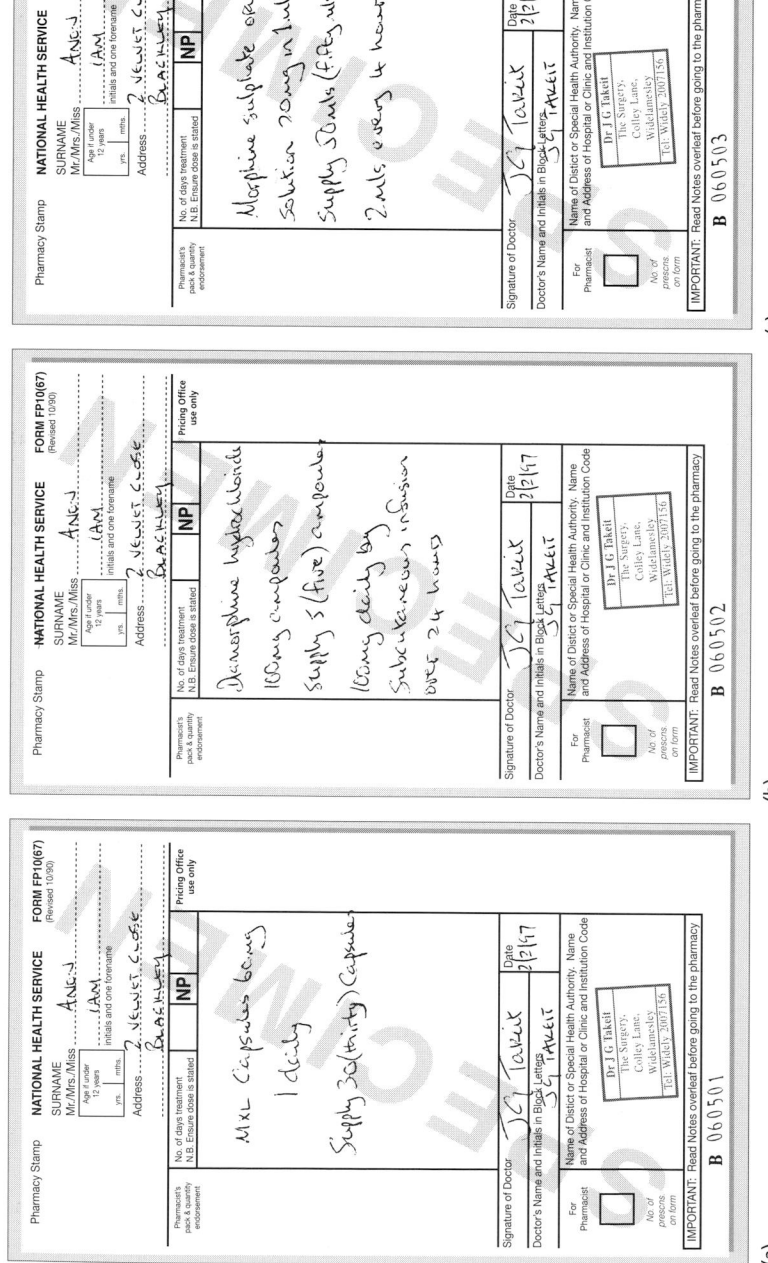

Fig. 3.1 Examples of controlled drug prescriptions.

Box 3.3 Details required for a controlled drug prescription

- The name and address of the patient
- In the case of preparations, the form (i.e. tablets, capsules, mixture, etc.) and where appropriate the strength (if there is more than one available) of the preparation
- The total quantity of the preparation, or the number of dosage units, in both words and figures
- The specified dose; for example, the instruction 'one as directed' constitutes a dose but 'as directed' does not

---

Exemptions to prescription requirements

Exemptions to the requirement for the prescriber's own handwriting include prescriptions for Schedule 3 drugs temazepam and phenobarbitone and controlled drugs in Schedule 4 (anabolic steroids and benzodiazepines). In addition temazepam prescriptions do not have to contain all the usual controlled drug requirements, such as 'total quantity in words and figures'. For the purpose of prescription writing temazepam can be written up as for any other prescription-only medicine.

Taking controlled drugs abroad

Patients who wish to holiday abroad and who need to take their own supply of Schedule 2 or 3 controlled drugs, such as morphine, with them, may need to seek a licence from the Home Office. Up to 15 days worth of opioids may usually be taken without licence unless the dose of opioids is particularly high (no clear definition of this is available). The patient's prescribing doctor will need to write a letter to the Home Office (see Useful Addresses, p. 377). The letter will need to include the following information:
- patient's full name and address and date of birth;
- country of destination;
- medication details, including; name, form, strength, and total quantity of each controlled drug to be taken out of the UK;
- departure date and return date.

The Home Office will, if the quantity or type of opioid requires it, issue a licence, allowing the patient to take the drug(s) through British customs. They will also issue, if necessary, the telephone number of the destination country's embassy. Ten days should be allowed for processing of the licence. It has no legal status outside the UK and does not ensure safe passage through the customs of the country of destination. The patient will need to contact that country's embassy to clarify the requirements for taking controlled drugs through the customs of the destination country.

Disposal of controlled drugs after a death at home

Controlled drugs can be returned to any pharmacist by a patient's representative for destruction.

Aids to compliance

Patients taking a large number of different medicines may have difficulty, for a variety of reasons, in adhering to the correct regimen. This is a complex issue and although compliance aids will be helpful to many patients other aspects of the prescribing and taking of medications should always be considered [11,12]. Patients who most depend on medicines to maintain their quality of life are often those least able to remember to take all their medicines exactly as prescribed. Compliance aids are available which may help some patients simplify and remember their particular medication regime, but funding for such aids is not straightforward. At present they are not prescribable on FP10 prescription (GP prescriptions). Special funding arrangements should be sought between health authorities and community pharmacists, so that patients do not have to bear the cost of the aids themselves.

There are a variety of compliance aids available such as charts and diaries, large print labels, and special memory aid packs and boxes [13].

Memory aid packs and boxes

These range from simple pill boxes to electronic programmable devices, but are suitable only for solid oral medications, i.e. pills. The simplest and most commonly useful are described below.

Blister packs. These are prepared by a pharmacist, and usually contain at least one week's medications. They are helpful when medication use is stable from week to week.

Daily pill dispensers. These contain the supply of pills for a single day in up to four dosage times. Each dosage time is labelled with the time, part of the day, and a number and/or 'braille' character. Some pill dispensers, such as Redidose (Fig. 3.2), come in sets of seven so that the system can be

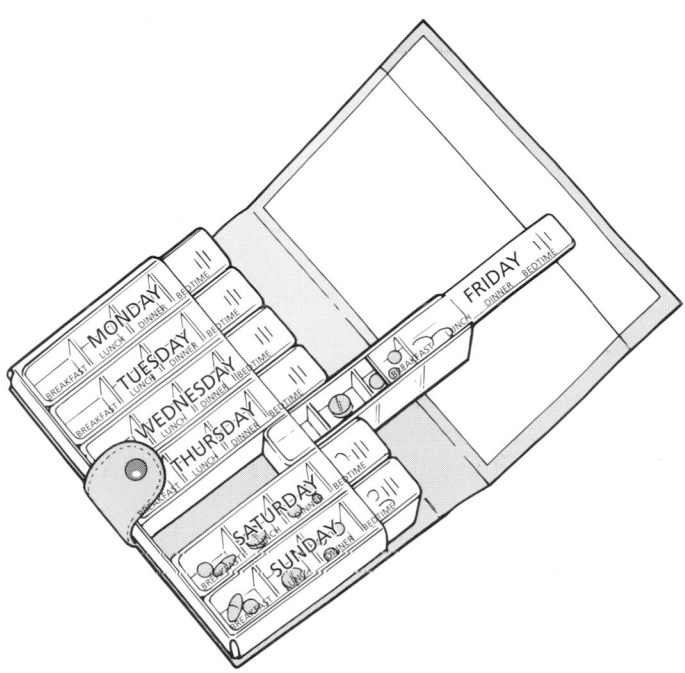

Fig. 3.2 The Redidose seven-day pill dispenser.

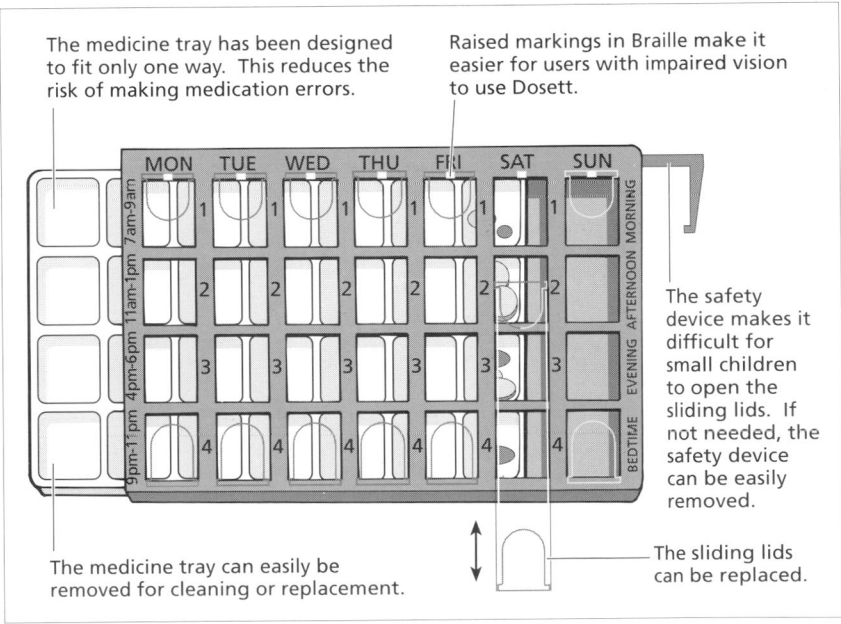

The medicine tray has been designed to fit only one way. This reduces the risk of making medication errors.

Raised markings in Braille make it easier for users with impaired vision to use Dosett.

The safety device makes it difficult for small children to open the sliding lids. If not needed, the safety device can be easily removed.

The medicine tray can easily be removed for cleaning or replacement.

The sliding lids can be replaced.

Fig. 3.3 The Dosett weekly pill dispenser.

recharged weekly but the tablets required for each day can be issued or carried separately.

Weekly pill dispensers. Weekly pill dispensers include the Dosett (see Fig. 3.3, p. 41). A tray of medicines for the week is accessed through clearly labelled compartments allowing up to four dosage times daily. These are available in a variety of size compartments to cope with patients on from two to as many as ten medicines. This system is used in many nursing homes.

Medi-wheel. The Medi-wheel allows patients to access their medicines for the day through a one-way rotation of compartments. Turning may be easier for some patients than lifting or sliding lids. The wheels can also be supplied in a week pack.

The future

Technological developments will continue to allow more patient care to be undertaken in the community. For example, the use of ambulatory infusion pumps has led to effective home-based chemotherapy and epidural infusion of analgesia for improved pain control. The RPSGB encourages community pharmacists to become involved with this specialist type of care [6]. Clearly there is a need for hospital, community, and hospice pharmacists to work together and for all to work closely with the primary health care teams and specialist teams to provide comprehensive care for patients [1].

The pharmaceutical needs of patients with advanced disease demand the development of specialist knowledge amongst pharmacists, particularly community pharmacists. A network of pharmacists with a particular role and expertise in palliative care could improve care for terminally ill patients in the community. To support pharmacists working in palliative care is the aim of the Hospice Pharmacists' Association (details found under Useful Addresses; see p. 377).

References

1 Marinker M (ed.). *Controversies in Health Care Politics: Challenges to Practice.* London: BMJ Publishing Group, 1994.
2 Bradley CP, Taylor RJ, Blenkinsopp A. Developing prescribing in primary care. *BMJ* 1997; 314: 744–747.
3 Blackshaw CA. An investigation into the current services available for the provisions and use of medicines in the care of terminally ill patients in the community. MSc Thesis, University of Keele, 1995.

4 Hepler CD, Strand LM. Opportunities and responsibilities in pharmaceutical care. *Am J Hosp Pharm* 1990; 47: 533–543.

5 Royal Pharmaceutical Society. Statement on pharmaceutical care. *Pharm J* 1996; 256: 345–346.

6 Royal Pharmaceutical Society of Great Britain. *Medicines Ethics and Practice, A Guide for Pharmacists*, No. 17. London: Pharmaceutical Press, 1996.

7 Royal Pharmaceutical Society of Great Britain. *Communication between Hospital and Community Pharmacists Concerning Patients' Medication and Pharmaceutical Needs (Guidelines on the Use of Hospital Admission and Discharge Forms)* London: Royal Pharmaceutical Society, 1994.

8 Allen M. What is palliative care? *Pharm J* 1995; 254: 193–194.

9 Chapman M. The community pharmacist's role in terminal care. *Pharm J* 1995; 254: 868–869.

10 The Misuse of Drugs Regulations 1985.

11 Aronson JK, Hardman M. Patient compliance. *BMJ* 1992; 305: 1009–1011.

12 Mullen D. Compliance becomes concordance. *BMJ* 1997; 314: 691–692.

13 Walker R. Which medication compliance device? *Pharm J* 1992; 248: 605–607.

Further reading

British National Formulary. Guidance on prescribing in terminal care (in the first section of the book).

Position paper on the pharmaceutical care of cancer patients in the community, in the light of the Health of the Nation and the Calman report. London: Royal Pharmaceutical Society, 1996.

Controlled dosage systems for residential homes. *Pharm J* 1990; 244: 385–386.

Jackson C, Rowe P, Lea R. Pharmacy discharge—a professional necessity for the 1990s. *Pharm J* 1993; 250: 58–59.

National Health Services Management Executive. Responsibility for prescribing between hospitals and GPs. Executive Letter EL(91) (27). London: Department of Health, 1991.

Royal Pharmaceutical Society. A domiciliary pharmaceutical service (working party report). *Pharm J* 1988; 241: 90–93.

Stewart BJ. *Terminal Care in the Community*. Oxford: Radcliffe Medical Press, 1996.

4: Needs Assessment and Audit in Palliative Care

IRENE HIGGINSON

Needs assessment

Introduction

As people live longer and acute illnesses become less common as a cause of death, progressive and chronic illnesses are becoming increasingly common. Patients with these illnesses, and their families, will need palliative care.

In an attempt to provide assistance for those purchasing palliative care services, an epidemiologically based needs assessment for palliative and terminal care has been produced for the NHS Executive [1]. The actual local numbers of patients dying from cancer and other diseases are available from the Office of National Statistics or local health authorities. GPs may also have data from their own records. Table 4.1 shows the number of deaths within a 1 000 000 population in England during one year for the most common causes. Roughly equal numbers of men and women would die and the numbers would be roughly constant over time.

Need among cancer patients and their families

Within a population of 10 000 people (e.g. a group practice) national estimates suggest that there are approximately 28 cancer deaths per year, many of whom would have a period of advancing progressive disease, when palliative care would be appropriate. The estimates of prevalence of symptoms and problems are based on population and other studies of patients with advanced disease and their families. Applying the population estimates to the 28 patients who would die from cancer suggests that during the year of their death 23 would have problems with pain, 13 with breathlessness, 14 with vomiting or nausea, 20 with anorexia, and 9 where the patient and 7 where the family had severe anxiety or worry that was seriously affecting their daily life and concentration (see Table 4.2).

Table 4.1 The number of deaths in the population during one year for the most common causes. (Note: a population of 1 000 000 is used to capture rare causes.)

Cause of death	Men	Women	Total
Neoplasms*	1464	1341	2805
Circulatory system	2429	2624	5053
Respiratory system	595	626	1221
Chronic liver and cirrhosis	34	26	60
Nervous system and sense organs**	88	88	176
Senile and pre-senile organic conditions	22	22	44
Endocrine, nutritional, metabolic immunity	187	123	310
Total of these diseases	4819	4850	9669
Total deaths from all causes	5356	5644	11 000
Neoplasms include:			
Lip, oral, pharynx, larynx	41	34	74
Digestive and peritoneum	449	339	788
Trachea, bronchus, lung	394	291	685
Female breast	0	255	255
Genitourinary	243	178	421
Lymphatic and haematopoietic	154	54	208
Other, unspecified	7	7	14
**Nervous system and sense organs include:*			
Parkinson's disease	37	28	65
Multiple sclerosis	1	1	2
Meningitis	4	4	8

Note: deaths in those aged under 28 days excluded * and ** for breakdown of main groups.

Current levels of use of specialist palliative care services can also be employed as an indirect estimate of need. However, these do not take account of unmet need and can only represent existing supply. Estimates of average service used nationally do not necessarily indicate that these levels of use are correct. In England, studies have estimated that between 15 and 25% of those dying of cancer received in-patient hospice care, with between 25 and 65% receiving input from a support team or Macmillan nurse. Applying these figures to a population of 10 000 would suggest that each year 7–18 cancer patients require support team care, and 4–7 require in-patient hospice care (see Table 4.3). Some patients will obviously require both services and some may be admitted to a hospice two or more times.

Table 4.2 Cancer patients: prevalence of problems (per 10 000 population).

Symptom	Symptom in last year of life (%)*	Estimated number in each year
Pain	84	24
Trouble with breathing	47	13
Vomiting or nausea	51	14
Sleeplessness	51	14
Mental confusion	33	9
Depression	38	11
Anorexia	71	20
Constipation	47	13
Bedsores	28	8
Loss of bladder control	37	10
Loss of bowel control	25	7
Unpleasant smell	19	5
Severe family anxiety/worries	33	9
Severe patient anxiety/worries	25	7
Total deaths from cancer		28

* Symptoms as per Cartwright and Seale studies [2][3], based on a random sample of deaths and using the reports of bereaved carers.
* Anxiety as per Field *et al.* [4], Bennett and Corcoran [5], Higginson *et al.* [6], Addington-Hall *et al.* [7].
Note: Patients usually have several symptoms.

Table 4.3 Cancer patients: need for specialist palliative services based on national and regional estimates of use (per 10 000 population)*.

	Number of adults	Percentage (%)
Deaths from cancer in one year	28	
Needing support team	7–18	25–65
Needing in-patient hospice care	4–7	15–25

* Studies used include: Bennett and Corcoran (1994) [5]; Cartwright (1991) [2]; Seale (1991) [3]; Higginson *et al.* (1992) [6]; Addington-Hall [8,9,10,11]; Frankel (1990) [12]; Eve and Jackson (1994) [13].

Need among non-cancer patients and their families

As for cancer patients, estimates of the prevalence of symptoms and other problems from existing studies can be applied to a population to determine

Table 4.4 Patients with non-cancer progressive illness: prevalence of problems (per 10 000 population).

Symptom	Symptom in last year of life (%)*	Estimated number in each year
Pain	67	46
Trouble with breathing	49	34
Vomiting or nausea	27	18
Sleeplessness	36	25
Mental confusion	38	26
Depression	36	25
Anorexia	38	26
Constipation	32	22
Bedsores	14	10
Loss of bladder control	33	23
Loss of bowel control	22	15
Unpleasant smell	13	9
Severe family anxiety/worries	33	22
Severe patient anxiety/worries	25	16
Total deaths from other causes, excluding accidents, injury and suicide, and causes very unlikely to have a palliative period		68

As per the Cartwright and Seale studies [2,3], based on a random sample of deaths and using the reports of bereaved carers.
Anxiety as per Field *et al.* [4], Bennett and Corcoran [5], Higginson *et al.* [6], Addington-Hall *et al.* [7].
Note: Patients usually have several symptoms.

the numbers of people with these problems in the last year of life (see Table 4.4).

The numbers of people affected are more than double those for cancer. Primary care plays a very important role for these patients and their families, as it does for those with cancer. In many of the illnesses it is more difficult to prognosticate; with the illness being sometimes acute, sometimes progressive, and sometimes chronic.

Traditionally specialist palliative care services have concentrated on, and gained experience with cancer patients, but this is changing. Such services see their role as increasingly providing expert symptom control and psychosocial advice and care for people with other illnesses. As specialist palliative care services move towards providing more home care, respite care, and short admissions to attend to symptom or other problems, they may become increasingly able to help in non-malignant disease. Therefore,

Table 4.5 Patients with progressive non-malignant diseases: need for specialist palliative services based on local studies of use or need (per 10 000 population)*.

	Number of adults	Percentage (%)
Deaths in one year	68	
Needing support team	4–14	0.5–1 times numbers of cancer patients needing care
Needing in-patient palliative care	2–7	0.5–1 times numbers of cancer patients needing care

* Studies used include: Hockley *et al.* (1988) [19], Severs and Wilkins (1991) [20]; Noble (1993) [21].

estimates of need based on the current patterns of use of specialist palliative care services by this group of patients (see Table 4.5) are likely to be inaccurate; although these may give an indication of those patients who need especial attention.

Home care

Five studies, in different developed countries, have found that between 50 and 70% of cancer patients would prefer to be cared for at home for as long as possible, and to die at home [14–18]. A longitudinal study of patients in the care of a domiciliary palliative care team suggested that as death approached patients changed their preferences: hospital and home became less preferred and hospice more preferred, although even one week before death 50% still wished to be cared for at home [12]. However, far fewer achieve care at home until death. The number of people who die at home has fallen in recent years (from 42% in 1969 to 24% in 1987); 29% of cancer deaths included in the Regional Study of Care for the Dying (RSCD) by Addington-Hall *et al.* died at home [8,9].

Need during bereavement

The primary care team is often the first point of contact for a bereaved person. For every person who dies there may be one or more bereaved carers who will have physical, emotional, social, and spiritual changes as a result of their loss. This will apply for both chronic and acute deaths. Grief is known to have a marked effect on mortality and morbidity. Mor *et al.* found that when age, sex, and prior health were controlled for, bereaved spouses were at increased risk of physician visits, hospitalization, use of anti-anxiety medication, and increased alcohol use compared with national averages [22]. In a study of bereaved older adults Norris and Murrell found that bereavement was followed by increased 'psychological distress' [23]. Bowling and Charlton showed an increase in mortality after bereavement [24]. All these effects will result in needs for care and support during bereavement, although the extent of this need in the primary care setting is not well researched.

Areas for improved care

Many studies have demonstrated deficiencies in conventional care for dying people both in hospitals and the community. A review of the literature from 1960 indicated that dying patients have suffered severe unrelieved symptoms, particularly pain, had unmet practical, social, and emotional needs, and suffered as the result of poor co-ordination of services and because health professionals appeared unwilling to share information [8]. In hospital studies, staff were observed to withdraw from patients and to pay little attention to their symptoms, emotional needs, or needs for care [8]. The Regional Study of Care of the Dying, which examined care in the last year of life for random samples of cancer and non-cancer deaths, demonstrated continued problems of unrelieved pain and other symptoms and that relatives bore the brunt of caring [9].

Families and carers also suffered because of poor communication by health professionals and had unmet needs for emotional, practical, and bereavement support [8]. Cancer patients were found to have depression and anxiety more commonly than in the 'normal' population, while their families also were at risk of developing social and psychiatric problems [8].

In national terms, areas for improved care can be summarized as follows:
- pain and symptom control;
- emotional, social, and spiritual support;
- communication;
- co-ordination of care;
- bereavement support;
- care for people in the place(s) of their choice;
- respite care and support for carers.

This may vary from area to area, and perhaps it is sensible for practices to consider the above list against their local circumstances.

Audit

Choosing measures and standards for audit

Palliative care audits have been described in detail in *Clinical Audit in Palliative Care* [25] along with full details of measures already tested in palliative care settings.

In primary care there are various options for measures and standards. The Support Team Assessment Schedule (STAS) was developed for palliative care and was used initially in home care and hospital support teams, but is now used more widely. Designed to assess mainly the outcomes of care, it includes aspects concerned with the patient's quality of life (e.g. pain, symptoms, anxiety, spiritual, and planning needs), the family, communication, and the needs of other professionals (see Box 4.1).

In England, a nationally representative project team with individuals representing all care settings, including primary care, is adapting this STAS for wider use. The group is seeking to develop a small core audit measure,

---

Box 4.1 Items in the Support Team Assessment Schedule (STAS). A patient is rated for each item, o (no problem) to 4 (overwhelming problems), with definitions for each point [25].

Nine patient and family items
- Pain control
- Symptom control
- Patient anxiety
- Family anxiety
- Patient insight
- Family insight
- Spiritual
- Planning
- Communication between patient and family

Seven service items
- Practical aid
- Financial
- Wasted time
- Communication from professionals to patient and family
- Communication between professionals
- Professional anxiety
- Advising professionals

which will work in primary care, hospital, day care, and other settings. Details of the measure are available from the authors.

In Cambridge Dr Todd and colleagues are developing CAMPAS (Cambridge Palliative Care Schedule). Although originally based on STAS, CAMPAS has evolved to examine the specific concerns of general practitioners and those in primary care. It includes a combination of process and outcome items [26].

A systematic review of outcome and quality of life measures which might be used in palliative care identified the Edmonton Symptom Assessment Scale, the McGill Quality of Life questionnaire [27–29] and the EORTC-QLQ C30 as reasonably short outcome measures which could be used in palliative care, particularly earlier stage disease [30,31]. The last two of these measures have been used in community settings although not primary care. It may be that these measures or standards are not suitable for some situations, but aspects may provide a catalyst to develop other more appropriate items.

An alternative approach might be to undertake topic audit [25], which would concentrate on one topic within primary care, and define the measures and assessments for this. Forms of a topic audit could be: review of communication [32] and/or a review of knowledge of services [33,34].

When performing such as audit the following actions could be taken.
1 Survey of the views of bereaved carers. A standardized questionnaire which has been used in studies since 1969 is being adapted for use as a postal questionnaire, or could be used in interview [35]. Alternatively, GPs could develop local questionnaires from those used in other studies [36].
2 Educational audit, where educational programmes for GPs and those in the primary care team are assessed [37].
3 Review of where patients die, or last reasons for admission, or whether the patients' and families' wishes for place of care or death were met [34], or review of place of death within a general practice [38].

In the UK, Medical Audit Advisory Groups (MAAGs) can provide advice, peer support, and resources for audits in primary care. In addition, monies for clinical audit are made available to the purchasers of health care. In most authorities money is allocated in each financial year. Some authorities examine bids; others make a payment to MAAGs, health services, or trusts; others will agree an audit programme through contracts.

National and international perspective

There are some sources of national and international information on audit and outcomes measures. The Outcomes Clearing House, an NHS Executive initiative, is designed to provide information on current work on health outcomes in the UK. Based in Leeds, the Clearing House encourages any individuals using health outcomes to register on their database. Any person can contact the outcomes centre and ask for a search on the database of projects of interest. The Cochrane collaboration, an international collaboration which aims to increase evidence-based health care, has developed a Pain and Palliative Care Group (PAPAS), to co-ordinate systematic reviews of evidence.

In addition the author has developed a database of STAS users and a newsletter for the STAS users which can provide information of new developments and adaptations of STAS.

Conclusions

Within a population of 10 000, a general practice might expect almost 100 deaths per year where there is some need for palliative care, including bereavement support. Most of these will have symptom, psychosocial, and spiritual needs that require support.

Clinical audit, evaluation, and studies of outcome are all means to improve the quality of care for patients and families. It is important that this aim is continually revisited, and that the audit or outcome studies do not become merely a paper exercise.

References

1 Higginson I. Palliative and terminal care. In: Stevens A, Raftery J, eds. *DHA Project: Research Programme. Epidemiologically Based Needs Assessment*, Series 2. Oxford: Radcliffe Medical Press, 1997.
2 Cartwright A. Changes in life and care in the year before death 1969–1987. *J Pub Health Med* 1991; 13 (2): 81–87.
3 Seale C. A comparison of hospice and conventional care. *Soc Sci Med* 1991; 32 (2): 147–152.
4 Field D, Douglas C, Jagger C, Dand P. Terminal illness: views of patients and their lay carers. *Palliat Med* 1995; 9: 45–54.
5 Bennett M, Corcoran G. The impact on community palliative care services of a hospital palliative care team. *Palliat Med* 1994; 8: 237–244.
6 Higginson I, Wade A, McCarthy M. Effectiveness of two palliative support teams. *J Pub Health Med* 1992; 1: 50–56.
7 Addington-Hall JM, MacDonald L, Anderson H, Freeling P. Dying from cancer: the view of bereaved family and the friends about the experiences of terminally ill patients. *Palliat Med* 1991; 5: 207–214.
8 Addington-Hall JM. *Regional Study of Care for the Dying. Feedback for District*

Health Authorities. Cancer Deaths Only. London: Department of Epidemiology and Public Health, University College London, 1993.

9 Addington-Hall JM. *Regional Study of Care for the Dying. Feedback for District Health Authorities. Non-cancer Deaths Only.* London: Department of Epidemiology and Public Health, University College London, 1993.

10 Addington-Hall JM, McCarthy M. Regional study of care of the dying: methods and sample characteristics. *Palliat Med* 1995; 9: 27–35.

11 Addington-Hall JM, McCarthy M. Dying from cancer: results of a national population-based investigation. *Palliat Med* 1995; 9: 295–305.

12 Frankel S. Assessing the need for hospice beds. *Health Trnd* 1990; 2: 83–86.

13 Eve A, Jackson A. Palliative care, where are we now? *Palliat Care Today* 1994; 3 (2): 22–23.

14 Dunlop R, Daviews RJ, Hockley JM. Preferred vs. actual place of death: a hospital palliative care support team study. *Palliat Med* 1989; 3: 197–201.

15 Townsend J, Frank AO, Fermont D *et al.* Terminal cancer care and patients' preference for place of death: a prospective study. *BMJ* 1990; 301: 415–417.

16 Ashby M, Wakefield M. Attitudes to some aspects of death and dying, living wills and substituted health care decision-making in South Australia: public opinion survey for a parliamentary select committee. *Palliat Med* 1993; 7 (4): 273–282.

17 Hinton J. Can home care maintain an acceptable quality of life for patients with terminal cancer and their relatives? *Palliat Med* 1994; 8 (3): 183–196.

18 Costantini M, Camoirano E, Madeddu L *et al.* Palliative home care and place of death among cancer patients: a population based study. *Palliat Med* 1993; 7: 323–331.

19 Hockley JM, Dunlop R, Davis RJ. Survey of distressing symptoms in dying patients and their families in hospital and the response to a symptom control team. *BMJ* 1988; 296: 1715–1717.

20 Severs MP, Wilkins PS. A hospital palliative care ward for elderly people. *Age and Ageing* 1991; 20 (5): 361–364.

21 Noble B. A snapshot survey of hospital and hospice patients. In: *Older Peoples: Palliative Care Strategy.* Sheffield: Family and Community Services, Health Authority and Family Health Services Authority, 1993, Appendix B.

22 Mor V, McHorney C, Sherwood S. Secondary morbidity among the recently bereaved. *Am J Psych* 1986; 143 (2): 158–163.

23 Norris FH, Murrell SA. Older adult family stress and adaptation before and after bereavement. *J Gerontol* 1987; 42 (6): 606–612.

24 Bowling A, Charlton J. Risk factors for mortality after bereavement: a logistic regression analysis. *J Roy Coll Gen Pract* 1987; 37 (305): 551–554.

25 Higginson I, ed. *Clinical Audit in Palliative Care.* Oxford: Radcliffe Medical Press, 1993.

26 Berkley S, Todd CJ. Audit of general practice based palliative care in Cambridge. *Palliat Med* 1997; 1: 11 (1): 68 (research abstract).

27 Cohen SR, Hassen SA, Lapointe BN, Mount BM. Quality of life in HIV disease as measured by the McGill quality of life questionnaire. *Aids* 1996; 10 (12): 1421–1427.

28 Cohen SR, Mount BM, Tomas JJ, Mount LF. Existential well-being is an important determinant of quality of life. *Cancer* 1996; 77(3): 576–586.

29 Cohen SR, Mount BM, Strobel MG, Bui F. The McGill Quality of Life Questionnaire: a measure of quality of life appropriate for people with advanced disease. A preliminary study of validity and acceptability. *Palliat Med* 1995; 9 (3): 207–219.

30 Hearn J, Higginson I. Outcome measures in palliative care for advanced cancer: a review. *J Publ Health Med* 1997; 19 (2): 193–199.

31 Bruera E, Kuehn N, Selmser P, Macmillan K. The Edmonton Symptom Assessment System (ESAS). A simple method for the assessment of palliative care patients. *J Palliat Care* 1991; 7: 6–9.

32 Todd C, Still A. General practitioners' strategies and tactics of communication with the terminally ill. *Family Pract* 1993; 10: 268–276.

33 Seamark DA, Thorne CP, Rones RV, Gray DJ, Searle JF. Knowledge and perceptions of a domiciliary hospice service among general practitioners and community nurses. *Br J Gen Pract* 1993; 43: 57–59.

34 Holden J. *An Audit of Terminal Care: The RCGP Audit Programme.* London: RCGP, Mersey Faculty Audit Group, 1993.

35 Addington-Hall J, McCarthy M. Audit methods: views of the family after the death. In: Higginson I, ed. *Clinical Audit in Palliative Care.* Oxford: Radcliffe Medical Press, 1993.

36 Jones RVH, Hansford J, Fiske J. Death from cancer at home: the carer's perspective. *Br Med J* 1993; 306: 249–251.

37 Nash A, Hoy A. Terminal care in the community – an evaluation of residential workshops for general practitioners and district nurses. *Palliat Med* 1993; 7: 5–17.

38 Holden JD. Auditing palliative care in one general practice over eight years. *Scand J Prim Health Care* 1996; 9: 14 (3), 136–141.

5: The Person, the Patient and their Carers

PATRICIA WILKIE

Introduction

There were lots of people in charge of different parts of Jack's body, but no-one was in charge of Jack.
John Hoyland, April 1997

A patient is a person who may be a mother or father, a parent, child, or partner. Patients belong to different age groups, and both sexes. Some patients may be deeply religious, while other patients have no particular faith. A patient is not a sarcoma or a Hodgkin's or an end-stage renal failure, or a motor neurone disease (MND), or an octogenarian but a person who is a member of a family and of the wider community and who has particular and individual needs.

The UK is made up of people from many varied cultural and social groups whose views about illness, suffering, pain, and death will also be many and various.

Patients with a medical condition that seriously affects their daily living and their families want to feel secure in the knowledge that as individuals they are receiving the best possible care. That is, relief of distressing symptoms, plus being helped to achieve the highest possible quality of life. Such patients need proper palliative support with skilled and compassionate care [1]. Such patients do not all have the same underlying illness. While there may be a tendency for members of the public and even some professionals to consider that palliative care applies only to those with cancer and perhaps HIV and AIDS, palliative care is appropriate for people with very different chronic conditions such as Huntington's disease and old age.

This chapter is intended as a short introduction to demonstrate that patients and particularly those requiring palliative care are not a homogeneous group of people holding the same views, having the same needs, and having the same expectations of care.

Palliative care: meeting the needs of the whole person

People with illnesses for which there is no further curative treatment, often face the following emotions:
- fear of the unknown;
- fear of pain and unpleasant symptoms;
- fear of dying;
- concern about how to cope;
- confusion and uncertainty;
- anger and bitterness;
- depression;
- loneliness;
- sadness.

They also have to try to cope with the manifestations of a terminal illness, which may include pain, breathing troubles, sleeplessness, loss of bladder and bowel control, and mental confusion. These symptoms of terminal illness can be frightening, distressing, and isolating.

Patients have also to deal with what could be described as the secondary effects of being ill, such as having to go into hospital or into respite care. Some patients may fear that they will not get home again. Patients may also be concerned about the extra demands made by their conditions on family and friends.

Older patients are often very concerned about the burden imposed by the illness on their husband or wife caring for them. Their partner, if still alive, will probably also be an aged person. Many older people are quite isolated as families do not live nearby and friends are also older and less able to help. The fact that the person's life is coming to an end may be distressing both for the patient and their partner.

Patients and their relatives can be overwhelmed by their situation. They will be considering some of the following questions:
- How am I going to manage?
- Who is going to help?
- Who is going to look after me?
- Where will I be looked after?
- How will this be paid for?

There are further questions that may be concerning the patient. Some people may wish to remain at home and die at home. For some that may be possible while for others it will not be possible. Many patients may be concerned about the changing relationship with their partner and/or their children that is brought about by their illness. Some people will not talk about their illness because they are trying to protect their loved one(s) from unnecessary distress or worry. This also applies to partners for the same reason. Some patients will not talk about their situation simply because they do not know how to express themselves. A wall of silence between partners can make the situation even more difficult for all concerned.

The patient still needs intimacy and the sexual relationship that they have had. However, chronic disease and disabling illnesses can have serious effects upon a person's sexuality, their sexual expression, and their sexual health [2]. Mutilating surgery and amputation can affect body image, and specific cancer treatments such as radiotherapy and chemotherapy can seriously affect sexuality [3]. Hence there are several reasons why patients receiving palliative care may have difficulties in maintaining a sexual relationship. These include: lack of libido; sexual dysfunction due to their illness; or depression. There may also be a breakdown in communication with their partner, or a lack of place or privacy to maintain intimacy. The subject of sexuality may be difficult for the patient and their partner to discuss. It may also be difficult for staff, who should be aware of this need in their patient. Staff who have this awareness will be able to encourage communication with the patient and thus enable the patient to have the intimacy that they need.

Palliative care or palliative treatment involves looking at the whole person and not just at one symptom. It is also clear that for the patient successful palliative care will, to a great extent, depend on good communication between the patient and his or her family, between the patient and different professionals, and between the different professionals looking after the patient.

Patient knowledge of palliative care

Professionals may understand the concept of palliative care and what can be offered to patients, but does the patient know or understand what the term 'palliative care' means? There are apparently no published studies on patients' understanding of palliative care.

Some cancer patients will know that for them active therapeutic treatment has been exhausted but that they will continue to be cared for with the relief of unpleasant symptoms and pain. Such patients may even know that they are going to attend the palliative care unit. While some cancer hospitals have a protocol which is followed when patients are to be admitted or transferred to the palliative care unit [4] and where patients are told what can be offered to them in the palliative care unit, it is less likely that such detailed procedures are yet followed in most general hospitals and in general practice.

Not all cancer patients will be aware of the availability of palliative care; and for the many people who do not have cancer and for whom palliative care is appropriate, will these patients know the difference between palliative care and terminal care? For some patients and their families palliative care may mean that death is imminent.

It is possible that there may be confusion in the mind of the patient, who is being offered palliative care, and their family as to what precisely is entailed. The transfer of a patient from therapeutic to palliative care, or the introduction of a patient to palliative care should involve:

• explanation of what is meant by palliative care;
• information about the services available;
• information about the range of people who will help;
• information about nursing home, hospice, and respite care;
• clarification and identification of the key worker;
• reassurance, where appropriate, that palliative care does not mean imminent death;
• information about relevant voluntary organizations.

It is likely that the ability to comprehend details of the consultation may be affected if the patient and their family believe that information about palliative care is synonymous with 'being a hopeless case'. As Speechley and Rosenfeld [5] state: 'Some people live for a number of years and have regular palliative treatment. Not being able to be cured does not mean that there is nothing that can be done to help you to continue to live as you usually do'.

Relationship with professionals

Your GP is an expert in health care but only you know exactly what and how you feel. The more openly you and your GP can talk together the better the service he or she will be able to give you [6].

The sentiment expressed here is in a leaflet produced jointly by patients and doctors at the Royal College of General Practitioners, London. In palliative care the ideal relationship between patients and those looking after them should be egalitarian, as well as complementary, with patients being able to state what their health needs are and what they expect of interventions. This is particularly important when the patient is part of a large team including carers and relatives. Neither patients nor professionals have a monopoly on wisdom but each need to recognize that within the limits of current knowledge it is the patient who should determine what is an acceptable outcome and what is an intolerable intervention.

In order to reach such a balance there must be informed decision-making and clear communication between the patient, their relatives, and all the professionals involved in the decision-making process. All involved in the patient's care should understand the aims of care. A team approach is needed. However, such an approach may initially cause confusion for the patient, who needs to know:

• which professional is going to look after them?
• who is going to co-ordinate these services?
• who does the patient contact when he or she needs help?
• who is going to see the patient regularly when the patient is no longer able to visit the surgery?
• who is going to be aware of changes in circumstances of the patient?
• how will information be transmitted to and between different members of the team?

It is important that, from the perspective of the patient and their family, care does not become fragmented, confusing, and overwhelming, with different people responsible for different parts of the care. For many patients and their families, the source of help and information has been the GP. If the key worker becomes a member of the team other than the GP, the patient may need to be reassured that they still have access to their GP, who remains interested in them.

Therefore the patient and their family need to know: which people are involved in the multidisciplinary team; the role of each member and their names and contact numbers. They also need assurance that patient and family confidentiality will be protected.

It is important to acknowledge that the patient and their family are also part of the team, and that by including the patient in decision-making, the need for clear and open communication among all members of the team is essential [7].

Problems in the management of palliative care

While it is possible to treat many of the physical symptoms of terminal illness, the optimal treatment of these symptoms should not be considered in isolation from other aspects of the patients' needs. Palliative care is often managed by attempting to deal with each particular problem as it arises. It can be argued that such an ad hoc policy has its advantages as it means that no inappropriate or rigid programme is adhered to if the illness is not following a typical course. Such a policy also means that there is no need to make predictions about the course of terminal illness. This approach may also be good practice when the illness is known to run a fluctuating or unpredictable course. However, the absence of an overall policy has disadvantages. If the terminal nature of the illness is not acknowledged a habitual pattern of treatments or investigations may be conducted with little benefit to the patient. Furthermore, those responsible for the treatment may not give the appropriate priority for the comfort of the patient and their family. A further and equally important consideration is that the lack of a co-ordinated policy may recognize the appropriate solution to each problem as it arises but the facilities to deal with the problem may not be available.

John Hoyland [8] highlights the need for the co-ordination of palliative care services. His article concerns the treatment of Jack Sutherland, a dignified octogenarian and the stepfather of the author. Jack had Parkinson's disease, arthritis, and an enlarged prostate. In the last 18 months of his life, Jack was treated 'by three different sets of specialists for these different ailments and was shunted back and forth between three different hospitals.' Communication between the hospitals was minimal with notes frequently lost or delayed or sent to the wrong hospital. As a result Jack often spent days or even weeks without being treated at all, and he lost out on the care of his ailments that were not the speciality of that particular hospital. As John Hoyland states, 'The problem was that while there were lots of people in charge of different parts of Jack's body, no-one was in charge of Jack.'

What Jack needed was someone or a team of people to be responsible for his care and to work with each other, and with Jack and his family, to provide the transition between hospital and community services and to mastermind the link between the different specialities. In other words to provide the 'seamless care'.

Hoyland identifies another problem, the need for planned treatment when caring for an elderly person with several chronic complaints: 'the NHS is not geared up to people dying and in particular that people have a tendency to die when they are old. The NHS is mainly concerned with patching up whatever seems to be wrong with people and sending them back to their normal lives as soon as possible. With younger people this often works. But old people don't recover from illness so easily, if at all. They require a different kind of care.' What happened to Mr Sutherland shows an absence of patient-centred care, and an absence of care with dignity for an elderly person.

Campbell [9] suggests that we feel cared for when our needs are recognized and when the help that is offered does not overwhelm us. Conversely a care which imposes itself on us forcing a conformity to someone else's idea of what we need merely makes us feel helpless and vulnerable. The recognition of a key worker with whom the patient and their family feel comfortable and with whom they will liaise, can help prevent the patient being overwhelmed.

Fragmentation of care

The situation of Mr Sutherland has illustrated how the emphasis on treating the symptoms and not the whole person resulted in fragmentation of care, leaving the patient and his family isolated and helpless. Similar situations can arise for patients with many other diseases, for example Huntington's disease. People with Huntington's disease (Huntington's chorea, or HC) have progressive chorea, progressive muscle weakness, and often dementia. The physical and mental suffering can be very severe. There is no effective therapy [10].

Voluntary organizations for HC suggest that people with Huntington's and their families are best helped by a team of experienced professionals, including neurologist, psychiatrist, nurse, dietician, social worker, speech therapist, family doctor, and geneticist [11]. Over 20 years ago, Marjorie Guthrie, founder and president of the US Committee to combat Huntington's Disease, submitted a plan for a diagnostic and referral centre to sustain a programme of continuous care for patients with chronic degenerative disorders. Such a centre was to serve as a model for a 'centre without walls', which would provide clinical and research facilities and would serve as the base for outreach teams to provide information, training, treatment, and care for patients and their families. In the UK the services for patients with Huntington's are still very fragmented.

Voluntary organizations

Many disease-specific voluntary organizations have been established to provide informal support for members, to educate the public and the professions about the respective conditions, to support relevant research, and to lobby for changes and improvement in services [12]. Most of these voluntary organizations now provide excellent information and advice for members about different aspects of the particular disease.

Sometimes it is the family or carer who needs the support offered by a voluntary organization—for example, in the UK, the Carers' National Association. Many disease-specific organizations are able to help members of the patient's family in discussions about problems associated with the illness, about their own feelings, about the burden of the illness on them, and about their concerns for the future [13].

Professionals should ensure that patients and their families are informed about appropriate voluntary organizations and are given help to get in touch when that is appropriate.

Research in palliative care

In medical research the primary intention is to advance knowledge so that patients in general may benefit. The individual patient participating in the research may or may not benefit directly from participating in the research.

Research in palliative care raises some specific issues of importance. Also, it is imperative to differentiate between innovative medical practice for an individual patient and research of more general applicability. Firstly, the informed consent of the patient must be properly obtained. Patients should be encouraged to discuss their participation with relatives and carers. Secondly, all members of the team involved in the care of the patient must know that the patient is involved in a research project. There must be a realistic assessment of the condition of the patient and the length of time available for the research when considering and setting protocols. Research which is primarily to advance the career of a health care worker should be discouraged. Also, administering a placebo is not justifiable in palliative care if there is a treatment known to be more effective than a placebo [14].

Some patients may very much wish to participate in a project even though their participation may cause them inconvenience or even discomfort. The patient may wish to help and to 'give'. In addition they may gain the knowledge that their participation in the research may benefit future patients.

The family may influence the patient's decision whether or not to enter a research project. Some families may wish the patient to participate in research and may encourage the patient to be involved, for example because the illness is genetic and the information may be useful to the other family members. Some people may think that if someone is troubling to involve the patient in research there is still hope. Conversely families may be disappointed when their relative agrees to participate because the time spent in research is precious time which is not being spent with them.

Conclusion

The provision of such a high-quality service requires great skill and commitment on the part of the professionals involved. It may also require the breaking down of traditional professional barriers between the different professional groups involved so that the person whom the patient finds most acceptable becomes the key worker. This is challenging.

We, the public, are the future patients who may benefit from palliative care; we need to be made more aware of palliative care and its great benefits. It is only with this knowledge that we can become real partners in the palliative care team.

References

1 Fallowfield L. *The Quality of Life*. London: Souvenir Press, 1990.
2 Grigg E. Issues of sexuality and intimacy in palliative care. In: Penson, J, Fisher, R, eds. *Palliative Care for People with Cancer*, 2nd edn. London: Arnold, 1995.
3 Thomson J. Sexuality, the adolescent and cancer. *Nursing Standard* 1990; 4: 26–49.
4 Travis S. Personal communication. Royal Marsden Hospital, London, April 1977.
5 Speechley V, Rosenfeld M. *Cancer Information at your Fingertips*. London: Class Publishing, 1996.
6 The Patients' Liaison Group, Royal College of General Practitioners. *You and Your GP During the Day*. London: RCGP, 1977.
7 Penson J, Fisher R, eds. *Palliative Care in People with Cancer*. London: Arnold, 1995.
8 Hoyland J. Thanks, NHS, for a rotten way to die. *The Independent Tabloid* 22 April 1997.
9 Campbell AV. *Moderated Love*. London: SPCK, 1984.
10 Pierce BA. *The Family Genetic Sourcebook*. Toronto, Canada: John Wiley & Sons, 1990.
11 Phillips DH. *Living with Huntington's Disease*. London: Junction Books, 1982.
12 *The Health Address Book*. London: The Patients' Association, 1992.
13 Multiple Sclerosis Resource Centre. *Putting People First*. Essex: Multiple Sclerosis Resource Centre, 1996.
14 Working Party of the National Council for Hospice and Specialist Palliative Care Services. Guidelines on research in palliative care. In: *Manual for Research Ethics Committees*. London: The Centre of Medical Law and Ethics, King's College, 1996.

6: Ethical Issues in Palliative Care

DAVID JEFFREY

Introduction

Ethics have a central role in clinical decision-making and involve the whole of a patient's care at all stages of their illness. Ethics and clinical medicine are inseparable. This chapter will focus on the issues arising at the very end of life.

Why ethics?

Palliative care demands that health professionals are both competent and compassionate. An ethical framework that clarifies complex issues can directly improve the quality of patient care. A high standard of care also requires: ethical sensitivity; an understanding of the legal dimension of a clinical situation; and good communication skills [1] (see Chapter 8).

Ethical dilemmas are an increasingly important part of health care for a variety of reasons. Firstly, advances in medical technology hailed by the media as 'breakthroughs' have raised patient expectations. Some patients believe that doctors can postpone death almost indefinitely, whilst others are wary of modern technology and fear a prolonged, undignified process of dying. Secondly, a managed market approach to health care has strained interprofessional relationships. Moreover, health care rationing is now explicit and has changed the public's view of doctors. Thirdly, 'patient's charters' emphasize the rights of patients and the duties of doctors while neglecting the responsibilities of patients and the rights of health care professionals. Patients are encouraged to complain, with a resulting dramatic increase in legal claims against health care providers. The situation is fuelled by the media, which exploits every opportunity to sensationalize the ethical dilemmas that arise.

Ethical theory

Ethics is a dynamic topic in which there is a tension between looking back to the wisdom of the philosophers of the past and looking to the future to forecast the consequences of the decisions and discoveries of today. There is a need to identify the ethical issues which arise in the care of patients and to develop ethical models to assist health care professionals to deliver appropriate palliative care [2].

Ethical principles

Four basic principles have been developed to guide medical care:
- respect for autonomy (self-determination);
- beneficence (to do good);
- non-maleficence (not to harm);
- justice (to be fair).

In addition there needs to be an understanding of the limits of each of these principles and how they operate and conflict in clinical practice.

Autonomy

Autonomy is the capacity to think, decide and act on the basis of such thought and decision, freely and independently [3].

In expressing autonomy an individual shapes and gives meaning to his/her life. In a situation where death is, or is thought to be, imminent, then respect for the patient's autonomy assumes a particular importance. Patients with advanced disease can appear physically frail and are therefore vulnerable to well-intentioned, but unwanted, medical intervention.

AUTONOMY VS. PATERNALISM

Paternalism is a denial of autonomy, and a substitution of an individual's judgements or action for his own good. A conflict may exist between a doctor's duty of beneficence—to do what is best for his patient—and his respect for the patient's autonomy. A claim that a duty of non-maleficence is of a higher priority fails when one considers a doctor's qualification to weigh the various 'harms' and 'benefits' in the proposed paternalistic act. Doctors may be medical experts but they are not 'experts' in the social, spiritual, or emotional aspects of the patient's life. These non-medical aspects may be of much greater significance to the patient than his or her illness. An essential part of the principle of autonomy is the respect for the individual, who has different priorities from those of the health care professional [4].

Paternalism seeks to treat patients as children; such treatment is inappropriate for adults and can lead to encouraging the patient to become over-dependent. Patient autonomy can best be respected by providing full honest information and ensuring that the patient has given his consent before any medical intervention. Patient consent thus acts as a mechanism to protect autonomy against paternalistic intervention.

INFORMED CONSENT

All medical interventions, whether diagnostic, therapeutic, or for research, carry the potential for violating patient autonomy. The central function of informed consent is to ensure a sharing of power and knowledge between doctor and patient.

Informed consent is thus much more than a granting of permission, and may be defined as:

> *a voluntary uncoerced decision, made by a sufficiently competent or autonomous person, on the basis of adequate information and deliberation, to accept rather than reject some proposed course of action that will affect him or her [3].*

Doctors should offer alternatives and discuss choices. This 'sharing' option is clinically and emotionally more demanding for doctors and involves a sensitivity to the ever-changing needs of the patient.

Compassion

For professionals to deny emotions and feelings of vulnerability in themselves and in their patients is to deny compassion, and to distance themselves from patients [5]. Compassion is an essential part of the doctor–patient relationship and the health team–patient relationship. A team approach allows health care professionals to share problems and to co-ordinate different skills for the benefit of the patient. There may be problems in reaching a moral consensus. The process of attempting to resolve ethical dilemmas may cause stress to doctors and nurses. There is a necessity for those working in palliative care to have time to meet together for mutual support and to reflect on their practice.

Euthanasia: the limits of respect for autonomy

A patient's request for assistance in ending his or her life presents the doctor with a moral challenge. Medical training instils a sense of responsibility to preserve life, yet there is a duty to relieve suffering. Recently there has been increased interest in the moral arguments surrounding euthanasia. A British Medical Association report concluded that euthanasia was 'intuitively wrong' [6]. These arguments were formally debated by a House of Lords select committee on medical ethics [7].

Active and passive euthanasia

A doctor who intends to end the life of a suffering patient or help a patient to commit suicide is engaging in active euthanasia. A doctor refraining from treating a potentially remediable condition which results in the death of a terminally ill patient is employing passive euthanasia. Passive euthanasia may involve physically neglecting the basic needs of the patient, such as food and water, or taking a decision not to prescribe futile treatments such as antibiotics or cardiopulmonary resuscitation, as the patient approaches death [8].

Active euthanasia: the issues in palliative care

Suffering. It could be argued that if palliative care was improved, and suffering controlled, requests for euthanasia would be eliminated, or rightly be regarded as irrational [9]. However, there remains a minority of patients in which suffering is not controlled despite the best efforts of specialist palliative care. Doctors are not qualified to judge that this suffering is always of negative value. The process of dying is unique for each individual. For some death is quiet and painless, others 'rage against the dying of the light' [10]. An ethical requirement at this stage is to help the patient find his own meaning to his life and not to abandon him.

Burden to others. Patients may feel that they are a burden to their families. The euthanasia request may be a test to see if their life is of value to others. Ethical care acknowledges the unique value of each individual [4].

Sanctity of life. Judaeo-Christian ethics emphasize the sanctity of human life. This doctrine is enshrined in the Hippocratic Oath, which forbids killing. Doctors have special duties of beneficence and non-maleficence, and to kill a patient is to neglect these moral obligations.

Limited resources. Economic pressures may tempt some doctors and health service managers to favour euthanasia as a cheaper, practical solution to the expensive problem of caring for the terminally ill. It is important that the ethical issues of rationing and euthanasia are clearly separated, especially when resources are scarce [11].

Respect for autonomy. A patient may feel that she is no longer in control and the only way of exercising her autonomy is to choose to die, and to do so sooner rather than later. Respect for autonomy, however, carries the limitation that such respect does not infringe the autonomy of others, including the doctor's and that of other patients in this dilemma. The terminally ill individual requires time to come to terms with symptoms, to assess the past, and to find meanings. The choosing of active euthanasia, however, precludes all these choices, thus limiting autonomy. Since the time span regarded as 'terminal' is variable, there is no way of predicting for certain when death will take place nor what important events for the patient and their family might take place in the last weeks or days of life. This time may be of great value for resolving unfinished business and restoring relationships.

Right to die. The law clearly prohibits all actions causing intentional death. The Suicide Act, in legalizing suicide, is a pragmatic response to the practical problem of administering sanctions to suicide victims rather than acknowledging the 'right to die'. Assisting suicide remains a serious crime.

Mistaken diagnosis. Patients with advanced disease may become clinically depressed. In such a situation feelings of low self-esteem and suicidal ideas are common. Chronic and advanced disease tend to isolate patients, and in that isolation a quick death may seem the best option. It is rather alarming to note that doctors often miss a diagnosis of depressive illness, particularly in the elderly [12]. If a doctor is unable to recognize treatable depression then his response to a depressed patient's request for assisted suicide may be based on his own fears about ageing, cancer, and dependency.

Death with dignity. Death with dignity is hard to define because the perception of indignity often lies with the observer. The moral challenge for doctors is to see that the life of a wasted, jaundiced, dying patient is still of infinite value. Devaluing and/or not supporting such a life on the basis of age, non-productivity, cost, or degree of physical handicap is not morally acceptable.

Slippery slopes. If doctors allow active voluntary euthanasia in certain specific 'hard cases' then imperceptible steps lead down a slope to involuntary euthanasia. Once on this slope, doctors may slide towards a reduced sensitivity to killing and then to a slackening of resolve to save life. For instance, although the Abortion Act stipulated strict guidelines on eligibility, the interpretation of these criteria have become more lax over time. Indeed, although not legalized, euthanasia can be carried out in the Netherlands providing strict rules are followed [13]. There is already concern that these rules are not always adhered to [14]. The existence of the choice for active euthanasia puts the elderly and terminally ill under some pressure to choose this alternative.

Passive euthanasia: letting die

Doctors owe patients a duty not to kill them, but feel less strongly that they have to 'strive officiously to keep alive' [15]. The traditional medical view that it is worse to kill than to let die reflects the Acts and Omissions doctrine derived from Roman Catholic theology. The doctrine argues that actions that result in some undesirable consequence are morally worse than a failure to act which has the same consequence. If doctors continue to actively treat a patient who has expressed a wish not to receive such treatment they are failing to respect the patient's autonomy. Withholding futile but life-prolonging treatments in such patients is not only permissible but morally required. There is a need to acknowledge the lethal power of terminal diseases. This concept has been summarized within the principles of palliative care adopted by the World Health Organization:

> *Affirms life and regards dying as a normal process. Neither hastens nor postpones death [16].*

Passive euthanasia in practical settings

Issues concerning passive euthanasia occur in three common palliative care settings.

Use of opiates to relieve pain

A person's intentions and obligations are as relevant, in a moral analysis, as the outcome. Some argue that we can clearly distinguish intended from unintended consequences of an action—the principle of double effect [3]. Thus a doctor who gives an injection of diamorphine with the intention of relieving the patient's pain is not morally culpable if, as a side-effect of this necessary treatment the patient becomes weaker and develops a fatal pneumonia.

Resuscitation

A locally agreed policy on cardiopulmonary resuscitation is necessary for two reasons: to enhance clinical care and respect for patient autonomy; and to protect doctors and nurses from criticism [1]. There is no duty to preserve life at all costs nor is there a duty to provide futile treatments. If the prospect of survival is virtually non-existent or if the patient is in terrible suffering which would only be prolonged by active treatment then resuscitation should not be attempted. Ordinarily a patient's consent should be obtained for withholding resuscitation. However, when a patient has terminal cancer and is dying from the disease, there is no moral or legal obligation on doctors to discuss any futile treatments. In a situation where attempts at cardiopulmonary resuscitation would be futile there should not be any duty for the doctor to have to inform the patient of this any more than saying, for example, 'you are not going to have a liver transplant', and to do so may be maleficent.

Withdrawal of feeding and fluids

The primary goal of terminal care is the comfort of the patient. In deciding whether to withdraw fluids and feeding of patients with advanced disease the doctor must consider the views of the patient and family.

A theological doctrine relevant to the debate is that of ordinary and extraordinary means. The statement is that the good of saving life is morally obligatory if its pursuit is not excessively burdensome or disproportionate to the expected benefit [17]. Ordinary means are morally obligatory, such as providing food and water; extraordinary means are morally optional (e.g. inserting gastrostomy tube).

There are differing opinions as to the appropriate management of terminally ill patients who are unable to eat and drink. Various issues need to be considered (see Chapter 20). For example, there is a difference between dying from dehydration and dehydration in dying patients [17]. Intravenous fluids may do little to relieve symptoms if the patient is not thirsty. Meticulous mouth care may be more beneficial for comfort and symptom relief. Intravenous infusions may give confusing messages to relatives, who may feel that the goal of care is to prolong the dying process. Intravenous infusions and nasogastric tubes may act as a physical barrier between the patient and his family. Rehydrating with intravenous fluids may worsen some symptoms, such as vomiting, respiratory secretions, and incontinence [18]. The perceived need for intravenous fluids by relatives may necessitate transfer of a dying patient to hospital and deprive him of his wish to die at home.

Each case needs to be considered on an individual basis, and the views of the patient, family, and nursing staff should be sought by the responsible physician. If the patient is heavily sedated and unable to make a decision then the views of the relatives must be considered alongside any further evidence of the patient's wishes, such as an advance directive.

The legality of withdrawing hydration and nutrition and hydration in the terminally ill has not been tested in the courts in Britain [19].

Advance directives: living wills

Some patients have made written directives known as 'living wills' or advance directives, which state their wish not to be resuscitated in certain clinical situations, for example advanced cancer. Living wills have a legal force in Britain (Airedale Hospital Trust vs. Bland) and should be respected by doctors [20] (see Box 6.1). They are not legal unless they describe the precise clinical situation in advance. A living will cannot force a doctor to carry out treatment which he feels is inappropriate [1].

Living wills (or advance directives) are not a substitute for good communication between patients and doctors. The honest approach is to take steps to elicit the patient's choice in a sensitive manner and to record this information in the records, and to communicate it to the rest of the team. Improved communication would do much to calm the anxieties of patients about unnecessary treatments and lead to a reduced demand for living wills. Living wills do not take into account the fact that patients may wish to change their minds during the course of their illness. The presence of a living will may be of some help in influencing a doctor's decisions, but it is a sad reflection on the quality of the doctor–patient

---

Box 6.1 The case of Anthony Bland

Anthony Bland was a 22-year-old who suffered hypoxic brain damage following a crush injury at the Hillsborough disaster. He was diagnosed as being in a persistent vegetative state and was kept alive by artificial feeding.

Three years later, no change in his clinical condition had occurred and expert opinion had agreed that his cerebral hemispheres were completely destroyed. Legal proceedings supported a request to discontinue artificial feeding, which resulted in the patient's death. As part of this process, Lord Goff supported the principle of advance directives as means of informing such decisions [7].

relationship that a resort to such a device is considered necessary in palliative care [20].

Ethical care

Improved communication between doctors, nurses, patients, and patients' families will lead to a better mutual understanding of the patient's wishes. Ethical dilemmas have no easy solution but using a framework of ethical principles and treating patients with respect and compassion may help pose the right questions. It is in the struggle with such questions that we define what lies at the heart of being a doctor or nurse.

Palliative care may be given in a hospital or in community settings, not only in hospices. Patients need doctors and nurses to listen to their views. A requirement for informed and understood consent serves to facilitate a partnership between patients and professionals. In the context of such a partnership both parties become more aware of each other's needs and can then work effectively together to achieve the best possible outcome for the one who is dying and the many who care.

References

1 Hope T, Fulford KWM, Yates A. *The Oxford Practice Skills Course.* Oxford: Oxford University Press, 1996: 28–29.
2 Jeffrey D. *There is Nothing More I Can Do.* Penzance: Patten Press, 1993.
3 Gillon R. *Philosophical Medical Ethics.* Chichester: John Wiley, 1985.
4 Higgs R. Shaping our ends: the ethics of respect in a well-led NHS. *Br J Gen Pract* 1997; 47: 245–249.
5 Alderson P. Abstract bio-ethics ignores human emotions. *Bull Med Eth* 1991; May: 13–21.
6 British Medical Association Working Party. Euthanasia. *BMJ* 1988; 296: 1376–1377.
7 House of Lords. *Report of the Select Committee on Medical Ethics.* London: HMSO, 1993.
8 Wilkinson J. The ethics of euthanasia. *Palliat Med* 1990; 4: 81–86.
9 Parker M. Moral intuition, good deeds and ordinary medical practitioners. *J Med Ethics* 1990; 16: 28–34.
10 Thomas D. Extract from 'Do not go gentle into that good night'. In: Heaney S, Hughes T, eds. *The Rag Bag.* London: Faber & Faber, 1982: 131.
11 Crispell KR, Comez CF. Proper care of the dying: a critical public issue. *J Med Ethics* 1987; 13: 74–80.
12 Conwell Y, Caine ED. Rational suicide and the right to die: reality and myth. *New Engl J Med* 1991; 325: 1100–1103.
13 Righter H, Borst-Eilers E, Leenon HJJ. Euthanasia across the North Sea. *BMJ* 1988; 297: 1593.

14 Fenigsen R. The case against Dutch euthanasia. Hastings Center Report. *Mercy, Murder and Morality: Perspectives on Euthanasia.* 1989: 22–30.

15 Clough AH. The latest decalogue. In: Glover J, ed. *Causing Death and Saving Lives.* Pengu, 1977 (in press).

16 *Cancer pain relief and palliative care.* Technical Report Series 804. Geneva: World Health Organisation, 1990.

17 Gillon R. Deciding not to resuscitate. *J Med Ethics* 1989; 15: 171–172.

18 Haas F. In the patient's best interests? Dehydration in dying patients. *Prof Nurse* 1994; November: 82–87.

19 Craig GM. On withholding nutrition and hydration in the terminally ill: has palliative medicine gone too far? *J Med Ethics* 1994; 20: 139–143.

20 Airedale NHS Trust v Bland. *Weekly Law Reports* 1993; 2: 316.

7: Adapting to Death, Dying, and Bereavement

RICHARD WOOF AND BRIAN NYATANGA

Introduction

Our fear of death and the loss of a loved one are two of the most monumental emotional challenges of human existence. This anxiety is usually suppressed and is only exposed when the reality of a possible death is confronted. Palliative care has recognized the power of this suffering and is concerned with helping people cope and adapt. This is incorporated into a philosophy of care that attempts to address needs holistically (see Chapter 1).

This chapter will review literature that has improved the understanding of the processes involved, the damaging consequences that can occur, and the role of health professionals in caring for the dying and the bereaved.

Death in society

Humanity's fear of death has interested artists and scientists alike. Philosophers have considered death in terms of fear of extinction and insignificance; psychologists have devised models that explain death-related emotion; and sociologists have observed how death anxiety can bind groups (e.g. religions, armies). It has even been suggested that politics are influenced by a desire to control the anxiety death provokes. This 'death anxiety' is said to be driven by three separate fears [1].
- Fear of what happens after death.
- Fear of the act of dying (e.g. pain, loss of control, rejection because of illness).
- Fear of ceasing to be.

These arguments may seem like stretching the point a bit: after all, people generally do not go around in a perpetual state of anxiety about their eventual demise. However, by assuming that fears can be neatly packaged in the subconscious, then death anxiety can be seen as hugely influential on behaviour without disrupting functioning. Concepts such as these illustrate the potency of death anxiety on thinking and help explain how people react when faced with death.

People differ in how they respond to the prospect of death. In caring for the dying and bereaved, it is useful to try to understand the different factors that influence this behaviour. Although personal factors are very important (e.g. gender, nature of disease and treatment, coping mechanisms, social support, personality, etc.), these partly relate to what is known as the 'death system' in a society. This phenomenon varies between societies and depends on the following four factors [2].

1   Exposure to death—prior experience of death has a strong influence on the approach to subsequent deaths, including our own.
2   Life expectancy—society holds an estimate for what is considered a reasonable life span, based on observations of the community. The more deaths in a community the greater the exposure, the shorter the life expectancy. Obviously different societies vary considerably in this respect.
3   Perceived control over the forces of nature—beliefs about the ability to influence destiny (fate vs. control) will affect perceptions of death.
4   Perception of what it means to be human—'meaning' in this context relates to a variety of belief systems that constitute spirituality. The clarity and conviction with which a society holds these views will influence the death system.

Each death will be influenced to varying degrees by a combination of personal factors within a particular cultural death system. For instance, an elderly Indian widow who sees illness in a religious sense, will respond differently from the young Western atheist who has never experienced death and believes in their own ability to control life events.

Personal spirituality

The spiritual component of health is an important theme in the philosophy of palliative care [3]. Spirituality is concerned with how individuals understand the purpose and meaning of their existence within the universe. It requires an individual to develop a harmonious intellectual connection between themselves and their spiritual thought. For some there may be a strong religious component to this aspect of their life, but for others such cultural norms are less relevant. These differences are readily seen in pluralistic Western societies such as the UK.

Death poses a challenge to these personally held belief systems. Some individuals possess a set of beliefs that adequately answer this challenge, but others can suffer as they strive to attain an inner peace. It is clear that a patient's individual spirituality can never be assumed. Carers must remain aware of this when considering the spiritual needs of patients.

Spiritual health can be encouraged in several ways. One important step is to eliminate the distraction of physical suffering. It is also helpful to encourage the expression of repressed emotion. Patients can be enabled to attain spiritual growth, either by personal reflection or with the help of an adviser (professional or lay). It is essential, though, to respect the individual and their culture in all interactions.

Adapting to dying

By understanding how societies deal with death, it is possible to explore the more specific issues of how patients cope, the problems that can arise, and how carers should respond. This includes care of both the patient and those important to them. This whole topic area has been termed 'anticipatory grief' by some authors.

Psychosocial theories

Various psychological models have been developed which provide insight into patients' responses to their impending death. The most celebrated work was performed by Kubler-Ross [4], who described a five-stage model of dying: denial, anger, bargaining, depression, and acceptance. Other authors have proposed different models that also contribute to our understanding [5–11]. The main advantage of these theories is that they allow us to make sense of people's behaviour more constructively.

> It is not enough for us to stay close and open our hearts to another person's suffering: valuable as this sympathy may be, we must have some way for stepping aside from the maze of emotion and sensation if we are to make sense of it [12].

However, these models have their limitations. They should only be used to assist in the understanding of patients and allow the carer not to be overwhelmed by the emotions observed. They are not universal truths and should not be applied dogmatically.

Particular problems in adapting to dying

The extent of the distress experienced by patients depends on a wide variety of factors. In many cases, the psychosocial needs of the patient and carers are met with honest information given sensitively. But in more complex instances, the debilitating effects of the adaptive process require more intense professional support. Physical symptoms can be influenced by the emotional state of patients. Concepts such as 'total pain' are at the core of the palliative care philosophy. Consequently emotional distress can be an important component in physical suffering and therefore in its management.

There is an array of emotional responses that can occur when facing death, which can be difficult for patients to bear. These include anger, anxiety, guilt, and depression. As patients grapple with all these emotions and the changing nature of their illness, feelings of isolation can also occur. This alienation compounds the many other losses that are experienced at this time.

Not surprisingly, the enormity of the adaptive process can be overwhelming and result in psychiatric morbidity. Although research has found it difficult to confirm, it is said that there is an increased prevalence of depression, anxiety, panic, and suicidal behaviour [13].

Although some patients do undoubtedly suffer in this way, it is important to remember that many adapt healthily. Research has revealed that patients achieve this by using techniques such as 'positive reappraisal' and 'cognitive avoidance strategies' [14]. To the professional observer, some of these strategies may seem like distortions or misinterpretations of the facts, but to the patient they insure against emotional overload. It is important not to dismantle individual adaptive processes.

The debilitating effect of the emotional consequences of a terminal illness compounds the physical deterioration to produce significant social costs. Social losses are closely related to quality of life issues and include such things as employment, recreation, relationships, and family.

The demands of caring for a terminally ill patient should not be ignored by professionals. Indeed, in some cases the multidisciplinary team's focus is more appropriately directed not so much at the patient but at the patient's family and friends. The need for constant nursing care at home can be physically draining and occasionally result in injury or illness to the carer. In addition, family and friends are subjected to a series of actual and potential losses that demand considerable emotional strength. Examples of these challenges include the following:

- loss of a certain future;
- loss of role within the family and the outside world;
- concerns about the burden of caring;
- issues about sexuality;
- loss of financial security.

In many cases these questions provoke emotions in carers that are similar to those experienced by their dying loved one. Such emotional strain can result in significant levels of sleeplessness, anxiety, and weight loss.

The social consequences of caring for a terminally ill loved one can be far-reaching. The time and energy required can impinge on employment, recreation, and relationships. Although society recognizes this in terms of respect for altruism, the economic burden can be considerable and only partially compensated for by statutory government allowances.

The multidisciplinary team has an important role in recognizing the potential dangers of caring for a loved one and should endeavour to intervene to prevent problems.

Management

Assessing the emotional needs of dying patients and their loved ones requires an empathic attitude complemented by adept communication skills and familiarity with the issues surrounding the subject. Research suggests certain factors may be inherently influential on the process of adaptation (age, gender, interpersonal relationships, the nature of disease, and culture) [15]. However, given the diversity of emotional responses, it is usually necessary to make a detailed individual assessment. In order to get an accurate picture of the patient, it may be necessary to meet on a series of occasions and incorporate the opinions of the multidisciplinary team.

Symptom control. Unremitting physical symptoms can be 'soul destroying'. Emotional needs are best tackled in a symptom-free environment.

Facilitating effective communication. These skills are pivotal to effective care. See Chapter 8.

Counselling and therapy. Counselling is concerned with enabling individuals to attain solutions to an emotional challenge by using particular techniques. This approach can be especially helpful in unusually difficult situations. This treatment can be achieved either through one-to-one work or as part of group therapy, and often needs the involvement of specialist help.

Maintaining hope. Patients require hope to be sustained. This is achieved either by setting achievable goals or by the use of intermittent or persistent denial.

Drugs. Appropriate use of psychotropic medicines (antidepressants, anxiolytics, or antipsychotics) is occasionally useful in palliative medicine. In some cases it is difficult to differentiate between clinical psychiatric morbidity, which may respond to pharmacological intervention, and the normal emotions of dying. In this circumstance a trial of medication is a reasonable approach.

Complementary therapies. Various complementary modalities can be helpful in relieving emotional distress. See Chapter 21.

Emotional crises

This subject cannot be discussed in sufficient depth here to do justice to the importance of this area. The reader is referred to Stedford (1984) [16], Vachon (1993) [13], and Stevens (1993) [17].

Emotional crises do not arise without a trigger and pre-morbid factors of vulnerability. Understanding *both* of these for patient and family will help in management of the distress. Vulnerable patients and families should be identified in order to try to prevent crises through proactive access to additional support.

Various risk factors have been identified:
- pre-morbid factors in the family at diagnosis;
- strong dependency issues; hostility, ambivalence;
- other stresses within the family, e.g. relationship problems, poor housing, debts;
- illness and bereavement history—previous experiences of death and loss are important both in the quantity and quality of experience and coping mechanisms developed (or not developed) with previous distress;
- poor coping mechanisms;
- psychiatric history;
- for the family, poor patient adjustment compounds their risk of distress;
- nature of illness—families of older male patients dying from lung cancer and of young women dying from cancer of the cervix are more at risk of becoming overwhelmed and distressed [18].

Management

It is useful to have a team approach, with more than one professional available to a family in acute distress, although one professional should take the lead role. The distress needs to be acknowledged and space must be given for the patient and/or family to regain control. In order to facilitate this the cause of the distress should be explored. The 'cues' to this may need to be picked up from the patient (see Chapter 8).

Once the background and the triggers have been understood a plan can be negotiated. Many crises arise because the patient and/or family feel trapped, with no control and with no choices. Discussing options that they have not perceived can diminish distress. Follow-up is essential to review the situation and plan, to modify the plan when necessary, and to explore any unresolved issues. A sense of security for the patient and family, and also trust in the professional team are important therapeutic components.

Adapting to bereavement

Although many people possess sufficient resources to cope with bereavement, for some the emotional challenge can be exacting and a risk to health. This observation has encouraged some health workers to develop patterns of care for the bereaved, most noticeably within the hospice movement [19] and voluntary sector.

Psychological theories

It might be tempting to view bereavement as a variant of depression and anxiety. But doing so would ignore a wealth of literature that enables us to understand more clearly the processes and emotions involved.

Freud's influential work in 1917 [20] described grief as a period of time where the reality of a death is repeatedly tested until attachment is withdrawn from the deceased. From observations made of bereaved people, Lindemann [21] describes five sub-groups of symptomatology: somatic distress; preoccupation with images of the deceased; guilt; hostility; and activity that appears restless and meaningless.

Bowlby, building on his psychoanalytical theories on attachment and loss, interpreted previous publications to devise a four-stage model for bereavement [22]. Although individuals can move back and forth between stages, there tends to be a progression through the following phases.
1 Phase of numbing.
2 Phase of yearning and searching.
3 Phase of disorganization and despair.
4 Phase of reorganization.
Stroebe [23] has developed an idea first discussed by Parkes [24] and has proposed the Dual Process Model of Coping with Loss. This theory describes a process where the bereaved oscillate from time to time between two psychological orientations (see Fig. 7.1). Individuals choose to change orientation to achieve relief from the emotional pain of the other.

Drawing from empirical and anthropological observations, Walter [25] has proposed that the bereaved need to talk about the deceased in order

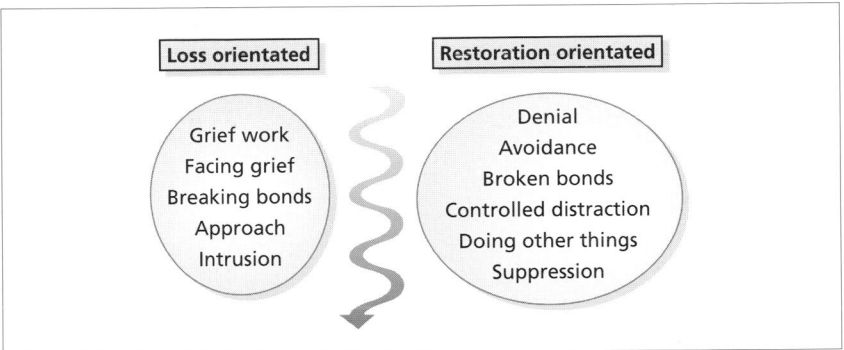

Fig. 7.1 A dual process model for coping with grief.

to construct a biography that they can integrate into their ongoing lives. This allows the creation of a new identity that includes the persistent and usually unobtrusive memory of the deceased.

Consequences of bereavement

There has been considerable research into the adverse health consequences of bereavement [26,27]. Studies have attempted to confirm the lay theory that patients can die of a 'broken heart'. In fact this has been very hard to prove, but it is probably true that the bereaved are at greater risk of death themselves, although this risk remains low in absolute terms. Other work has examined the psychiatric morbidity following a bereavement. This research has been difficult to perform, but it seems to suggest that the bereaved are at risk of the following complications [26,27]:

- depression;
- anxiety;
- alcohol use;
- increased use of prescribed drugs;
- suicidal behaviour.

The evidence for an increase in physical morbidity is less conclusive, as research has failed to confirm any association between grief and physical disease.

PATHOLOGICAL BEREAVEMENT

The boundary between the normal emotions of grief and those exaggerated responses that would constitute abnormality, has been the subject of

Table 7.1 Examples of abnormal bereavement reactions.

Absent
Individuals show no evidence of the emotions of grief developing, in spite of the reality of the death. This can appear as an automatic reaction or the result of active blocking.

Delayed
This initially presents in a similar way to absent grief. However, this avoidance is always a conscious effort and the full emotions of grief are eventually expressed after a particular trigger. This may be seen in more compulsively self-reliant individuals.

Chronic
In this instance, the normal emotions of grief persist without any diminution over time. It is postulated that this is most often seen in relationships that were particularly dependent.

considerable debate. For severe psychiatric disease, the notion of abnormality is straightforward (suicidal activity, alcohol abuse, etc.). However, for more minor affective disorders (e.g. depression, anxiety), it could be said that the symptoms represent normal bereavement. Various authors have proposed means to differentiate the normal from the abnormal. Time has been suggested as a useful, if arbitrary discriminator. Unfortunately no consensus appears to have been agreed and times ranging from 2 to over 12 months have been suggested [26,27].

Other research has concerned itself with describing symptoms that combine to produce particular bereavement syndromes. It is hoped that in defining new conditions in this way, clinicians will be able to develop care for those bereaved individuals who present with particular problems. Consequently an array of terms have been devised which has led to some confusion. Recently an attempt to reach some international consensus was made, and three conditions seem to have achieved some recognition as pathological bereavement reactions (see Table 7.1) [28].

Management

Although there are known adverse health consequences of bereavement, many bereaved individuals adapt to their loss with minimal assistance from health professionals. Indeed, there are potential dangers in over-medicating grief. For instance, a bereavement can promote emotional growth within individuals and families. However, suffering does exist and services have been developed in the UK to answer this need. Accurate assessment of risk is the key component of appropriate bereavement care [29].

ASSESSMENT

As in other aspects of palliative care, accurate assessment is a necessary part of management. This could be performed by any member of the multidisciplinary team and is best achieved by someone with the following attributes.
- Good communication skills to facilitate expression of emotion.
- An ability to screen for psychiatric disease (e.g. depression, anxiety, suicidal intent).
- Familiarity with events surrounding death.
- An understanding of the social background.
- An awareness of risk factors of pathological grief (see Box 7.1).

Other needs should also be considered when assessing the bereaved. These include social needs, i.e. the social consequences of a bereavement that may need attention and occasionally the assistance of a social worker (e.g. rehousing, benefits, day care) (see Chapter 2, p. 21). In some circumstances there are also physical needs; for example where a death results in unmet nursing needs in the bereaved. This is most likely in an elderly couple and may require the input of district nursing services or the geriatric health visitor (see Chapter 2, p. 18).

BEREAVEMENT SERVICES

As a result of the assessment it may be necessary to provide some emotional support. This could involve brief intervention by the professional making

---

Box 7.1 Risk factors for pathological bereavement

- Younger age
- Poor social support
- Sudden death
- Previous poor physical health
- Previous mental illness
- Poor coping strategies
- Multiple losses
- Stigmatized death
- Economic difficulties
- Previous unresolved grief

the assessment or by using the array of bereavement services available. The services listed below do not include the very important help provided by religious advisers, but focus more on the work of health professionals and allied workers. Besides the bereavement services, various communities have developed social groups designed to overcome loneliness.

Written information

For those with low risk, providing written information may be all that is needed. This could range from pamphlets on where to get help should problems arise, to practical guides on what to do after a death and self-help books that normalize the bereavement process. There are some useful books that can be particularly helpful when explaining death to children.

Primary care team

The fact that patients are registered with personal general practitioners (GPs) promotes continuity of care and encourages primary care involvement in bereavement support. Although bereavement visits are made, GP input tends to be variable and in many cases is only reactive to requests for help. GP bereavement care could include such things as a bereavement visit, brief emotional support, referral to practice counsellor, use of psychotropic drugs, or the involvement of other services.

Palliative care team

The hospice movement has seen bereavement care as integral to its service and has adopted a proactive approach. In some instances, these teams are considered as specialists within this field. They can provide an array of services, including: one-to-one support; telephone contact; written information; anniversary letters; social activities; group work; and memorial services [19]. In general, this work is performed by trained volunteers who are supervised by hospice staff.

Voluntary services

In the UK the main voluntary service is CRUSE Bereavement Care. This national organization takes referrals from any source and can provide one-to-one or group work. It is staffed by trained volunteers and functions with a system of formal supervision. They prefer to take self referrals and are contractable by phone (see Useful Addresses, pp. 377–381). The experience of some volunteers makes them able to tackle complex bereavement reactions.

Other organizations can provide support for parents who have lost a child (e.g. Compassionate Friends).

Hospital-based services

Naturally, psychiatric teams are involved in the more damaging bereavement reactions, particularly those resulting in major psychiatric illness. Other hospital services have traditionally been less involved in bereavement care, although casualty departments are becoming increasingly aware of their role following sudden deaths brought to them. Similarly, maternity units are beginning to provide support to their patients who suffer loss.

Some hospitals are providing bereavement officers to assist with certain aspects of the arrangements following the death of an in-patient.

Funeral directors

Some funeral directors are beginning to consider bereavement support as part of their service.

BEREAVEMENT COUNSELLING/THERAPY

Supporting the bereaved involves the application of the communication skills outlined elsewhere in this book (e.g. active listening, empathy, setting limits, clarification). Specialist authors have gone further and formulated approaches that provide greater guidance on bereavement counselling, either as general principles or in particular situations. Generally these have been based on the concept of 'grief work', of which Worden's book has

Table 7.2 Worden's four tasks of mourning.

Task 1
To accept the reality of the loss.

Task 2
To work through the pain of grief.

Task 3
To adjust to the environment in which the deceased is missing.

Task 4
To emotionally relocate the deceased and move on with life.

been the most influential [30]. He suggests that it is helpful to separate counselling (helping people facilitate normal grief) from therapy (specialist techniques that help with abnormal grief). Central to his approach is the need for the bereaved to work through the four 'tasks of mourning', (see Table 7.2).

This model has recently been criticized for not allowing denial, lacking evidence of effectiveness, and inconsistencies with cross-cultural or historical perspectives. While this theoretical controversy continues, readers may find some of Worden's suggestions helpful.

Summary

Death, dying, and bereavement challenge the fundamental values and meaning of the human experience. Such a threat has the potential to provoke considerable distress and has therefore interested today's health professionals. As a consequence, it has been possible to identify maladaptations and formulate patterns of care in response. This chapter has detailed some of the literature on this subject, with an aim to improve understanding of the processes involved and the role of professionals in providing care.

References

1 Chonon J. *Death and the Modern Man*. New York: Macmillan, 1974.
2 Kastenbaum R, Aisenberg R. *The Psychology of Death*. New York: Springer Publishing Company, 1972.
3 Narayanasamy B. *Spiritual Care: A Resource Guide*. Nottingham: BKT Information Services, 1991.
4 Kubler-Ross E. *On Death and Dying*. New York: Macmillan, 1969.
5 Glaser BG, Strauss AL. *Awareness of Dying*. Chicago: Adeline, 1965.
6 Timmermans S. Dying awareness: the theory of awareness revisited. *Sociol Health Ill* 1994; 16: 322–337.
7 Glaser BG, Strauss AL. *Time for Dying*. Chicago: Adeline, 1968.
8 Pattison EM. The living-dying process. In: Garfield CA, ed. *Psychological Care of the Dying Patient*. New York: McGraw-Hill, 1978.
9 Greer S. Psychological response to cancer and survival. *Pyschol Med* 1991; 21: 43–49.
10 Copp G. Facing impending death: the experiences of patients and their nurses in a hospice setting. In: *Conference Proceedings—Palliative Care Research Forum* UK. Coventry: Palliative Care Research Forum, 1996.
11 Noyes R, Clancy J. The dying role: its relevance to improved patient care. In: Corr CA, Corr D, eds. *Hospice Care—Principles and Practice*. London: Faber & Faber, 1983.
12 Parkes CM. Bereavement as a psychosocial transition: process adaptation and

change. In: Dickinson D, Johnson M, eds. *Death, Dying and Bereavement*. London: Sage, 1993.

13 Vachon MLS. Emotional problems in palliative medicine: patient, family and professional. In: Doyle D, Hanks G, MacDonald N, eds. *The Oxford Textbook of Palliative Medicine*. Oxford: Oxford University Press, 1993: 577–605.

14 Jarrett SR, Ramirez AJ, Richards MA *et al*. Measuring coping in breast cancer. *J Psychosom Res* 1992; 36: 593–602.

15 Neimyer RA, Van Brunt D. Death anxiety. In: Wass H, Neimyer RA, eds. *Dying—Facing the Facts*. Washington: Taylor Francis, 1995.

16 Stedford A. *Facing Death*. Oxford: Heinemann Medical Books, 1984.

17 Stevens MM. Family adjustment and support. In: Doyle D, Hanks GWC, Macdonald N, eds. *Oxford Textbook of Palliative Medicine*. Oxford: Oxford University Press, 1993: 707–717.

18 Wellisch DK, Fawzy F, Landsverk J, Pasnau RO, Wolcott DL. Evaluation of psychosocial problems of the homebound cancer patient: the relationship of the disease and the sociodemographic variables of patients to family problems. *J Psychosoc Oncol* 1983; 1: 1–15.

19 Payne S, Relf M. The assessment of need for bereavement follow up in palliative and hospice care. *Palliat Med* 1994; 8: 291–297.

20 Freud S. Mourning and melancholia. In: *Collected Papers Vol IV*. London: Hogarth Press, 1925.

21 Lindemann E. Symptomatology and the management of acute grief. *Am J Psych* 1944; 101: 141–148.

22 Bowlby J. *Loss: Sadness and Depression (Attachment and Loss)*, Vol. 3. New York: Basic Books, 1980.

23 Stroebe M. Helping the bereaved come to terms with loss. In: *Bereavement and Counselling—Conference Proceedings*. London: St George's Mental Health Sciences, 1994.

24 Parkes CM. *Bereavement Studies of Grief in Adult Life*. London: Tavistock Publications, 1972.

25 Walter T. A new model for grief: bereavement and biography. *Mortality* 1996; 1: 7–25.

26 Woof WR, Carter YH. The grieving adult and the general practitioner; a literature review in two parts (part 1). *Br J Gen Pract* 1997; 47: 443–448.

27 Woof WR, Carter YH. The grieving adult and the general practitioners: a literature review in two parts (part 2). *Br J Gen Pract* 1997; 47: 509–514.

28 Middleton W, Moylan A, Raphael B *et al*. An international perspective on bereavement and related concepts. *Aus NZ J Psych* 1993; 27: 457–463.

29 Parkes CM. Bereavement counselling—does it work? *BMJ* 1980; 281: 3–10.

30 Worden JW. *Grief Counselling and Grief Therapy*. London: Routledge, 1992.

8: Communication Skills in Palliative Care

DAVID JEFFREY

Introduction

A patient who wants to make plans, needs to have information about the diagnosis, prognosis, treatment options and side-effects, and sources of support. Therefore, good communication is central to quality of palliative care.

Communication between patients, family, and professionals extends throughout care and it is important to acknowledge the value of listening to the patient's story and of discovering ways of helping patients to find meaning to their lives and to be able to place their illness in the context of their own life values and plans.

Good communication is necessary for the following reasons [1]:
- to maintain trust;
- to reduce uncertainty;
- to prevent unrealistic expectations;
- to allow the patient to adjust;
- to prevent a conspiracy of silence.

Barriers to communication

Many patients with serious illness are unhappy with the quality of communication that takes place between themselves and their professional carers. Indeed, poor communication is the commonest reason why patients complain about doctors [2–4]. What is it that makes it difficult for professionals to communicate with people faced with life-threatening disease?

The sources of difficulty in talking to dying patients can be divided into three groups [5].

Social

Lack of experience of death and dying at home. The large increase in palliative care resources in the community over the last two decades has not resulted in any change in the pattern of place of death: 65–70% of patients still die in institutions. Consequently death is commonly medicalized and professionals may find caring for dying patients at home frightening and at odds with a strict biomedical paradigm. Thus, pressures exist that perpetuate the myth that hospital is 'the best place to be if you are ill'. Yet, paradoxically, most people wish to die at home.

Death denial. Death remains a taboo subject and people discussing it are often accused of being morbid. For example, perhaps some people's reluctance to make a will is due to the irrational feeling that just by talking about death we might help to bring it about [6]. Indeed, media claims of breakthroughs and cures help to persuade people that death can be postponed indefinitely.

Secular society. There has been a change in the role of religion, and less emphasis is placed on spiritual needs in health care.

Patient

Fear of death and dying. It is not simply the prospect of a 'premature' death, but the likelihood of an undignified, painful process of dying which frightens patients, especially those with cancer. Once the patient becomes aware of their impending death, the world becomes unpredictable. People need a sense of control and uncertainty is difficult to bear.

Professional

Shared distress. The professional may feel distressed at sharing the bad news and feel some of the pain that the patient is experiencing.

Fear of blame. Traditionally there is a tendency to blame the messenger for the news he brings. Our society has such high expectations of good health and a long life that it seems that if someone is ill and deteriorating, it must be the fault of the doctor [5]. This can be felt by the doctor as a sense of failure.

Fear of the patient's reaction. Many doctors and nurses feel reluctant and unprepared to deal with the patient's reaction on hearing the news. Some doctors may still perceive that upsetting the patient does them harm.

Fear of our own reaction. Doctors and nurses may feel worried that they will show emotion. Indeed medical training highlights the need to control emotions such as anger or panic. Paradoxically, the doctor who expresses no emotion in this area of practice is likely to be perceived as insensitive [5].

Not knowing what to say. Doctors and nurses are trained to be active doers and may be uncomfortable when the appropriate response is to admit uncertainty, and sit and stay with a patient who is struggling to come to terms with his own mortality.

Own fears of illness or death. Personal fears of death and dying may make it especially difficult for the professional to communicate with patients with whom he or she identifies.

Fear of criticism from our seniors. Junior doctors and nurses may not be sure what the consultant or general practitioner has already said to the patient, and fear criticism if they are honest with the patient.

Not enough time. Doctors and other professionals may feel that time spent talking may be keeping other patients waiting inappropriately.

Communication skills

How not to react

Faced with the inherent difficulties of the situation for both patient and professional, it is not surprising that health care professionals commonly adopt distancing or blocking tactics in an effort to avoid some of the stress of caring [7,8]. These include the following:
- avoiding the patient or 'hiding' behind physical barriers, e.g. a desk;
- small talk;
- ignoring cues;
- dealing only with the positive;
- false or premature reassurance;
- switching the topic;
- passing the buck;
- use of jargon.

Listening to the patient's story

A careful assessment is essential; skilled communication not only allows an exchange of information between patient and professional but the telling of the story is in itself of great therapeutic benefit. Listening to the patient's story is a powerful way of respecting their autonomy [1,7].

PREPARATION

It is important at the outset to set aside enough time and try not to be disturbed. The patient should be asked whether they wish to be seen alone or with a relative. It is also important to ensure privacy if possible. Think about the way the chairs/bed are arranged so that the patient feels at ease. Make sure that you have any factual information which the patient may require, for example notes or results of recent tests. Think about support for the patient, either a relative or nurse.

COMMUNICATION

A few basic guidelines for structuring the opening of the interview are useful. Introduce yourself, explain who you are and the reason for the interview. Notify the patient of the time available, and check with the patient that they are happy to talk. Follow the patient's agenda—it will save time. Check for any missing details on the professional agenda.

INTERVIEWING SKILLS

The use of certain techniques can greatly assist the interviewing process. Use appropriate eye contact. Ask open questions; enquire about feelings and encourage the expression of emotion. Make sensitive use of prompting, summarizing, and clarifying, and try to pick up cues. Ask questions about mood and fears, and feel comfortable about silence. Appropriate use of touch can be helpful. Allow the appropriate display of your own emotions. Follow your hunches and do not make assumptions. These skills will not only allow you to cover the patient's agenda, but also the details required for your palliative care history.

ENDING THE ASSESSMENT INTERVIEW

Just as the way the interview opens is important, so it is necessary to cover particular items at the conclusion of the interview.
• Summarize current problems.
• Clarify treatment goals.

- Agree a plan of action.
- Arrange follow-up and give contact number.

Common communication problems in palliative care

BREAKING BAD NEWS

The general principles of good communication outlined above apply. Breaking bad news is a process not a single event. The sensitive professional will assess the patient's current level of knowledge and find out how much the patient wants to know. The patient needs to be warned that bad news is coming and the information needs to be given in stages. At each stage it is vital to check what the patient has understood. As in the assessment, follow the patient's agenda and explore fears and emotions. This process has been well described by Kaye in his 10 steps to breaking bad news [1] (see Box 8.1).

Follow-up

This can be a time to check what has been understood from the initial interview. Offer further explanation, perhaps with the use of diagrams, literature, tapes, or videos. Outline local resources and services. Check for emotional adjustment to the news, and offer to speak to relatives. Try to see the whole family, and include the children in this process.

The patient's emotional reaction to bad news

The individual patient's reaction varies enormously, and the doctor or

---

Box 8.1 Ten steps to breaking bad news (from Kaye 1996) [1]

1 Preparation
2 What does the patient know?
3 Is more information wanted?
4 Give a warning
5 Allow denial
6 Explain
7 Listen to concerns
8 Encourage feelings
9 Summary and plan
10 Offer continued support and availability

nurse should be aware of the possible range of emotions which can be felt. There is no rigid sequence which the patient follows; adjustment to loss takes time, and in many ways mirrors the grieving process [1].

Fear. This may be shown as denial or later with anxiety.

Anger. This may take the form of blame, and may be directed against doctors, as complaints.

Despair. Feelings of helplessness are frequently experienced. However, these points of crises can lead to the setting of new priorities [1].

Isolation. The patient may withdraw from family or friends.

Faith. The religious beliefs of the patient can be questioned.

Depression. Although sadness is common, it can occasionally present as clinical depression [8]. Alternatively, it may be directed in a positive way as a fighting spirit. This is a healthy response but care should be taken to help the patient if at a later time things go wrong and they blame themselves: 'if I had fought harder I would have beaten the cancer'.

'HOW LONG HAVE I GOT?' EXPLAINING A POOR PROGNOSIS

Doctors and nurses are not good at estimating how long an individual with advanced disease will live. As with all difficult questions the professional must be thinking 'why has this person asked this question?'. A suitable beginning might be to acknowledge that this is a difficult area and there is a great deal of uncertainty. The conversation could then go on to explore underlying concerns or future events that the patient is worried that he/she will miss.

In such a way the patient and professional can learn much from each other and set some realistic goals. Part of this task may be to reduce unrealistic expectations. It is best to avoid giving dates, since even the vaguest mention of a time will often be reported back to the family as 'The doctor gave me three months to live'.

For those who really press for a time limit it may be appropriate to give them some sense of control. This might be achieved by informing the patient of the sort of signs they might expect when death is approaching.

'THE NEWS WOULD KILL HIM—YOU MUST NOT SAY ANYTHING.'
DEALING WITH COLLUSION

Every doctor and nurse is familiar with this situation, which occurs when a relative is told the diagnosis or bad news before the patient is informed. A relative reacts initially by trying to protect their loved one from harm, arguing from the 'ignorance is bliss' standpoint. The situation may worsen if the doctor insists that it is his duty to inform the patient and then ignores the relative's concern. Alternatively, doctor and relatives enter into a collusive relationship and begin a conspiracy of silence, which serves only to isolate the patient, cause family disruption, and leads to a poor standard of health care.

It is vital to acknowledge from the outset that this distressing dilemma is almost always avoidable if patients are always consulted first about the diagnosis in the ways described earlier. If, however, the relative has been told first and then insists that the patient should not be told, how can the doctor or nurse unravel the situation and promote openness?

Promoting openness

This process starts with speaking to the relative. It may be the first time that anyone has attended to their concerns rather than those of the patient. The aim of the interview is to gain their trust. While following the basic principles of the assessment interview, following the relative's agenda, the doctor or nurse should cover several areas in particular. At the outset it is appropriate to acknowledge the difficulty of the situation for the relative, and that he or she is the person closest to the patient. Assess the relative's understanding of the disease and its impact on the family. Review the relative's reasons for not telling the patient; acknowledge that some of these are good and come from the best of motives, i.e. not to harm a loved one. Consider then the consequences and potential harms of not telling. Focus on the personal cost to the relative of maintaining a deception, the isolating effect of collusion, and the likely angry reaction from the patient when he eventually discovers.

Ask what the relative thinks is the patient's level of understanding. Suggest that the research evidence indicates that most patients are aware that something serious is happening. Seek permission to speak to the patient alone to clarify their understanding. At this point it is helpful to offer to confirm to the patient any ideas that they might hold about the severity of the situation. This approach affirms to the relative that you are respecting their concerns. Review the patient with a focus on their concerns and views on communication within the family. Occasionally the relative is right and the patient gives clear signals that they do not wish to know. In this case it would be an infringement of their autonomy to force unwanted information upon them. Finally, see the patient and family together to share the information, to offer support and follow-up, and to start setting realistic goals for the future.

Sometimes it is the doctor who initiates the collusion. The ideal should be a situation where all doctors respond to the differing information needs of the patient in the appropriate way. Communication is a changing dynamic process. This could involve accepting denial at the outset but checking afterwards that the patient's need for information had not changed.

'I'M SURE I'M GETTING STRONGER'—DENIAL

Denial is common when patients first hear the bad news. It should be expected and accepted. Denial is an effective coping strategy which has been associated with prolonged survival in some studies [9]. When in denial the patient gives a strong signal that they do not wish to talk about their diagnosis or prognosis in a realistic way. Although research indicates that the majority of patients do want to be fully informed it is important to respect the view of the small percentage who do not want to know [10].

A patient who denies his illness with one doctor may confide his fears with another member of staff. It may be that health care professionals who use denial as a coping strategy for themselves encounter denial more frequently in their patients. It is important to check whether the patient wants to talk [1].

- How do you feel things are going?
- Do you ever worry that things might be worse?
- What things have you been thinking about your illness?

These questions are framed in the context of a trusting relationship, never in a confrontational manner. Patients in denial are frightened; they need patience and sensitive communication.

COMMUNICATING WITH CHILDREN

Children are pragmatic and often demand information in a direct way. Older children have the same information needs as adults but require it in easily understandable forms. Young children may need to assimilate information through the use of play, painting, videos, and books. Parents often need help to allow them to break bad news to their children. An offer to help often involves little more than sitting, listening, and being with a family as they struggle to share bad news. Generally the child will pick a favourite member of the professional team in whom they wish to confide. Children require and should receive the same ethical standards of honest information. It is important not to allow natural feelings of protection to generate situations of collusion.

THE ANGRY PATIENT

Anger is a common emotion in patients with serious physical disease. It is a response to the perceived loss of control that accompanies a diagnosis of a terminal illness. In helping the angry patient it is often possible to explore the feelings associated with the anger. Often there is accompanying guilt or depression which may need attention. It is easy to react to angry patients and perceive them as demanding and uncooperative. It is more helpful if the professional can resist this and instead view anger as a symptom for which there is an underlying cause. Anger and aggression can be productively defused, allowing the patient or relative to move towards acceptance. The key to dealing with anger is to allow expression of the emotion. This can be facilitated by using the principles of open questions and acknowledging the distress.

It takes time to allow patients or relatives to ventilate strong emotions. It is time which is well spent and is therapeutic in itself. It is also emotionally draining for the health care professional.

ADVOCACY

The doctor–patient relationship is unequal with regard to medical knowledge. The doctor may be perceived as knowledgeable and competent yet distant from emotions and suffering. One way of equalizing the power in the relationship is a requirement for informed consent; another mechanism is advocacy. Advocacy implies representing the cause of another person. Often nurses have this role of presenting problems to the doctor. In a team which is communicating this will be accepted. In some teams, however, advocacy can be seen by the doctor as a threat or obstructive interference and may thus contribute to team conflict.

Communication between health care professionals
(see also Chapter 2)

Doctors are not good at communicating with each other, particularly if the patient is transferring from one setting to another, for example from hospital to home [5]. It is important to clarify issues relating to the future management of the patient and family, level of awareness of the patient and family, nursing involvement, arrangements for follow-up, and establishing who is the key professional for a particular patient.

Coping with conflict and stress

There are various ways in which the health care professional can be equipped to cope better with the conflicts and stresses arising from this highly demanding work.

Taking time. Many health care professionals do not value time for reflection.

Talking to colleagues. Talking to colleagues can help personal awareness. We all bring our own fears and anxieties to this work. It is easy to feel indispensable. A colleague can help to place work in perspective and give an opportunity to ventilate our own emotions.

Defining areas of conflict. Plan how to move forward with the team members. This will include organizational strategies to reduce conflict in the future.

Seeking a balance. Work needs to be balanced with outside interests.

Education. Keeping up to date in the professional field is stimulating and affirms our skills. Education should be a continuing experience and may be facilitated by a clinical supervisor.

Conclusion

Honest, sensitive, and skilled communication lies at the core of palliative care. The message that health care professionals communicate should include:
- concern and support for the patient and family;
- information about the illness and treatment choices;
- a commitment to do the best to relieve suffering;
- a respect for the patient's individuality and involvement in decision-making;
- availability to listen to the patient's view;

- approachability to allow expression of emotions and fears;
- continuity of care—the patient will never be abandoned.

No matter how experienced the doctor or nurse, talking to patients and relatives can be challenging. By accepting this challenge and reflecting upon contact with patients and their loved ones, professionals will continue to develop communication skills, which in turn will improve their care of patients and job satisfaction. Indeed, for many professionals it is often in the context of this close personal interaction that the professional defines the meaning of their work and can reflect on their failures and successes.

References

1 Kaye P. *Breaking Bad News: A Ten Step Approach*. Northampton: EPL Publications, 1996: 3–25.
2 Reynolds M. No news is bad news: patient's views about communication in hospital. *BMJ* 1978; 1: 1673–1676.
3 Fletcher C. Listening and talking to patients. 1: the problem. *BMJ* 1980; 281: 845.
4 Dunkelman H. Patient's knowledge of their conditions and treatment: how it might be improved. *BMJ* 1979; 2: 311–314.
5 Buckman R. Communication in palliative care: a practical guide. In: Doyle D, Hanks GWC, Macdonald N, eds. *Oxford Textbook of Palliative Medicine*. Oxford: Oxford University Press, 1993: 47–61.
6 Boston S. *Merely Mortal*. London: Methuen, 1987.
7 Faulkner A, Maguire P. *Talking to Cancer Patients and Their Relatives*. Oxford: Oxford University Press, 1994.
8 Stedeford A. *Facing Death*. London: Heinemann, 1984.
9 Greer S. Cancer and the mind. *Brit J Psych* 1983; 143: 535–543.
10 Meredith C, Symonds P, Webster L, et al. Information needs of cancer patients in west Scotland: cross sectional survey of patients' views. *BMJ* 1996; 313: 724–726.

9: The Principles of Pain Management

KAREN FORBES AND CHRISTINA FAULL

Introduction

The successful management of pain requires careful assessment of the nature of the pain, an understanding of different types and patterns of pain, and a knowledge of how best to treat it. Good initial pain assessment will act as a baseline against which subsequent interventions can be judged. The multidimensional nature of pain means that the use of analgesics may be only part of a multiprofessional team strategy addressing physical, psychological, social, and spiritual distress, and, at times, the need for behavioural change. Negotiation of a management plan is a vital part of the process and requires good communication with patients and their carers.

Pain occurs in up to 75% of patients with advanced cancer [1] and in about 65% of patients dying from all other causes [2]. Of patients dying from heart disease, 78% are reported as having pain in the last year of life [3]. Despite considerable scientific and pharmacological progress, pain continues to be substantially undertreated [4–6]. The use of opioids remains an area of major concern for many clinicians, and the increasing variety of available formulations may compound this. This chapter will discuss the nature and experience of pain for patients, particularly those with cancer. A framework for the effective use of drugs and other interventional techniques in pain management will be discussed.

The nature of pain

Pain is an unpleasant sensory *and* emotional experience. Pain is essentially subjective since it can only be identified and quantified as 'what the patient says hurts' and is individual to the person experiencing it. Observation of behaviour and physical signs may provide some additional information but it must be recognized that the correlation between observer- and patient-reported pain may be poor. One person's response to the same painful stimulus will differ from another's according to a variety of circumstances. The observation of behavioural responses to pain is, however, particularly important where language is limited or absent, for example in neonates, infants, the mentally incompetent, and those deprived of language (e.g. following a stroke).

The concept of total pain

The experience of pain is influenced by physical, emotional, social, and spiritual factors. The concept of total pain acknowledges the importance of all of these dimensions of a person's suffering, and that good pain relief is unlikely without attention to all of these areas [7] (Fig. 9.1).

Patients with chronic or advanced disease face many losses: loss of normality; loss of health; and potential loss of the future. Pain imposes limitations on lifestyle, particularly in terms of mobility and endurance. In addition, the pain can be interpreted as an ever-present reminder of the underlying disease and its present and possible consequences. The significance of pain for patients with advanced disease will vary according to the person, their circumstances, and the illness. Pain due to muscle spasm in chronic degenerative neurological disorder may be distressing and frustrating; however, a patient with ischaemic heart disease may believe each episode of chest pain signifies imminent death.

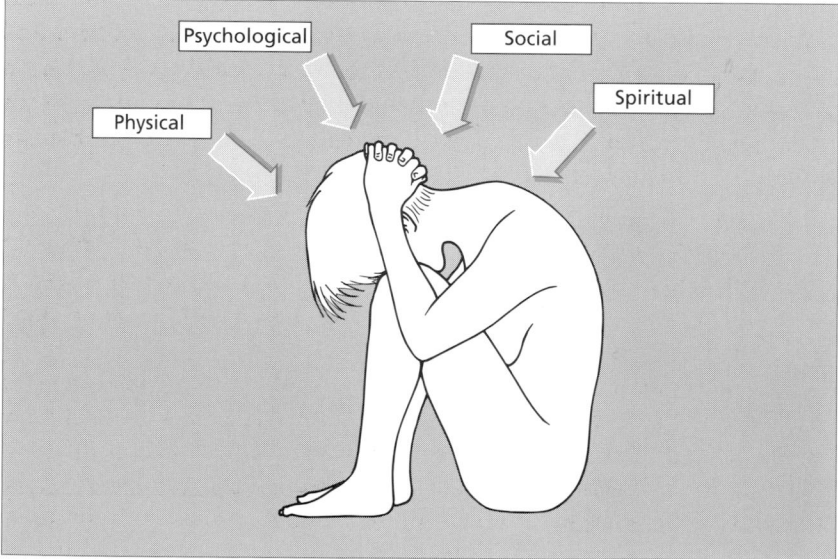

Fig. 9.1 The concept of total pain.

Many people feel that severe pain is inevitable in cancer, and this may lead to fear, suffering, and reluctance to ask for help. Pain may be erroneously interpreted by patients as an indication of progression of their cancer and therefore a signal of their approaching death.

Neuroanatomy and neurophysiology of nociception and analgesia

Nociception is the detection of noxious stimuli by specialized nerve endings known as nociceptors. Activation of nociceptors by mechanical, thermal, or chemical stimuli leads to the perception of so-called nociceptive pain. An understanding of the physiology that underlies this will allow improved pain assessment and management. A simplified schema of the neuroanatomy and site of action of a variety of analgesic modalities is shown in Fig. 9.2.

Nerve fibres are classified as A, B, or C fibres, with alpha, beta, delta, and gamma subcategories. A-beta, A-delta, and C are sensory fibres and therefore have a role in pain perception. A-delta nociceptors respond to pricking, squeezing, or pinching and lead to the 'fast', sharp pain of an injury. They are involved in the analgesia produced by acupuncture-like transcutaneous electrical nerve stimulation (TENS) (see below). 'Polymodal' C fibres respond to many noxious stimuli to produce 'slow', throbbing, more diffuse pain. These nociceptive afferent fibres synapse with neurones within the dorsal horn of the spinal cord; these project on, via interneurones, to the thalamus and cortex. A-beta and other sensory afferent nerve fibres also synapse with these dorsal horn neurones and may inhibit the transmission of the painful stimulus to the thalamus and cortex. This is known as gate control and is the mechanism of action of conventional TENS (see below).

Descending inhibitory neural pathways from the brain to the spinal cord also modulate incoming nociceptive information. The major neurotransmitters involved in these descending inhibitory pathways are serotonin and noradrenaline. This is the probable site of action of many adjuvant analgesics.

Opioid receptors occur throughout the spinal cord and in many areas of the brain. There are at least three types of opioid receptor that subserve opioid analgesia (see Box 9.1). The analgesia produced by acupuncture is thought to be due to the release of endogenous opioids (endorphins, dynorphins, and enkephalins) in the spinal cord.

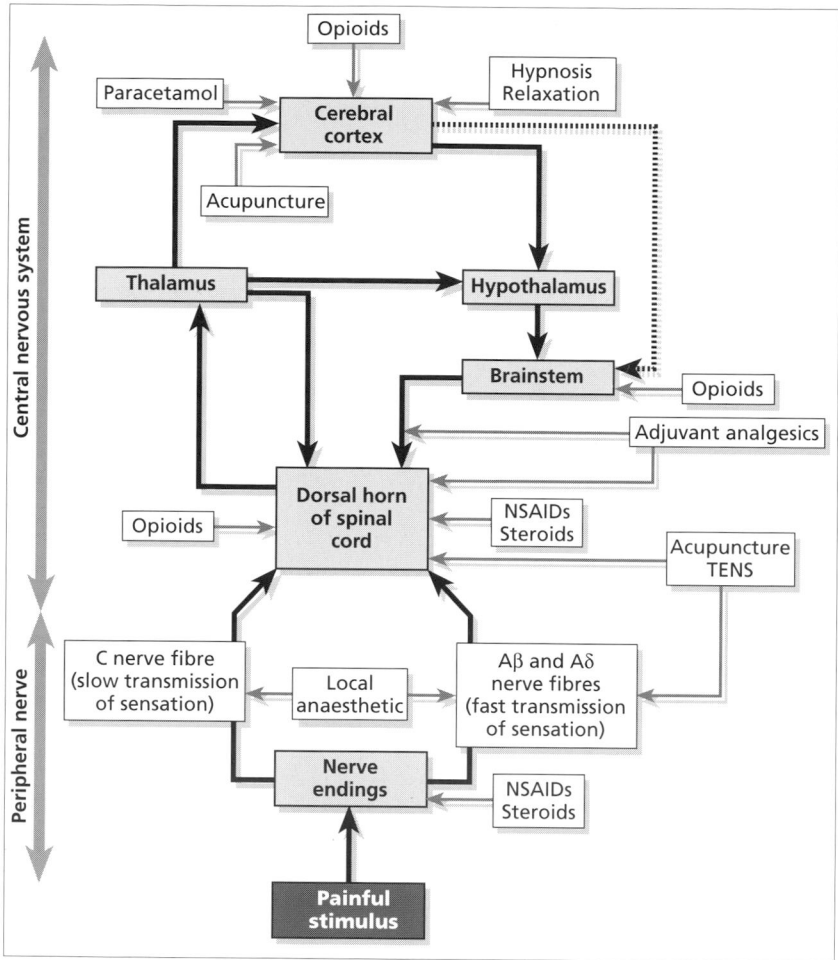

Fig. 9.2 A schema of the neuroanatomy of pain and the sites of action of different analgesic modalities.

Box 9.1 Opioid receptors	
Opioid receptor subtype:	**Effect of agonist:**
Mu	Analgesia, respiratory depression, reduced gastrointestinal motility, hypotension
Kappa	Analgesia, sedation, psychomimetic effects; some respiratory depression
Delta	Analgesia, respiratory depression

Patterns and types of pain

The classification of pain is not an esoteric exercise, since the type of pain may suggest its underlying cause and guide treatment decisions.

Acute and chronic pain

Whilst acute pain provokes a 'fight or flight' (sympathetic) response with tachycardia, hypertension, and pupillary changes, chronic pain allows adaptation to this. Many patients mount this physiological response only during acute exacerbations of pain, with few if any such signs at other times.

Chronic pain is not simply prolonged acute pain. Repeated noxious stimulation leads to a variety of changes within the central nervous system (CNS). For example, repeated C-fibre stimulation leads to accentuated neuronal responses in the dorsal horn of the spinal cord, leading to increased and prolonged pain perception. This is termed 'wind up', which is thought to be mediated via the excitatory amino acid N-methyl-D-aspartate (NMDA) receptor.

Somatic and visceral pain

Somatic and visceral pain are both nociceptive pains. Somatic pain arises from damage to the skin and deep tissues. It is usually localized and of an aching quality. Visceral pain arises from the abdominal and thoracic viscera. It is poorly localized and described as 'deep' and 'pressure'. Visceral pain is sometimes 'referred' and is felt in a part of the body distant to the site of noxious stimulation – for example, the visceral pain of diaphragmatic irritation is felt in the shoulder tip, and the pain of ischaemic heart disease radiates into the neck and arms. Visceral pain is often associated with other symptoms such as nausea and vomiting. Both types of pain usually respond to the non-opioid or opioid analgesics (see section on WHO analgesic ladder on p. 110).

Neuropathic pain

Neuropathic pain arises as a consequence of a disturbance of function or pathological change in a nerve or the nervous system [8]. It may arise from a lesion within the peripheral or central nervous system, and may follow nerve damage due to trauma, infection, ischaemia, degenerative disease, compression, tumour invasion, or chemical- or radiation-induced injury. The primary injury may sometimes be trivial.

Deafferentation pain is a type of neuropathic pain, for example following brachial or lumbosacral plexus avulsion injuries. Phantom limb pain is the classic example of deafferentation pain. Central pain is neuropathic pain following damage to the CNS, for example pain following stroke. Sympathetically maintained pain (e.g. reflex sympathetic dystrophy) is diagnosed in the presence of neuropathic pain in association with autonomic dysfunction such as swelling, changes in sweating and temperature, and trophic changes such as thinning of tissues, loss of hair, and abnormal nail growth. It is thought to be sustained by efferent activity in the sympathetic nervous system. Neuropathic pain often occurs in an area of abnormal or absent sensation [9].

Neuropathic pain may be improved but is often not completely relieved by non-opioid or opioid analgesics. Adjuvant analgesic drugs are often required (see p. 126).

ABNORMAL SENSATIONS IN NEUROPATHIC PAIN

Various abnormal sensations are associated with neuropathic pain.
• Dysaesthesia: spontaneous and evoked abnormal sensation.
• Hyperaesthesia: an increased sensitivity to stimulation.
• Hyperalgesia: increased response to a stimulus that is normally painful.
• Allodynia: pain caused by a stimulus that is not normally painful.
• Hyperpathia: explosive and often prolonged painful response to a stimulus.

The assessment of pain

Successful pain management relies on careful assessment to elucidate possible underlying causes and the effect the pain is having on the patient's life, plus the psychosocial and spiritual factors which might be influencing the pain and its impact on the patient. A full pain history (see Box 9.2) and a clinical examination are vital, and laboratory or radiographic investigations may then be necessary. It may be useful to use a specific assessment and monitoring tool.

Pain is a uniquely personal experience. There is no standard language of pain. Descriptions of pain will vary within families and cultural groups. It may be extremely difficult for a patient with advanced disease to find the language to describe his pain since it may be unlike anything he has previously experienced not least because of its emotional, social, and spiritual components.

Box 9.2 Taking a pain history

1   When did the pain start?
2   Where is it, and does it go anywhere else?
3   What does it feel like (nature and severity)?
4   Is it constant or does it come and go?
5   Does anything make it better or worse?
6   Are there any associated symptoms?
7   Is it limiting the patient's activities?
8   What does the patient think the pain is due to?
9   What does the patient feel about the pain (emotional impact)?
10 Which analgesics have been tried and what effect did they have?
11 What are the patient's expectations of treatment?
12 What are the patient's fears?
13 What is the patient's previous experience of pain and illness?

Pain and behaviour

Pain impinges on and alters people's lives, turning their focus inwards and potentially isolating them. This behavioural response may be graded by an observer—for example, grimacing or crying in a child—or reported by the patient—for example, alterations in behaviour such as:

- pain at rest, but pain can be ignored;
- in pain, but can carry out tasks;
- in pain, but with concentration can carry out tasks;
- pain overwhelming, dominating everything.

Pain assessment tools

Pain assessment tools will aid initial understanding of the nature of pain for the individual and will allow clear assessment of the effect of analgesics and other interventions. A report that the pain is 'better' is ambiguous and without such records may mean either improved or cured. Most patients can grade their pain out of 10. If this concept is difficult, a simpler categorical scale can be chosen in discussion with the patient (see Box 9.3).

VISUAL ANALOGUE SCALES

A visual analogue scale (VAS) is a 10 cm line labelled at each end to denote

Box 9.3 **Simple verbal and numerical scales for pain assessment**

- Present/absent
- Good/bad
- None/mild/moderate/severe
- None/mild/moderate/severe/excruciating
- Graded out of 10, where 0 = no pain and 10 = worst pain ever

the minimum and maximum extremes of whatever is being measured (in this case pain). The line is usually horizontal but some patients find vertical lines more understandable.

Least

possible —————————————————————————— Worst

pain   possible

    pain

    The patient puts a mark on the line corresponding to the intensity of the pain and the observer then measures its position. VASs are simple, reproducible, and reliable and correlate well with scores derived from categorical scales. They can be used in both clinical and research settings.

BODY CHARTS

Body charts can be used to evaluate the site and nature of pain. Body charts may emphasize that a patient has pain at several sites, possibly of different aetiologies and therefore requiring different treatments (Fig. 9.3).

PAIN QUESTIONNAIRES

There are numerous pain questionnaires but many are suitable for research only. The McGill Pain Questionnaire (Fig. 9.3) is used extensively in pain research [10] and can be a useful clinical tool for patients with difficult pain management in a specialist setting.

USEFUL TOOLS FOR CHILDREN

Children may be more comfortable drawing their pain on a body chart than describing it. Their use of colour at various sites can be discussed and related to the nature and severity of each pain. A pain thermometer can be used in the same way as a VAS, i.e. the child marks the intensity of

McGill pain questionnaire

Patient's name .... Date .... Time .... am/pm

PRI: S............ A............ E............ M............ PRI(T)............ PPI............
      (1–10)   (11–15)   (16)   (17–20)   (1–20)

1 Flickering Quivering Pulsing Throbbing Beating Pounding	**8** Tingling Itchy Smarting Stinging	**16** Annoying Troublesome Miserable Intense Unbearable	Brief —— Momentary —— Transient —— Rhythmic —— Periodic Intermittent ——
	9 Dull Sore Hurting Aching Heavy	**17** Spreading Radiating Penetrating Piercing	
2 Jumping Flashing Shooting			Continuous —— Steady Constant
3 Pricking Boring Drilling Stabbing Lancinating	**10** Tender Taut Rasping Splitting	**18** Tight Numb Drawing Squeezing Tearing	
4 Sharp Cutting Lacerating	**11** Tiring Exhausting	**19** Cool Cold Freezing	
	12 Sickening Suffocating		
5 Pinching Pressing Gnawing Cramping Crushing	**13** Fearful Frightful Terrifying	**20** Nagging Nauseating Agonizing Dreadful Torturing	
	14 Punishing Gruelling Cruel Vicious Killing	**PPI** **0** No pain **1** Mild **2** Discomforting	
6 Tugging Pulling Wrenching		**3** Distressing	
7 Hot Burning Scalding Searing	**15** Wretched Blinding	**4** Horrible **5** Excruciating	E = External I = Internal

Comments:

Fig. 9.3 The McGill Pain Questionnaire. The descriptors fall into four major groups: sensory, 1–10; affective, 11–15; evaluative, 16; and miscellaneous, 17–20. The rank value for each descriptor is based on its position in the word set. The sum of the rank values is the pain rating index (PRI). The present pain intensity (PPI) is based on a scale of 0–5. (Reproduced with permission from [10].)

the pain on the thermometer and the observer then measures the position of the mark. The shading of the thermometer from blue to red provides visual cues for children, who may not grasp the concept of a VAS.

Faces scales have been developed for the assessment of pain in children. Children rank their pain against a series of drawings or photographs of faces showing varying facial expressions of pain. They may also be useful when language presents a barrier between patient and professional.

Management of cancer-related pain

The remainder of this chapter will concentrate largely on pain due to cancer although many of the principles can be extrapolated to the management of chronic pain in other illnesses. It should not be assumed that cancer will lead inevitably to pain; some patients with cancer do not experience pain, and not every pain experienced by a patient with cancer is due to the cancer itself (see Box 9.4).

Principles of pain management in patients with cancer

The management of pain in cancer patients should be undertaken in a systematic manner, based on certain principles. Firstly, assess each pain separately, and ascertain if the pain is related to the cancer. If so, consider three main types of cancer-related pain.
- Somatic/visceral pain:
  usually opioid sensitive;
  use the WHO analgesic ladder (see below, p. 110).
- Bone pain:
  usually NSAID sensitive;

Box 9.4 Pain due to cancer

Thirty percent of people with cancer do not develop pain.
Those with pain may have four or more different types:
- related to the cancer
- related to the treatment
- related to consequent disability
- due to a concurrent disorder.
A patient who feels cared for may cope better with pain.
A patient who is free of pain is better placed to face the illness.
Cancer pain can be controlled in 80% of patients. If a patient's pain is not controlled within a week consider specialist advice.

may be poorly opioid sensitive;
radiotherapy often helps.
- Neuropathic pain:
may respond poorly or not at all to opioids;
adjuvant drugs have a key role (see below, p. 126);
often difficult pain to manage;
may need *early* specialist referral for best results.

It is also important to consider if the pain is incident pain, i.e. pain occurring on movement, which is best managed by treating the underlying cause where possible. Different analgesic doses are required for rest pain and movement-related pain to avoid excess sedation at rest, i.e. give extra analgesics before movement in anticipation of pain. Spinal routes of analgesic delivery may be useful (see below, p. 130).

Treatment of the underlying cause

For some patients it may be possible to treat the underlying cancer and thus reduce pain. There are three main approaches to this. One is chemotherapy; for example, palliative chemotherapy may reduce liver capsule pain by shrinking hepatic metastases. Another is radiotherapy; for example, a single fraction of radiotherapy for bone metastases provides good pain relief in up to 80% of patients. The third approach is hormone therapy. For example, bone pain related to metastatic prostatic cancer may be reduced by the commencement of antiandrogen treatment.

For other patients an orthopaedic procedure to stabilize a fracture or decompress the spinal cord, whilst not affecting the cancer, may relieve pain, particularly incident pain. For example, pain in the thigh due to a femoral metastasis may be relieved by internal fixation.

The use of analgesics

Patients with advanced disease usually have constant pain and therefore require regular analgesics taken at dosage intervals according to the pharmacokinetics of the drug. Regular analgesics taken before pain returns are likely to lead to smaller total doses of analgesics and smoother pain control with fewer adverse effects. However, patients with chronic pain will experience exacerbations of pain, for instance on movement, during changes of wound dressings, or at unpredictable times. This is known as *breakthrough pain*. Analgesics for these episodes should be available to the patient in addition to their regular analgesics, normally as an extra dose of their regular analgesic, or its equivalent.

The World Health Organization (WHO) analgesic ladder for cancer pain

The Cancer Pain Relief Programme of the WHO advocated a three-step 'analgesic ladder' in an attempt to improve the management of pain due to cancer worldwide [11,12] (Fig. 9.4). The underlying principle is that, following good pain assessment and with a thorough knowledge of a small number of analgesics, a simple approach should produce pain relief in the majority of patients.

Although the WHO analgesic ladder was developed for use in cancer pain, a stepwise approach using a limited number of drugs is equally applicable to the management of chronic pain due to other causes and has the potential to simplify prescribing (Fig. 9.4).

Opiates, opioids, and non-opioids: terminology

An *opiate* is a drug derived or synthesized from the opium poppy, such as morphine. The term *opioid* includes naturally occurring, semisynthetic, and synthetic drugs which, like morphine, combine with opioid receptors to produce their effects. These effects are antagonized by naloxone.

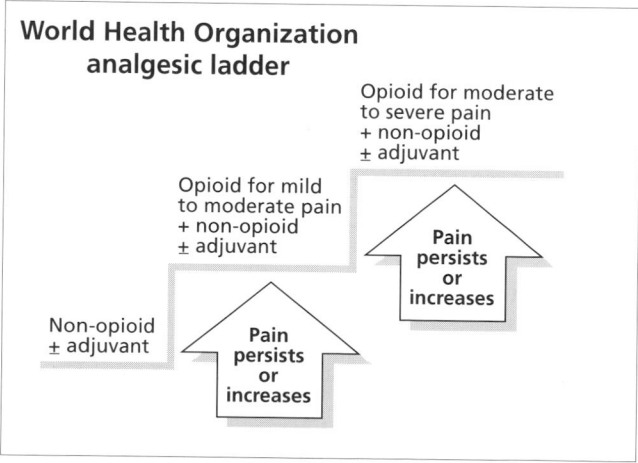

Fig. 9.4 The WHO analgesic ladder. The ladder has no 'top rung' as there is no maximum dose for strong opioids. If pain is still a problem with doses of morphine > 300 mg/day reconsider the underlying cause of the pain and/or seek specialist advice. (Adapted from [12].)

The *non-opioid* analgesics available in the UK are paracetamol and the non-steroidal anti-inflammatory drugs (NSAIDs), which include the salicylate, aspirin.

Opioids for mild to moderate pain

This term replaces 'weak opioids' in the 1996 revision of the WHO analgesic ladder. Opioids for mild to moderate pain are used in combination with a non-opioid analgesic such as paracetamol, at the second step of the ladder. There are numerous combination step-two analgesics available, many of which have subtherapeutic doses of the opioid, e.g. paracetamol 500 mg with codeine 8–10 mg per tablet (e.g. Co-dydramol). Such combinations probably increase side-effects without significantly increasing efficacy. More useful combinations are shown in Box 9.5.

If regular, maximum doses of opioids for mild to moderate pain do not achieve adequate analgesia they should be replaced with an opioid for moderate to severe pain such as morphine. There is no advantage in changing to an alternative opioid for mild to moderate pain.

Opioids for moderate to severe pain

These drugs, known previously as 'strong opioids', are at step three of the WHO analgesic ladder. There are many opioids available. Their relative potencies and potential areas of use are shown in Table 9.1. In the UK, morphine is the drug of choice for oral administration, and diamorphine for parenteral administration. The legal requirements governing the prescription of morphine and its availability in different countries vary, sometimes making prescribing problematic (see Chapter 1). Diamorphine is not available in some countries, such as the USA.

Box 9.5 Useful step 2 analgesics

Co-codamol 30/500	Codeine 30 mg + paracetamol 500mg per tablet
	Dose: 2 tablets 6-hourly
Co-proxamol	Dextropropoxyphene 32.5 mg + paracetamol 325 mg per tablet
	Dose: 2 tablets 4–6-hourly
Dihydrocodeine	Dose: 30–60 mg 4–6-hourly
Tramadol	Dose: 50–100 mg 4–6-hourly (relatively high potency; see Table 9.1)

Table 9.1 The relative potencies of opioids.

| Drug | Approximate equivalence to *repeated* doses of 10 mg of oral morphine sulphate | | Indication |
	Oral dose	s.c./i.m. dose	
Morphine	10 mg	5 mg (10 mg p.r.)	Oral strong opioid of choice in the UK
Diamorphine	10 mg	3 mg	strong opioid of choice in the UK
Dextromoramide	5 mg	–	Dressing changes and painful procedures
Hydromorphone	1.3 mg	0.5 mg	As for morphine
Methadone (chronic use)	3 mg	2 mg	Specialist use
Oxycodone	7.5 mg	15 mg (20 mg p.r.)	As for morphine
Buprenorphine	0.2 mg (s.l.)	–	Possible alternative to low dose morphine (has a ceiling effect)
Phenazocine	2 mg	–	As for morphine
Tramadol	70 mg	100 mg	Potent step 2 analgesic
Pethidine	160 mg	40 mg	Unsuitable for chronic pain
Codeine	120 mg	80 mg	WHO step 2 analgesic
Dihydrocodeine	100 mg	–	WHO step 2 analgesic
Dextropropoxyphene	100 mg	–	WHO step 2 analgesic

The reader may find slight variations in equivalence in other texts. However, the table is designed to be useful in clinical practice.

Morphine

Morphine is a natural derivative of the opium poppy. It is readily absorbed after oral administration, mainly in the upper small bowel, and is metabolized in the liver and at other sites to morphine-3-glucuronide (M3G) and morphine-6-glucuronide (M6G). M6G is an active metabolite, and is a more potent analgesic than morphine. Morphine and its glucuronides are excreted renally and so may accumulate with impaired renal function.

Four-hourly administration by any route is necessary to achieve constant, therapeutic blood concentrations unless the preparation is modified for sustained release of morphine (i.e. controlled release preparation).

MORPHINE PREPARATIONS AVAILABLE IN THE UK

Various preparations of morphine are available in the UK.

Oral preparations. For oral administration with immediate release there is a choice of either tablets or liquid, while for oral controlled release the alternatives are: 12-hourly controlled-release tablets or capsules; 12-hourly controlled-release suspension; and 24-hourly controlled-release capsules.

Rectal suppositories. These may be useful in the short term in a patient who cannot take oral morphine because of vomiting or a decreased level of consciousness. Absorption from the rectum can be variable, although the same dose and a 4-hourly dosing interval are recommended. Immediate- and controlled-release oral preparations of morphine are not suitable for rectal use.

Injection. Morphine has poor solubility, which results in large-volume, and therefore uncomfortable, intramuscular or subcutaneous injections. Diamorphine is the preferred drug in those countries in which it is available.

Gaining control of pain: titration of oral morphine to achieve analgesia

The European Association for Palliative Care published guidelines on the use of morphine in cancer pain in 1996, which expanded the principles of the WHO analgesic ladder [13].

Patients who are not pain controlled on a step-two analgesic should be commenced on 5–10 mg oral immediate-release morphine scheduled 4-hourly. (Occasionally a starting dose of 2.5 mg is advisable in elderly or frail patients.) Pain occurring between regular doses of morphine is termed breakthrough pain. Patients should have 'rescue' immediate-release morphine for breakthrough pain, at a dose equivalent to the regular 4-hourly dose.

> **Box 9.6 Titration of oral morphine**
>
> *Example 1*
> Drug: Immediate-release morphine
> Dose: 20 mg 4-hourly + 20 mg for breakthrough pain
> Previous 24 h: Three doses taken for breakthrough pain
> New dose: (20 mg × 6) + (20 mg × 3) = 180 T mg/24 h = 30 mg 4-hourly +
>   30 mg for breakthrough pain
>
> *Example 2*
> Drugs: Immediate-release morphine
> Dose: 30 mg 4-hourly + 30 mg for breakthrough pain
> Previous 24 h: One dose taken for breakthrough pain
> New dose: (30 mg + 30%) × 6 = 240 mg/24 h = 40 mg 4-hourly + 40 mg
>   for breakthrough pain

Regular doses should be taken 4-hourly even if a rescue dose has been necessary. After 24 hours, the total dose of morphine taken (regular plus rescue doses) should be calculated and divided by six to give a new 4-hourly dose. If patients are reluctant to take rescue medication but remain in pain, their regular medication should be increased by 30–50% at each review. In either situation the rescue dose should be increased to be the same as the new 4-hourly dose. A common error is to forget to increase the rescue dose so that medication for breakthrough pain becomes increasingly inadequate. This process of reviewing the daily dose allows the morphine to be 'titrated' against the patient's pain (see Box 9.6). Two-thirds of patients with cancer need up to 30 mg of morphine 4-hourly (180 mg/day). One-third of patients may need higher doses in the course of their illness.

Maintenance of pain control: the choices

Once a patient's four-hourly morphine dose has been titrated to gain good pain control, the patient may wish to have their analgesia maintained by a controlled-release preparation of an opioid for moderate to severe pain. This may have the advantage of greater convenience, easier compliance, and fewer peak-and-trough effects. In addition some opioids may have a different spectrum of adverse effects compared to morphine, and this may be an advantage for some patients.

The choices for the patient are:
- continue 4-hourly immediate-release morphine;

- convert to 12-hourly controlled-release morphine preparation;
- convert to 24-hourly controlled-release morphine preparation;
- convert to fentanyl patches;
- convert to other opioid controlled-release preparation.

The choice of preparation will depend on several factors, including: patient preference; professional experience, confidence, and preference; the tailoring of the side-effect profile to the patient's needs; and the ease of administration and patient compliance.

There is no evidence that one strong opioid preparation is superior to any other in analgesic effect at equivalent dose. For example, fentanyl, delivered by patch, will not improve pain control given in an equivalent dose to morphine. However, if the patient forgets to take tablets or has marked constipation, application of a fentanyl patch may provide indirect improvement in pain control through improved compliance and the side-effect profile may be altered.

Several important practical points must be borne in mind. Firstly, patients must be given very clear instructions (preferably orally *and* in writing) about the use of controlled-release and immediate-release preparations. Particular note should be made of prescribing controlled-release preparations by time interval not frequency (e.g. '12-hourly' *not* 'b.d.'); the use of rescue immediate-release medication for breakthrough pain; and the need to continue regular medication even when breakthrough medication is used.

Secondly, rescue immediate-release morphine (or occasionally other immediate-release opioid) at a dose equivalent to the 4-hourly dose should always be available. If rescue medication is required regularly, the total 24-hour opioid requirement should be calculated and the dose of the controlled-release preparation and rescue medication increased accordingly.

Finally, patients should *never* be prescribed more than one controlled-release opioid preparation at a time.

Patients with cancer-related pain require regular review. If further pain develops the cause and treatment should be assessed as above. It is unwise to assume that any new pain is also cancer related and/or that opioids are necessarily the most appropriate form of management for the new pain.

Titration with controlled-release morphine

Ideally, immediate-release morphine should be used to titrate to pain control. This procedure is relatively simple in hospitals and in-patient units but may be impractical in a community setting. In this situation, it is common practice to commence patients on a controlled-release opioid preparation. However, the longer the therapeutic effect of a preparation, the more inflexible it is. This sometimes makes titration to pain relief more difficult and there is an increased risk of toxicity for patients.

If this method is thought to have an advantage, the recommended starting dose is equivalent to 60 mg morphine daily; however, most practitioners reduce this to 40 mg or even 20 mg in the frail or elderly, given as 20 mg 24-hourly or 10 mg 12-hourly of the relevant controlled-release preparation. Patients still require access to immediate-release morphine for breakthrough pain, at a dose equivalent to the 4-hourly dose.

Diamorphine

Diamorphine is highly soluble. It is a prodrug and its analgesic effect depends on metabolism to morphine and M6G. Diamorphine should be given 4-hourly or by continuous infusion. Administration by injection is more potent than oral morphine. A dose of 1 mg parenteral diamorphine is equivalent to 3 mg of oral morphine. Diamorphine is *not* a more effective analgesic. Pain not controlled on oral morphine will not be improved by conversion to an equivalent dose of injectable diamorphine. Diamorphine mixes with many other drugs, such as antiemetics, if parenteral use is necessary and is therefore useful in a syringe driver (see Chapter 22).

Diamorphine may be given orally in which case it is approximately equipotent to oral morphine. The suspension has a much shorter shelf life than morphine liquid, which limits its use.

Fentanyl

Fentanyl is a synthetic opioid analgesic used in anaesthesia because of its short half-life. A patch system is available for transdermal delivery of fentanyl for chronic cancer pain (Fig. 9.5). Transdermal fentanyl has not been *shown* to be a more effective analgesic than other opioids although for some patients it may have advantages. Pain not controlled on oral morphine will not be improved by conversion to an equivalent dose of transdermal fentanyl. Fentanyl causes the same side-effects as morphine; however, constipation, sedation, and nausea are considered to be less severe with transdermal fentanyl in some patients. Like morphine, the effect of fentanyl can be reversed with naloxone.

The availability of transdermal fentanyl has offered a new pain-control option for patients. However, as with all controlled-release opioids, fentanyl patches present potential problems when prescribed by those unfamiliar with their appropriate use or when insufficient information is given to

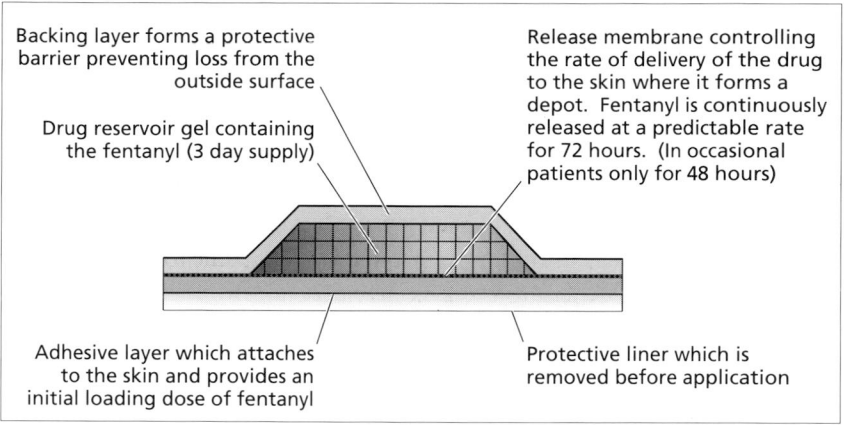

Backing layer forms a protective barrier preventing loss from the outside surface

Drug reservoir gel containing the fentanyl (3 day supply)

Release membrane controlling the rate of delivery of the drug to the skin where it forms a depot. Fentanyl is continuously released at a predictable rate for 72 hours. (In occasional patients only for 48 hours)

Adhesive layer which attaches to the skin and provides an initial loading dose of fentanyl

Protective liner which is removed before application

Fig. 9.5 The fentanyl transdermal system. Fentanyl patches are available in four sizes: 25, 50, 75, and 100. The amount of fentanyl delivered is proportional to the patch size; i.e. a '25' patch delivers 25 µg of fentanyl per hour. After application of the first patch, plasma levels rise for 24 h, analgesic levels are reached by 6–12 h, and a steady state is reached by the time of application of the second patch. The patch should be replaced every 3 days. On removal, a depot remains in the skin for 24 h, falling by 50% by 17 h.

patients. For this reason the indications, practicalities and difficulties in their use will be discussed in some detail.

The use of transdermal fentanyl may be considered for patients with opioid-responsive pain that is *stable* as an alternative to morphine (i.e. as a second-line opioid for moderate to severe pain). It is most appropriate in the following situations.

1   Where the patient is: unable to tolerate morphine (i.e. a patient who has intolerable side-effects, including constipation); unable to take oral medication (e.g. dysphagia); is requesting an alternative method of drug delivery, *or*

2   Where pain control might be improved by enhanced compliance.

The results of a trial of titration to pain control with fentanyl patches are awaited.

Transdermal fentanyl is *not suitable* for acute pain, where rapid dose titration is required, nor is it suitable for patients whose total daily requirement of opioid is equivalent to <30 mg/24 h of oral morphine. In addition those patients taking 30–60 mg/24 h of oral morphine or its equivalent may find the lowest-dose fentanyl patch too potent, leading to drowsiness.

Another group of patients in whom fentanyl should be avoided are those that are pyrexial, as the rate of absorption may be increased.

STARTING TRANSDERMAL FENTANYL

Convert from the oral morphine dose according to Table 9.2. Patients converting from immediate-release morphine will require continued regular morphine until peak plasma levels of fentanyl are reached, i.e. for the first 12–24 h. Patients converting from twice-daily controlled-release morphine should apply the patch at the same time as taking the final 12-hourly tablet. Patients converting from once-daily controlled-release morphine should apply the first patch 12 h after the final 24-hour capsule.

An immediate-release opioid preparation should always be available for breakthrough pain in the correct dose (see Table 9.2). The patient should be warned that they may experience more breakthrough pain than usual in the first 1–3 days. Laxatives should be reduced by up to 50% and then titrated to need.

The dose of the fentanyl patch should not be changed within the first 2 days of the first application or of any change in dose. Adequate analgesia can be achieved using rescue medication as needed. If needed, the dose should be titrated up in 25 µg/h steps.

PRACTICALITIES WHEN USING FENTANYL PATCHES

Fentanyl patches should be replaced at the same time every 3 days, although the site of application should be varied with each patch change. Each patch is designed to give 72 h of analgesia. In a few patients analgesia decreases on the third day and patches need to be changed every 48 h. The patches should be stuck to a flat, clean, dry area of hairless skin, usually on the trunk or back or on the upper outer arm. Men may need to cut, not shave, body hair, but the skin integrity must be preserved. The patches *should not* be cut.

Table 9.2 The relationship between oral morphine dose, s.c. diamorphine, and transdermal fentanyl patch size.

4-hourly oral morphine (mg)	24-hourly oral morphine (mg)	Fentanyl patch size (µg/h)	24-hourly s.c. diamorphine (mg)
5–20	30–130	25	10–40
25–35	140–220	50	50–70
40–50	230–310	75	80–100
55–65	320–400	100	110–130

Patients are able to shower with the patches in place, but hot baths and directly applied heat will rapidly increase absorption. Used patches should be folded sticky side together, and disposed of safely or best returned to a pharmacist.

In 10% of patients a physical and/or depressive opioid withdrawal syndrome occurs on changing from morphine to transdermal fentanyl. This is short lived (usually a few days) and easily treated by the use of immediate-release morphine when symptoms occur.

DISCONTINUING TRANSDERMAL FENTANYL

Transdermal fentanyl may need to be discontinued because a patient has rapidly changing pain or because of side-effects. A subcutaneous depot of drug remains for up to 24 h after the patch has been removed and therefore care is required in converting to other analgesics.

Different strategies are adopted depending on whether or not a patient's pain is under control.

Discontinuation in a patient whose pain is controlled

When discontinuing fentanyl patches in a patient whose pain is controlled, two options can be considered.

1 Changing to 12-hourly controlled-release morphine:
   calculate the dose of morphine required from Table 9.2 above;
   remove patches 6–8 h before the first controlled-release morphine dose;
   ensure an adequate dose of immediate-release oral morphine is available for breakthrough pain.
2 Changing to subcutaneous diamorphine infusion:
   calculate the equivalent dose of diamorphine required from Table 9.2 above;
   set up the syringe driver about 8 h after removing the fentanyl patches;
   ensure an adequate dose of immediate-release oral morphine or parenteral diamorphine is available for breakthrough pain.

Discontinuation in a patient whose pain is not controlled

In a patient whose pain is not controlled, the steps of fentanyl discontinuation are to:
• calculate the equivalent dose of diamorphine required from Table 9.2 above;
• increase this dose by 30%;

- administer a 4-hourly equivalent dose of diamorphine immediately;
- set up the syringe driver 8 h after removing the fentanyl patch.

It is vital to review the patient regularly during this changeover period.

Other opioids for moderate to severe pain

DEXTROMORAMIDE

Dextromoramide is twice as potent as morphine by mouth. It produces rapid analgesia when given sublingually, but this is of a shorter duration than morphine and therefore this drug has no role in chronic pain. However, it can be useful to cover painful procedures such as dressing changes.

HYDROMORPHONE

Hydromorphone is pharmacologically similar to morphine, but is five to six times more potent. It is available for oral (both immediate- and controlled-release preparations), rectal, and parenteral use in the USA and Ireland; and for normal and controlled-release oral use in the UK and many other European countries. The concentrated injection is useful where high-dose opioids need to be given to cachectic patients. Like other strong opioids, in some patients it may have a preferential side-effect profile when compared with morphine.

METHADONE

Methadone is well absorbed by mouth. Its average half-life is 24 h, although this may vary between 10 and 75 h in different individuals. Methadone should be used with extreme caution, particularly in the elderly, because its long half-life means that accumulation may occur. Patients may require up to six doses per day initially, but the dosing interval will subsequently be more prolonged so that one or two doses per day may be sufficient for maintenance.

Methadone may be useful in some patients who do not respond to or are intolerant of morphine (i.e. as a second line opioid). Specialist advice should usually be sought because of its complex pharmacokinetics and its use in patients with complicated pain.

OXYCODONE

Oxycodone can be given orally, by injection, or rectally. Only the latter preparation is currently available in the UK although other preparations may soon be introduced. Oxycodone pectinate suppositories may be used as an alternative to morphine suppositories because of their longer duration of action (6–8 h). In the USA oxycodone is available in combination with paracetamol and has proved a very useful drug for both cancer and non-malignant chronic pain.

BUPRENORPHINE

Buprenorphine binds to opioid receptors but has a lower intrinsic analgesic activity than morphine. It may therefore displace morphine from receptor sites if they are used together, and thus decrease analgesia. Buprenorphine is taken sublingually as 200 µg tablets 6–8-hourly. The maximum recommended dose is 1600 µg per day; dose escalation is limited by the number of tablets patients can dissolve sublingually. Vomiting is more of a problem than with morphine.

PHENAZOCINE

Phenazocine may be a useful alternative when patients are unable to tolerate morphine. A 5 mg tablet is equivalent to 25 mg of morphine. Whilst the tablet can be halved, this dose may be too high for some patients.

TRAMADOL

Tramadol has been available in Europe for many years and was introduced in the UK in 1995. It is one-tenth as potent as morphine given parenterally, and may have an analgesic effect unrelated to stimulation of mu opioid receptors. Tramadol is used for mild to moderate pain. It is available by mouth (immediate-release and controlled-release) and by injection. The oral dose is 200–400 mg daily and the maximum 24-hour dose by injection is 600 mg.

Tramadol has the usual opioid side-effects, although constipation appears less marked. It may precipitate convulsions in epileptic patients.

PETHIDINE

Pethidine is unsuitable for use in chronic pain. It is one-eighth as potent as morphine, given parenterally. Pethidine's non-analgesic metabolite, norpethidine, has a much longer half-life and therefore accumulates with repeated use. Norpethidine produces central nervous system effects which can lead to mood change, myoclonus, and fitting. Oral pethidine is one-quarter as potent as parenteral pethidine, so it leads to four times as much toxic metabolite for the same analgesic effect.

Fears about morphine and other opioids

Both professionals and patients have fears about the use of strong opioids, particularly morphine (see Box 9.7). These fears are largely unfounded and with careful, knowledgeable use there are few problems. However, since these fears are common and may lead to poor pain management, the professional will need to discuss these issues with the patient when commencing strong opioids.

ADDICTION

Addiction does not occur when opioids are used for the management of pain. If the cause of the pain is removed (e.g. by a nerve block or radiotherapy) then opioids can generally be reduced or withdrawn with no psychological problems. Occasionally there is a degree of *physical* dependence, with a physical withdrawal syndrome apparent upon withdrawal of the drug. However, with withdrawal of opioid in staged decrements this is easily managed.

RESPIRATORY DEPRESSION

Respiratory depression is unusual but may occur in opioid-naive patients given a large dose of an opioid for acute pain, or due to a drug error or accumulation of morphine metabolites in renal failure. In chronic use, tolerance to the respiratory depressant effects occurs rapidly and provided the dose is titrated against the patient's pain, morphine can be used safely, even in patients with chronic lung disease.

Box 9.7 Fears about opioid use

Professional's fears:	Patient's fears:
Addiction	Addiction
Respiratory depression	Side-effects
Excess sedation	Impending death
Confusion	Tolerance
	Decreased options for future pain relief

Sedation is common when commencing morphine and after the dose has been increased. It usually wears off after 2–3 days at the same dose, and patients on stable doses of morphine can be allowed to drive. Hallucinations, confusion, and vivid dreams may necessitate a dose reduction or a change to an alternative opioid; alternatively they can be managed with a small dose of haloperidol (1.5–3 mg) at night.

Other side-effects of morphine and other opioids

Side-effects should be discussed with patients before they decide to commence opioids. The majority of patients experience initial sedation on starting opioids or for 2–3 days after increasing the dose. All opioids can cause nausea (30–60% of patients), vomiting (10% of patients), and constipation (95% of patients). All patients commenced on opioids should be prescribed softening and stimulant laxatives and have access to an antiemetic (see Chapter 10).

Other well-recognized side-effects are dry mouth, itching, sweating, myoclonic jerks, and occasionally hypotension.

TOLERANCE

'If I take it now, it won't work later, when I really need it.' This fear is unfounded. An increase in analgesic requirement is usually due to an increase in pain due to advancing disease rather than to tolerance. Increasing experience of the use of opioids in both cancer and non-cancer-related pain confirms that tolerance is rare. There is much topical debate about tolerance and its apparent mechanisms, and specialist advice should be sought about a patient who appears to have tolerance to the effects of opioids.

Non-steroidal anti-inflammatory drugs (NSAIDs)

The NSAIDs are a group of chemically unrelated drugs which have analgesic, anti-inflammatory, and antipyretic properties through inhibition of the enzyme cyclo-oxygenase (Cox), involved in prostaglandin synthesis (Table 9.3).

There are two forms of Cox. Cox-1 is involved in normal prostaglandin synthesis, including the protective effect of prostaglandins in the gastrointestinal tract. Cox-2 is found in normal tissues only in the presence of

Table 9.3 Types and recommended doses of NSAIDs.

NSAID	Recommended dose			
	Oral i.r.	Oral m.r.	Rectal	Parenteral
Salicylates				
Aspirin	600 mg q.d.s.	–	600 mg q.d.s.	–
Diflunisal	500 mg t.d.s.	–	–	–
Acetates				
Diclofenac	50 mg t.d.s.	75–100 mg b.d.	50 mg t.d.s.	75 mg b.d.
Indomethacin	50 mg t.d.s.	75 mg b.d.	100 mg b.d.	–
Sulindac	200 mg b.d.	–	–	–
Propionates				
Flurbiprofen	50 mg t.d.s./q.d.s.		200 mg o.d.	100 mg b.d.
Ibuprofen	600 mg t.d.s.	–	–	–
Naproxen	500 mg b.d.	–	500 mg b.d.	–
Ketorolac	10 mg q.d.s.	–	–	30–90 mg s.c.
Fenamates				
Mefenamic acid	500 mg t.d.s.	–	–	–
Oxicams				
Piroxicam	10–30 mg o.d.	–	–	–
Pyrazolanes				
Phenylbutazone	Ankylosing spondylitis only			
Butazones				
Nabumetone	1 g nocte	–	–	–

Key: i.r. = immediate-release preparation; m.r. = modified-release preparation.

inflammation. The anti-inflammatory and analgesic effects of NSAIDs are related to inhibition of Cox-2. NSAIDs that are relatively Cox-2-specific, such as nabumetone, naproxen and diclofenac, do have fewer gastrointestinal side-effects. Selective Cox-2 inhibitors are under clinical trial.

The role of NSAIDs

NSAIDs are analgesic in their own right and can be used in conjunction with analgesics from all three steps of the WHO analgesic ladder. If one NSAID is ineffective or produces side-effects, another NSAID from a different chemical class is worth trying.

They are used in the following situations:

- for pain due to bony metastases, which may respond poorly to opioids;
- where pain has an inflammatory aetiology, e.g. pleuritic chest pain;
- for musculoskeletal pain, rheumatoid arthritis, and osteoarthritis;
- for the pain of soft-tissue injuries and fractures and for dysmenorrhoea, dental pain, and headache.

Side-effects of NSAIDs

NSAID prescriptions are numerous and it is estimated that there are 3000 NSAID-related deaths in the UK each year. NSAIDs and aspirin will precipitate symptomatic bronchospasm in 5% of asthmatic patients, and a few individuals develop allergic reactions such as anaphylaxis, rashes, and urticaria.

GASTROINTESTINAL EFFECTS

Up to 20% of people given any particular NSAID will develop dyspepsia, nausea, or vomiting, and some will develop peptic ulceration, haemorrhage, or perforation. Various steps can be taken to avoid or reduce these side-effects. For example, the prostaglandin E_1 analogue, misoprostol, prevents and heals NSAID-associated ulcers ($200 \mu g$ two to four times daily). The H_2 receptor antagonists prevent duodenal, but not gastric, ulcers on NSAIDs, and may help ulcer healing.

Patients at high risk of ulceration are those with a history of dyspepsia or ulceration, and particularly those taking both NSAIDs and steroids. Patients with advanced disease, whatever the aetiology, are likely to be at increased risk of peptic ulceration.

RENAL EFFECTS

NSAIDs increase sodium and water retention and can lead to oedema and even congestive cardiac failure. NSAID-mediated reduction of renal prostaglandins may lead to acute renal failure, particularly in the elderly, those on diuretics and antihypertensives, and those with impaired renal function. Renal function should be monitored in those at risk. Sulindac is relatively safe with impaired renal function.

HAEMATOLOGICAL EFFECTS

Aspirin and the NSAIDs inhibit platelet aggregation. This is clinically significant only if patients are also taking anticoagulants. Patients on anticoagulants who require an NSAID should be started on misoprostol and a low dose of an NSAID with relatively fewer gastrointestinal side-effects.

Parenteral NSAIDs

Diclofenac and other NSAIDs are available for deep intramuscular injection. Due to injection site problems the subcutaneous route should generally not be used.

Ketorolac may be delivered by the subcutaneous route when diluted with water, but has a high risk of gastrointestinal side-effects. A loading dose of 30 mg can be given intravenously or intramuscularly prior to commencing a subcutaneous infusion. The patient should be commenced on 30 mg over 24 h, increasing to 60 mg and 90 mg if necessary. If pain does not respond within 48 h the infusion should be stopped.

Adjuvant analgesic drugs

Adjuvant analgesics are drugs which are not analgesic in their own right and are primarily used for other indications, but can produce analgesia in certain situations. They have also been called co-analgesics. They can be used in combination with drugs from all steps of the analgesic ladder, and are particularly useful for neuropathic pain which has not responded sufficiently to opioids.

Antidepressants as adjuvant analgesics

The tricyclic antidepressants (TCAs) are useful for pains with constant, aching, burning, or paraesthetic qualities, although they also have a role in lancinating neuropathic pain. Amitriptyline has an established role but other TCAs such as dothiepin, imipramine, and clomipramine are also useful.

Usage

Amitriptyline 10 mg (or dothiepin 25 mg) is commenced at night. The dose should be increased by up to 25 mg weekly, as side-effects allow, to a dose of 150 mg, or until the pain is improved. If there is no improvement after 2–3 weeks at 150 mg, or side-effects are intolerable, then the drug should be stopped.

If sedation is troublesome and the patient wishes to pursue a trial of antidepressants, a less sedative drug (imipramine or lofepramine) can be substituted. Dry mouth, blurred vision, constipation, urinary retention and postural hypotension and confusion may limit dose escalation.

HOW DO ANTIDEPRESSANTS IMPROVE PAIN?

Antidepressants do not produce pain relief by reversing coexisting depression since pain relief occurs at lower doses and more rapidly than the anti-depressant effect. In some patients, improved sleep or lightened mood improves the ability to cope with pain, but this is not the primary effect in most patients. Many of the neurotransmitters involved in nociception are affected by TCAs, particularly the presynaptic reuptake of serotonin and noradrenaline. The selective serotonin reuptake inhibitor (SSRI) antidepressants are not as effective as analgesics as the TCAs. TCAs may also improve analgesia by increasing plasma morphine levels.

Anticonvulsants as adjuvant analgesics

Anticonvulsants such as carbamazepine, sodium valproate, and clonazepam are used for neuropathic pain, particularly of a lancinating or shooting nature, for example trigeminal neuralgia, postherpetic neuralgia, and the paroxysmal pain associated with multiple sclerosis and spinal cord trauma.

In patients with end-stage disease, the choice of drug used will be dictated by likely side-effects. In some patients, full anticonvulsant doses may be required to relieve pain. Frail patients are often unable to tolerate therapeutic doses of carbamazepine. Sodium valproate can be used as an alternative. A starting dose of 200 mg twice a day (100 mg b.d. carbamazepine) can be increased by 200 mg every 2–3 days up to a maximum of 400 mg four times daily (400 mg t.d.s. carbamazepine), or until side-effects such as tremor and sedation develop.

The benzodiazepine, clonazepam, can be commenced at a dose of 0.5 mg at night. This can be increased up to 8 mg per day in divided doses; however, doses above 2 mg are rarely necessary or tolerated. It may be delivered by subcutaneous infusion or injection.

Other membrane-stabilizing drugs as adjuvant analgesics

In some patients' neuropathic pain responds to intravenous lignocaine and pain relief can be maintained by the use of oral agents such as mexiletine. Oral anti-arrhythmic agents can be introduced without an initial trial of intravenous lignocaine and both mexiletine and flecainide have produced responses in neuropathic pain. Patients must be aware of the cardiac risks of flecainide and must have stopped tricyclic antidepressants. Usually such drugs are initiated with specialist advice.

Corticosteroids as adjuvant analgesics

Steroids can decrease oedema associated with inflammatory conditions and tumour growth. They may be beneficial for a patient whose pain is caused by tumour exerting pressure on structures sensitive to pain, for example cerebral metastases, or liver metastases causing liver capsule pain. They are also useful for neuropathic pain due to nerve compression by a tumour mass, for example sacral root compression from a pelvic mass causing sciatic pain. Steroids may also act as analgesics by decreasing local prostaglandins involved in inflammation and nociception.

Usage

Dexamethasone 6–16 mg daily is given, depending on the urgency of the problem. If the patient responds the dose should be reduced by 25% after 5–7 days and then by a further 2 mg every 3–5 days to a maintenance dose of 2–4 mg or to the dose below which symptoms recur.

Side-effects

Steroids have mineralocorticoid, glucocorticoid, and anti-inflammatory effects. Mineralocorticoid effects may lead to sodium and water retention, potassium loss, and hypertension. These effects are fewer with dexamethasone than with prednisolone. Glucocorticoid effects may lead to diabetes and osteoporosis.

Other side-effects of steroids are appetite stimulation, mental disturbance (euphoria, depression, or occasionally steroid psychosis), muscle wasting (less marked with prednisolone) and peptic ulceration.

Skeletal muscle relaxants

Pain due to spasticity can be treated with benzodiazepines or other muscle relaxants such as baclofen and dantrolene sodium. Sedation is the dose-limiting factor; initial doses should be low, increasing slowly to symptom relief or side-effects.

Antispasmodics

In patients with colic, for instance with intestinal obstruction, pain can be relieved by drugs which relax smooth muscle spasm. Hyoscine butylbromide is poorly absorbed orally; it can be given as a 20 mg i.m. or s.c. injection, or added to a s.c. infusion via a syringe driver at a dose of 60–120 mg per day. It causes less sedation than hyoscine hydrobromide, but similarly dries secretions.

Other adjuvant drugs

Other drugs which are used in the specialist setting for difficult pain include:
- bisphosphonates, given orally and intravenously for bone pain;
- the NMDA receptor antagonist ketamine, used subcutaneously for pain which responds poorly to opioids;
- the alpha$_2$ adrenergic agonist, clonidine, which has been used in the treatment of neuropathic pain, given orally, transdermally, or spinally.

Nerve blocks

In a patient with pain that is not responding to drug treatment, which is localized or appears to be within the distribution of a single nerve root, referral for consideration of a nerve block may be indicated. Nerve blocks are usually carried out initially with local anaesthetic to assess response. Injection of local anaesthetic plus steroid may then provide pain relief for some weeks. Neuroablation using phenol, cryotherapy, or radiofrequency lesions is indicated when pain improves initially but recurs.

Nerve blocks commonly used include:
- intercostal nerve blocks for chest wall pain (rib metastases or pleural infiltration);
- lumbar/caudal epidural for low back or sacral root pain;
- coeliac plexus block for the pain of carcinoma of the pancreas, liver metastases, or chronic pancreatitis;
- brachial plexus block for pain, particularly with axillary recurrence of

breast cancer. It may be necessary to infuse local anaesthetic via a fine catheter;
• dorsal root ganglion blocks may help local or radicular back pain, particularly the acute, severe pain of an osteoporotic crush fracture;
• patients with advanced disease may have coexisting osteoarthritis, and facet joint injections and injections into painful sacroiliac joints or shoulders may provide relief;
• lumbar sympathectomy for tenesmus and pelvic visceral pain;
• cordotomy is occasionally useful for unilateral body pain.

Spinal analgesia

Spinal analgesia encompasses the epidural and intrathecal delivery of drugs for pain relief. Spinal catheters are usually sited by pain clinic anaesthetists.

Various factors influence the suitability of a particular patient for spinal analgesia. Firstly, the likely candidate will have pain that is not controlled by escalating doses of opioids, or will have intolerable side-effects from opioids. Secondly, other possible measures to produce pain relief, for example surgery and radiotherapy, will have been explored. Thirdly, the patient's major sites of pain will generally be in the lower half of the body.

If the patient can be at home, facilities must be available in the community setting for care of the spinal catheter and for replenishing the syringe driver or pump. Specialist advice must be available for problems outside normal working hours.

Suitable drugs

Opioids, local anaesthetics, and other adjuvant drugs for neuropathic pain can be given spinally. The choice of epidural or intrathecal route depends usually on operator preference.

Opioids can be given spinally, usually as diamorphine (100 mg diamorphine s.c. = 10 mg epidurally = 1 mg intrathecally). Patients should have immediate-release oral opioids available for breakthrough pain or an 'on demand' spinal route delivery system (i.e. patient-controlled analgesia). Other opioids, apart from rescue medication, should be stopped.

The local anaesthetic bupivacaine can be given spinally for neuropathic pain. Concentrations of 0.125% and 0.25% usually produce pain relief. Concentrations of 0.375% and 0.5% often produce sensory change and then motor block. If the dermatomal spread of pain relief is inadequate then the rate of infusion is increased. Intrathecal infusions run at 0.5–

2 ml/h, the epidural range generally is 2–6 ml/h. Patients should be monitored for side-effects after a dose change or an increase in the rate of the infusion. Side-effects are sedation, respiratory depression, hypotension, sensory loss, weakness, and itch. Spinal analgesia may mask spinal cord compression.

Clonidine, ketamine, and fentanyl have also been used as spinal analgesics.

Transcutaneous electrical nerve stimulation (TENS)

TENS was originally used to select patients who were suitable for implantation of dorsal column stimulators for pain relief. It has since been used widely to relieve pain in its own right.

Electrical stimulation is achieved by attaching a TENS machine to electrodes on the skin. For conventional TENS, the waveform of the stimulator is set so as to stimulate large myelinated afferent (A-beta) fibres. This reduces the input from nociceptors via C fibres to the spinal cord and brain (gate control of pain). For acupuncture-like TENS, high-intensity, low-frequency stimulation produces muscle twitching. The A-delta fibres so stimulated induce pain relief by releasing endogenous opioids in the spinal cord (see Fig. 9.2).

In patients with chronic pain 70% respond to TENS initially. However, only 30% still find TENS effective after 1 year. Electrodes may be placed over the painful site, but greater pain relief is usually gained by stimulating over the nerve proximal to the area. Successful use of TENS requires a thorough explanation of the principles of TENS and a patient's willingness to experiment with pad positions and stimulation waveforms and intensities.

Other approaches to pain relief

Some patients may seek the techniques of complementary medicine to control their pain. The use of acupuncture is discussed in Chapter 21. It has well-documented analgesic effects. In most patients, but especially in those that are anxious, relaxation techniques may improve pain. Patients may be helped by visualizing their pain decreasing. Hypnotherapy can also be a powerful analgesic tool. Some patients find that aromatherapy massage decreases pain by relieving muscle spasm and producing relaxation. Homeopathic remedies may also be helpful.

Severe pain as an emergency

Usually this arises in an acute on chronic pattern: there is usually a warning as pain builds up over days and also an understanding of the underlying aetiology of the pain.

Acute, unanticipated pain may be due to:

- fracture;
- haemorrhage (e.g. haemorrhage into liver tumours);
- infarction or thrombosis;
- perforation of a viscus;
- nerve compression or inflammation;
- obstruction with colic.

Assessment of the likely cause of the pain is essential in management. Severe pain is an emergency which requires constant attention until the pain is controlled. Specialist referral and in-patient admission are often needed to provide sufficient observation and intervention for the patient.

Immediate management

The immediate management of severe pain is strong opioid analgesia, usually given parenterally for fast effect: for example, diamorphine i.m. s.c. equivalent to the 4-hourly dose or 10 mg in an opioid-naive patient. This is repeated after 30 minutes if the effect is insufficient. There may be added benefit from sedation with diazepam (5–20 mg p.r. or titrated i.v.) or midazolam (2.5–10 mg s.c. or titrated i.v.).

Ketamine 20–100 mg (0.5–2 mg/kg) i.v. or i.m. may be useful as a rapidly acting (minutes), analgesic and sedative, especially in severe nerve-related pain (e.g. haemorrhage into the spinal canal). It may require coadministration of midazolam or other benzodiazepine to avoid dysphoric side-effects. It is available in the community only on a named patient basis.

Simple nerve blocks with lignocaine 2% or bupivacaine 0.5% may be useful for fracture-related pain: a femoral nerve block can be used for a fractured femur, and an intercostal nerve block for a fractured rib.

Nitrous oxide (carried in ambulances) may have some role in fracture- or movement-related pain. Hysocine butylbromide 20–40 mg s.c. or i.m. may be useful for colic.

Conclusion

In patients with advanced disease, successful management of pain requires evaluation to assess the likely cause of the pain and the impact that pain is having on the patient's physical and emotional life. A thorough knowledge of a small number of drugs and a simple stepwise approach to their use will improve pain in the majority of patients. Continued reassessment and re-evaluation will allow a treatment regimen to be modified according to side-effects or changing circumstances. A minority of patients will have more difficult pain. Adjuvant drugs can then be introduced according to the probable cause of the pain. In patients whose pain persists despite these measures, referral for specialist advice is indicated.

References

1 Bonica JJ. Cancer pain: current status and future needs. In: Bonica JJ, ed. *The Management of Pain*, 2nd edn. Philadelphia: Lea & Febiger, 1990: 400–445.
2 Seale C. Death from cancer and death from other causes: the relevance of the hospice approach. *Palliat Med* 1991; 5: 12–19.
3 McCarthy M, Lay M, Addington-Hall J. Dying from heart disease. *J Roy Coll Phys* 1996; 30: 325–328.
4 Larue F, Collequ SM, Brasser L, Cleeland CS. Multicentre study of cancer pain and its treatment in France. *BMJ* 1995; 310: 1034–1037.
5 Cleeland CS, Gonin R, Hatfield AK, *et al*. Pain and its treatment in outpatients with metastatic cancer. *New Engl J Med* 1994; 330: 592–596.
6 Addington-Hall J, McCarthy M. Dying from cancer: results of a national population-based investigation. *Palliat Med* 1995; 9: 295–305.
7 Saunders CM. *The Management of Terminal Illness*. London: Hospital Medicine Publications, 1967.
8 International Association for the Study of Pain Subcommittee on Taxonomy. Classification of chronic pain. *Pain* 1986; Suppl. 3: 216–221.
9 Glynn C. An approach to the management of the patient with deafferentation pain. *Palliat Med* 1989; 3: 13–21.
10 Melzack R. The McGill Pain Questionnaire. In: Melzack R, ed. *Pain Measurement and Assessment*. New York: Raven Press, 1983: 41–48.
11 World Health Organization. *Cancer Pain Relief*. Geneva: WHO, 1986.
12 World Health Organization. *Cancer Pain Relief*. Geneva: WHO, 1996.
13 Hanks GW, de Conno F, Ripamonti C *et al*. Morphine in cancer pain: modes of administration. *BMJ* 1996; 312: 823–826.

Further reading

Doyle D, Hanks GW, MacDonald N (eds). *Oxford Textbook of Palliative Medicine*, 2nd edn. Oxford: Oxford University Press, 1997.
McGrath PA. *Pain in Children: Nature, Assessment and Treatment*. New York: The Guildford Press, 1990.
Twycross RG. *Pain Relief in Advanced Cancer*. Edinburgh: Churchill Livingstone, 1994.

10: The Management of Gastrointestinal Symptoms

MARIE FALLON AND JOHN WELSH

Introduction

Symptoms related to the gastrointestinal tract are such a common problem for patients with advanced disease that questions regarding dry and sore mouth, appetite, nausea, and constipation should always be considered. Many patients who suffer unrelenting nausea find this more disabling than pain, and adequate management requires a logical, systematic, and persistent approach. Constipation can cause considerable distress, which can be prevented for most patients, but this is often neglected. Most of the authors' understanding and experience is gained from patients with cancer but the principles outlined are mostly equally applicable to patients with non-malignant disease.

It should be remembered that the gastrointestinal tract represents the physical and psychological focus of continued health, and all symptoms relating to dysfunction carry enormous significance for the patient and carers. The importance of this in caring for patients should never be underestimated.

Nausea and vomiting

Nausea and vomiting are very unpleasant symptoms, often described by patients as 'worse than pain'. They can be a major cause of poor quality of life in patients with both malignant and non-malignant diseases. Nausea and/or vomiting occurs in 40–70% of patients with advanced cancer [1,2].

Management involves a very careful assessment of the patient, in particular the identification of possible aetiologies and the recognition of syndromes. It is vital to have knowledge of the emetogenic pathways and understanding of the mechanism of action of antiemetic drugs (Fig. 10.1).

The route of administration of antiemetic and other drugs should be carefully considered. Many patients will not absorb oral medication well because of vomiting or gastric stasis. Rectal or parenteral administration

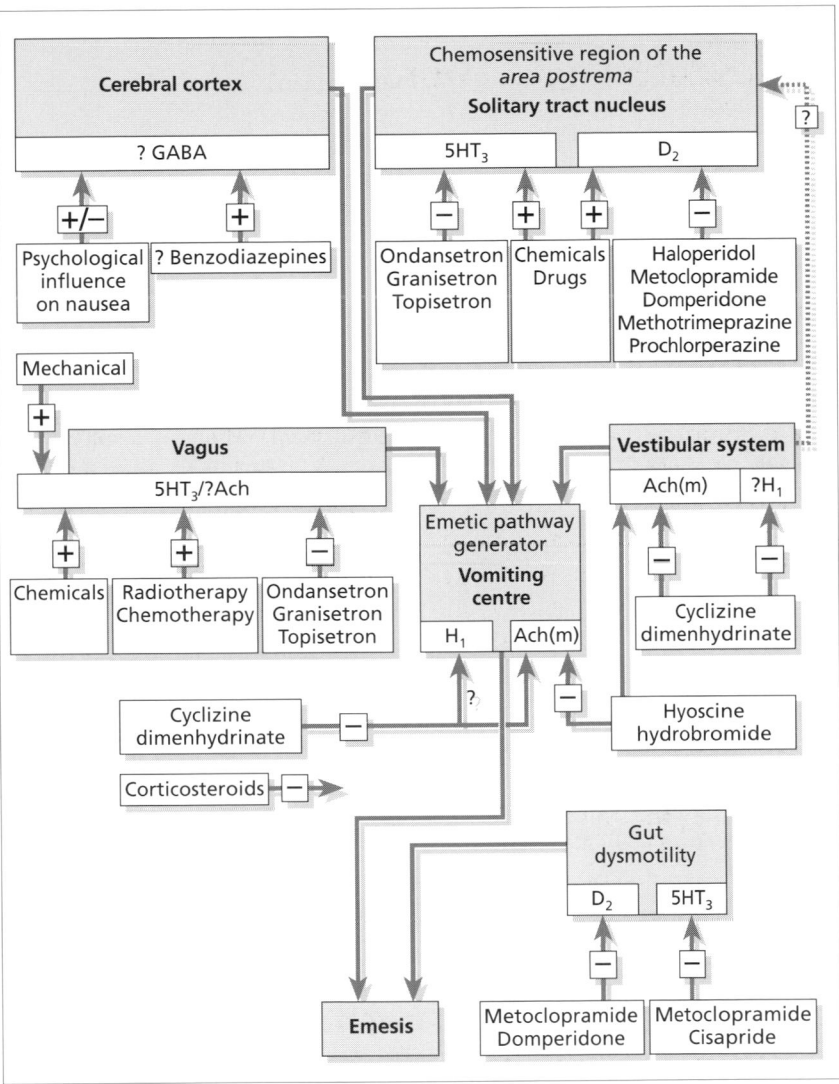

Fig. 10.1 A schema of the pathways of emesis (nausea and vomiting), important neurotransmitters, and site of antiemetics. Receptor types—GABA: gamma-amino-butyric acid, H: histamine, D: dopamine, Ach(m): acetylcholine muscarinic, 5HT: serotonin (5-hydroxytryptophan). Subscript denotes receptor subtype: + denotes agonist or enhancing stimulus; – denotes antagonist or blocking stimulus.

may be required until plasma drug levels control symptoms well enough to allow oral administration. The subcutaneous (s.c.) route is the preferred parenteral route in most situations.

Treatment can be appropriately tailored for the individual, and control of symptoms using one antiemetic is possible in 60% of patients. However, about one-third of patients require concurrent administration of a second antiemetic. These may be patients who have emesis of more than one origin. In these patients antiemetics of different mechanisms of action should be combined (e.g. cyclizine and haloperidol). This is discussed further below under 'Persistent vomiting' (see p. 141).

Non-pharmacological interventions for nausea and vomiting

Acupuncture and ginger are two commonly used complementary techniques (see Chapter 21). Other approaches such as relaxation therapy and hypnotherapy are invaluable for patients with a high degree of anxiety or to combat the anticipatory nausea induced by chemotherapy treatments.

Common syndromes of nausea and vomiting

GASTRIC STASIS AND GASTRIC OUTFLOW OBSTRUCTION

Causes

The causes of gastric stasis and gastric outflow obstruction generally fall into the following categories.
- Drugs (anticholinergic effect):
  hyoscine and other anticholinergics;
  opioids;
  amitriptyline and other tricyclic antidepressants;
  cyclizine;
  broad-spectrum neuroleptic agents (e.g. chlorpromazine).
- Autonomic failure:
  nerve infiltration;
  paraneoplastic (rare);
  diabetes.
- Ascites.
- Hepatomegaly.
- Tumour infiltration of gastric mucosa.
- Tumour infiltration or compression of gastric outlet or upper small bowel.
- Peptic ulcer.

- Gastritis:
  stress;
  drugs (e.g. NSAIDs);
  radiotherapy.

Clinical features

Stasis and outflow obstruction may give rise to a range of clinical features. The patient often complains of epigastric discomfort that is exacerbated by eating and relieved by vomiting. In other cases there may simply be epigastric fullness and early satiety. Nausea is of varying intensity and often relieved by vomiting. The vomitus can be of considerable volume and may contain undigested food. Vomiting may be provoked by movement of the torso. Further common symptoms include flatulence, hiccup, and acid reflux and regurgitation of stomach contents. A succussion splash may be present. Other features of autonomic failure may be present.

Management

Various management strategies should be considered in order to ease symptoms and make life more tolerable for the patient. A useful maxim is 'reverse the reversible'; for example, perform paracentesis to control the build-up of ascites. The prokinetic agents of choice are:

metoclopramide 10–20 mg t.d.s. p.o. or 40–80 mg s.c./24 h; *or*
cisapride 20 mg b.d. p.o.

The acidity and volume of gastric secretions is reduced by using: H_2 antagonists or a proton pump inhibitor. Rarely, octreotide may be beneficial (see 'Obstruction', p. 143). Flatulence can be relieved with dimethicone. Steroids may occasionally improve the dysfunction induced by tumour infiltration of nerve plexuses (e.g. dexamethasone s.c./i.m./i.v. 8–16 mg/24 h).

If prokinetic agents are unsuccessful, blockade of Achm receptors by hyoscine butylbromide (or cyclizine) may be necessary to reduce vagal-stimulated gastric and small bowel secretions (see section below on obstruction, p. 143. Both drugs will, however, worsen gastric stasis.

A nasogastric tube may help to relieve symptoms and is appropriate for some patients with obstruction or profound gastroparesis. Many patients decline a nasogastric tube and tolerate intermittent vomiting if nausea is controlled. A venting gastrostomy or palliative surgical bypass is occasionally helpful [3].

CHEMICALLY INDUCED NAUSEA

Causes

The causes of chemically induced nausea generally fall into three categories.
- Drugs (see Box 10.1)
- Metabolic:
  renal failure;
  liver failure;
  hypercalcaemia;
  hyponatraemia;
  ketoacidosis.
- Toxins:
  ischaemic bowel or traumatized bowel, e.g.
  gastrointestinal (GI) obstruction;
  food poisoning;
  possible tumour effects;
  secondary to infection.

Clinical features

The nausea is usually constant, but the vomiting is variable in volume and timing. With drug-related nausea there are associated features of the specific drug toxicity. Other features of the underlying disease may be apparent.

Management

Again, the first objective is to reverse the reversible; for example, it may be possible to stop or decrease any drug-related aetiology by altering

---

Box 10.1 Drugs which commonly cause nausea

- Antibiotics
- Opioids
- Anticonvulsants
- Digoxin
- Selective serotonin reuptake inhibitor
- Digoxin
- Theophylline
- Non-steroidal anti-inflammatory drugs

the medication. Various antidopaminergic agents may be employed; these include:

- haloperidol 1.5–5 mg o.d. p.o./s.c.;
- domperidone 10–20 mg t.d.s p.o. or 30 mg t.d.s p.r.;
- metoclopramide 10–20 mg t.d.s. p.o. or 40–80 mg s.c./24 h;
- methotrimeprazine 6.25–50 mg o.d. p.o./s.c.

$5HT_3$ antagonists are useful for highly emetogenic chemotherapy and perhaps in cases of intractable vomiting of metabolic cause, but their cost-effectiveness in other circumstances is not yet established.

Opioid-induced nausea and vomiting

This side-effect occurs in 10–30% of patients on initiation of treatment. It usually settles within 3–4 days but can reappear with an escalation of dose. An anti-D_2 antiemetic such as haloperidol 1.5–3 mg nocte is helpful. If delayed gastric emptying is also a feature then metoclopramide should be the drug of choice; 10 mg t.d.s. p.o. half an hour before meals.

STRETCH/IRRITATION OF VISCERAL AND GASTROINTESTINAL SEROSA

Causes

Stretch or irritation of the visceral and gastrointestinal serosa can be attributed to a number of causes.

- Liver metastases.
- Ureteric obstruction.
- Retroperitoneal lymph nodes or tumour deposits.
- Constipation.
- Bowel obstruction (see below).

Clinical features

Nausea is usually constant but vomiting is less common (except in bowel obstruction). Pain is frequently an associated feature. Other features may reflect the underlying cause.

Management

All simple steps should be taken to reverse the reversible; for example, constipation is relieved with enemas and stimulant laxatives as needed. Steroids may reduce tumour bulk through reduction of peri-tumour oedema (e.g. dexamethasone 8–16 mg/24 h p.o./s.c./i.m./i.v.). Cyclizine is also beneficial; typical dosage regimens are: 25–50 mg t.d.s. p.o.; or 100–150 mg s.c./24 h; or 50 mg t.d.s. p.r.

RAISED INTRACRANIAL PRESSURE AND MENINGISM

Causes

Raised intracranial pressure and meningism can be attributed to various causes.
- Intracranial tumour.
- Cerebral oedema.
- Intracranial bleeding.
- Meningeal infiltration by tumour.
- Skull metastases.
- Cerebral infection.

Clinical features

Nausea may be worse in the morning, and the vomiting can be projectile in nature. Nausea and/or vomiting provoked by head movement is associated with vestibular pathway aetiology.

There is headache, which may be worse in the morning, although neurological signs may be absent. Various features, including neuropathic pains, dizziness, and ear or throat symptoms, are associated with metastases at the base of the skull.

Management

Take steps to reverse the reversible. For example high-dose steroids may reduce cerebral oedema and/or tumour mass (e.g. dexamethasone 16 mg/day p.o./s.c./i.m./i.v.). Again, cyclizine is beneficial; typical dosage regimens are: 25–50 mg t.d.s. p.o.; or 100–150 mg s.c./24 h; or 50 mg t.d.s. p.r.

If there are signs of vestibular pathway aetiology, administer one of the following: hyoscine hydrobromide 0.8–3.6 mg s.c./24 h; or Kwells, one tablet (hyoscine hydrobromide 300 µg) q.i.d. p.o.; or Transcop patches, one patch (hyoscine hydrobromide, 1.5 mg) per 72 h.

NAUSEA AND VOMITING THAT PERSISTS DESPITE SPECIFIC TARGETING OF EMETIC PATHWAY

Thirty percent of patients require the concurrent use of two antiemetics. These should be selected for different mechanisms of action which are compatible in effects. Haloperidol with cyclizine is a good choice. Cyclizine and hyoscine hydrobromide will counteract the prokinetic (but not the central, direct antiemetic) effect of metoclopramide and domperidone (and cisapride) but will not counteract the central antiemetic effect of metoclopramide.

Low-dose methotrimeprazine, 5–12.5 mg p.o. or s.c. over 24 h, can also be useful. It is a 'broad-spectrum' antiemetic (Achm, D_2 and 5HT antagonist activity) and in low doses does not generally cause troublesome sedation.

Corticosteroids are potent antiemetics although their mechanism of action is not fully understood. Dexamethasone at 2–6 mg o.d. is useful to add to an antiemetic regimen for patients with resistant problems.

Malignant gastrointestinal obstruction

Malignant gastrointestinal obstruction occurs most commonly in patients with advanced abdominal or pelvic cancers: in 25% of patients with a primary bowel cancer; in 6% of patients with a primary ovarian cancer; and in about 40% of advanced ovarian cancer patients.

Where surgery is technically not possible, is inappropriate, or is not acceptable to the patient, medical management of malignant gastrointestinal obstruction can offer good symptom control. Patients may live for surprisingly long periods of time (sometimes months) and be able to take small quantities of food and fluids as desired, usually without the need for a nasogastric tube or parenteral fluids. Most patients can be cared for at home.

Evaluation

Clinical evaluation must consider non-malignant causes of obstruction in cancer patients which may be amenable to surgical or other appropriate intervention. These include:
- adhesions;
- constipation;
- drugs;
- unrelated benign conditions.

Box 10.2 Classical features of complete intestinal obstruction

- Large-volume vomits
- Nausea worse before vomiting
- Nausea relieved by vomiting
- Nil per rectum or per stoma
- Abdominal distension
- Visible peristalsis
- Increased bowel sounds, classically tinkling, but may be absent
- Background abdominal pain
- Colicky abdominal pain

The clinical scenario may only have some of the classic features of complete bowel obstruction outlined in Box 10.2. Malignant obstruction may present acutely but more commonly is gradual in onset, intermittent, and variable in severity. Gross distension is often absent, even in lower bowel obstruction since the bowel may be constricted at several points.

Patients with lower bowel obstruction will often have infrequent, faeculent vomiting, while those with high bowel obstruction may vomit undigested food.

It is always useful to determine whether colic is present or absent since this will affect the management strategy (see below).

Investigations can be helpful and may include a biochemical profile (hypokalaemia may cause ileus, hypercalcaemia may cause pseudo-obstruction due to constipation). A plain abdominal X-ray will demonstrate constipation, but can be misleading when multiple levels of obstruction are present. A CT/MRI scan can be indicated if surgery is to be considered.

Management

Chemotherapy may offer a palliative option for some patients with ovarian carcinoma. Any surgical or oncological intervention should run in parallel with more immediate symptomatic treatment.

SURGICAL INTERVENTION

Surgery should always be considered in malignant gastrointestinal obstruction. However, it will often be inappropriate or technically impossible. Surgical intervention is unlikely to be successful in the following situations:

- radiological or previous surgical evidence indicating that a surgical procedure will not be technically possible;
- a stiff, doughy abdomen with little abdominal distension [4];
- diffuse intra-abdominal carcinomatosis;
- massive ascites which reaccumulates rapidly after paracentesis;
- poor general physical status [5];
- previous radiotherapy to the abdomen or pelvis, in combination with any of the above.

MEDICAL MANAGEMENT OF MALIGNANT GASTROINTESTINAL OBSTRUCTION

A nasogastric tube and intravenous fluids are rarely necessary if the following strategy is used.

Pain

Analgesia for background pain is obtained by using a continuous s.c. infusion of diamorphine (dose: 1/3 total daily morphine dose ± 30–50% increment as dictated by the pain). If opioid naive, start on a diamorphine dose of 10 mg/24 h. Not all patients require opioid analgesia if no background pain is present and colic can be relieved by more appropriate drugs (see below).

Gut motility

If colic is present avoid all drugs which could worsen this (i.e. prokinetic drugs, bulk-forming, osmotic, and stimulant laxatives). If colic persists, add hyoscine butylbromide s.c., starting at 60 mg/24 h (up to 200 mg/24 h as needed).

If colic is absent a trial of metoclopramide s.c. 40–80 mg/24 h, with or without dexamethasone s.c./i.m./i.v. 6–16 mg daily, may allow resolution of partial obstruction or pseudo-obstruction due to dysfunction of the nerve supply to the gut. In the absence of colic, incomplete obstruction in the large bowel may be helped by a stool-softening laxative, such as docusate sodium 200 mg b.d.–q.d.s.

Nausea

The choice of antiemetic depends on whether the patient is experiencing colic. If colic is not a feature, metoclopramide is administered s.c. 40–

80 mg/24 h (see above). If colic is present, give haloperidol (s.c. 5–20 mg/24 h) or cyclizine (s.c. 100–150 mg/24 h). A combination of haloperidol and cyclizine is sometimes necessary.

5HT$_3$ antagonist antiemetics may have a role in relief of the nausea induced by bowel distension and stimulation of the vomiting centre through vagal afferents (see above) but this is unclear.

Vomiting

Reduction in the volume of gastrointestinal (GI) secretions will reduce colic, nausea, pain, and the need to vomit. This can usually be adequately achieved with hyoscine butylbromide (s.c. 60–200 mg/24 h [6]) with or without an H$_2$ antagonist or proton pump inhibitor.

If large-volume vomiting persists despite hyoscine butylbromide, the somatostatin analogue, octreotide, will further decrease the volume of intestinal secretions in the gut lumen [7]. A trial of octreotide, given at a rate of 300 µg/24 h by s.c. infusion, should be performed. The dose can be titrated over 2–3 days to 600 µg/24 h; If there is no benefit at 600 µg/24 h it should be stopped. The dose should be reduced daily by 100 µg/24h to the lowest effective dose (mean dose 300 µg/24 h) [8].

In some cases octreotide is not effective, particularly in high obstructions such as gastric outlet obstruction. It may then be helpful to use a nasogastric tube or consider a venting gastrostomy to allow the patient to continue to drink and eat as desired without the fear of provoking immediate vomiting. Venting gastrostomy can be performed under local anaesthetic.

Studies of the compatibility of many drugs are not available (see Chapter 22). Some patients may require the use of two subcutaneous infusions to ensure efficacy of drug administration. Clinical observation, however, suggests the following are compatible and maintain efficacy:
• diamorphine, haloperidol, and cyclizine;
• diamorphine, haloperidol, and hyoscine butylbromide;
• diamorphine, cyclizine, and hyoscine butylbromide;
• diamorphine and octreotide;
• diamorphine, haloperidol, and octreotide.

Diet and hydration

Sensitive, pre-emptive discussion of the situation is a vital part of care for the patient and family. Many patients with obstruction can eat and drink in modest amounts when symptoms are controlled. A liquid, low-residue diet may be the least problematical.

Hydration should be considered on an individual basis. Oral discomfort and dryness can largely be relieved by frequent, attentive mouth care, ice to suck, and drinks as desired and tolerated. Profound thirst is not common but some patients may benefit from parenteral fluids, for example s.c. infusion of 1–2 l 0.9% saline/24 h or i.v. fluids.

Palliation of oesophageal obstruction

Swallowing may be difficult for patients with oesophageal cancer for several common reasons:
- oesophageal compressive and/or obstructive lesions;
- functional dysphagia;
- odynophagia (painful swallowing);
- oro-oesophageal thrush.

INTERVENTIONS TO RELIEVE OBSTRUCTION

The treatment of oesophageal obstructive lesions is outlined in Box 10.3. The insertion of a plastic tube can be carried out endoscopically and allows rapid relief of symptoms. Perforation, however, occurs in 10% of patients with a rigid tube, and tubes commonly block with food debris and regrowth of tumour. Migration of tubes is an additional problem and many patients have symptomatic reflux and discomfort from the presence of a rigid tube in the oesophagus [9]. They are very useful for relief of symptoms due to broncho- and tracheo-oesophageal fistulae.

Self-expanding metal stents are individually expensive but are highly flexible and require little oesophageal dilatation prior to insertion. Perforation

---

Box 10.3 Treatment options for obstructive lesions of the oesophagus

- Surgery (not for disease with metastatic spread)
- External beam radiotherapy
- Brachytherapy
- Chemotherapy
- Endoscopic injection of absolute alcohol
- Laser therapy
- Bouginage
- Celestin or Atkinson tube
- Self-expanding stents
- Pharmacological palliation alone or in combination with any of above

may occur in 1–5% of patients. Covered metal stent insertion is often highly effective in alleviating symptoms due to broncho- and tracheo-oesophageal fistulae [10]. Following insertion of a stent, radiotherapy or chemotherapy may be administered to augment the improvement by means of tumour shrinkage.

Per-endoscopic injection of absolute ethanol is often dramatically successful in achieving tumour shrinkage and stopping bleeding. There is a minimal risk of perforation. Injections are repeated weekly initially, then as needed.

Laser therapy results in good resolution of dysphagia and probably has fewer complications than the placement of tubes or stents. Perforation rates are lower in this technique. However, the procedure must be repeated 3–4 times weekly and commonly necessitates an overnight hospital admission.

SYMPTOMATIC MANAGEMENT

General symptom control is vital whatever the cause of obstruction or possibility of intervention. Mucaine, an antacid containing the local anaesthetic agent oxethazaine and used as often as necessary, may be useful for pain when swallowing. Standard titration through the analgesic ladder should be adopted. Strong (non-oral) opioids, such as sub-cutaneous diamorphine or transdermal fentanyl, may be required to control background pain (the latter only in stable pain syndromes; see Chapter 9).

In total obstruction of the oesophagus, coping with saliva and secretions can be distressing for the patient. The following may be helpful:
• hyoscine hydrobromide (Kwells), 1–2 tablets sublingually q.d.s.;
• hyoscine hydrobromide s.c. 1.2–3.6 mg/24 h;
• hyoscine butylbromide s.c. 40–80 mg/24 h (less sedating than hydrobromide).

Biliary stenting has significantly improved the quality of life of many patients with pancreatic and cholangiocarcinomas. If a localized stricture or obstruction of the bile duct is identified on ERCP then endoscopic (or occasionally percutaneous) placement of a stent may allow return of flow of bile. Stents may block after 3–4 months but can be replaced as required [10]. Diversion of bile flow may be considered in some patients.

Radiotherapy may reduce obstruction due to lymph nodes in the porta hepatis. Steroids (dexamethasone 4–16 mg daily) may reduce peritumour oedema.

Steatorrhoea is best managed with a low-fat diet. Opioids may be required to reduce its frequency, and pancreatic enzyme supplements may be useful particularly in patients with pancreatic cancer. Vitamin D, E, and K supplements should be considered in those living with profound malabsorption for several months.

Palliation of rectal obstruction

Rectal obstruction (usually incomplete) can be very distressing, extremely painful and severely affect quality of life. Rectal bleeding, faecal incontinence, and offensive discharge occur in addition to pain. Treatment options include:

- radiotherapy with or without chemotherapy;
- palliative surgery with stoma formation;
- endoscopic injection of absolute alcohol;
- laser therapy and diathermy;
- metal stent [11] alone or in combination with laser or alcohol;
- pharmacological palliation.

Pharmacological palliation of pain and obstructive symptoms is important for all patients. The stool should be kept very soft to pass through the obstructive lesion. Docusate sodium is given at a dose of 200 mg at least q.d.s. but titrated to stool consistency; it can be combined with a stimulant laxative, such as Co-danthrusate. Careful insertion of softening enemas may be useful.

PAIN AND TENESMUS

Pain from a rectal lesion may be troublesome in a number of ways. Constant nociceptive, visceral and bone which may be worsened by movement. In some cases sitting may be impossible. The pain may be present only on, or worsened by, either standing or defecation. Neuropathic pains can result from infiltration of the lumbosacral plexus. Some patients experience tenesmus: a painful sensation of rectal fullness and an urge to defecate.

The WHO ladder (see Chapter 9) will be helpful for all of these pain syndromes. Type 4 pain will be additionally helped by keeping the faeces soft. For some patients a palliative colostomy will be the best form of pain relief.

Neuropathic pain, of which tenesmus is one type, may be helped by opioids but will probably require adjuvant analgesics such as amitriptyline 10–150 mg nocte. Tenesmus may also be helped by:

- steroids—dexamethasone 4–16 mg daily;
- calcium channel antagonists—nifedipine 10–20 mg b.d.–t.d.s; smooth muscle relaxant;
- radiotherapy;
- bupivacaine enema;
- sacral epidural injection of steroid and local anaesthetic;
- bilateral lumbar sympathectomy;
- intrathecal 5% phenol to posterior sacral nerve roots.

Occasionally epidural delivery of opioids and local anaesthetic may be appropriate for relief of pain at rest and on defecation, particularly if the obstructive lesion is very low in the bowel. In the ill, dying patient, the most appropriate option is to achieve complete constipation with opioids and hyoscine butylbromide.

RECTAL BLEEDING AND DISCHARGE

While radiotherapy, alcohol injection, diathermy, or laser therapy is being planned, or if these are not possible or helpful, other measures may be needed to reduce the distress and discomfort from rectal bleeding. Enemas may be performed using various active ingredients, including: tranexamic acid (2–4 g/day made up in KY jelly) [12]; and aluminium coating via an enema (1% alum or sucralfate g in KY jelly) [13]. Distress or discomfort due to rectal discharge may be alleviated by steroid enemas and metronidazole suppositories.

Constipation

More than 50% of patients admitted to hospices in the UK complain of constipation [14]. Physical illness, immobility [15], poor oral intake, opioids, and many other drugs are risk factors for constipation. Other causes of constipation in patients with cancer and other illnesses are shown in Box 10.4.

Constipation can be prevented in the majority of patients by prescription of appropriate laxatives and careful review. All patients prescribed a weak or strong opioid should be advised to also take a stimulant laxative unless a contraindication exists. The dose of laxative will usually need to be increased as the dose of opioid is increased. It is not appropriate to wait until (predictable) constipation occurs before commencing laxative treatment. The vicious cycle of inappropriately treated abdominal pain and constipation should be anticipated in all patients with cancer or others taking opioid analgesics (see Fig. 10.2).

Box 10.4 Causes of constipation in patients with cancer and advanced illness

Direct effects of cancer
- Intestinal obstruction
- Damage to lumbosacral spinal cord, cauda equina, or pelvic plexus
- Hypercalcaemia

Secondary effects of advanced disease
- Poor dietary intake*
- Poor liquid intake*
- Weakness and immobility*
- Poor/unfamiliar toileting arrangements
- Confusion

Drugs
- Opioids*
- Drugs with anti-cholinergic effects:
  tricylic antidepressants
  anti-parkinsonian agents
  phenothiazines
  hyoscine
  diuretics
  anti-convulsants
  iron
  anti-hypertensive agents.

Concurrent disease
- Hypothyroidism
- Hypokalaemia
- Diabetes
- Diverticular disease

Local anal/rectal pathology
- Haemorrhoids
- Anal fissure/stenosis
- Rectocele
- Colitis

* Commonest causes.

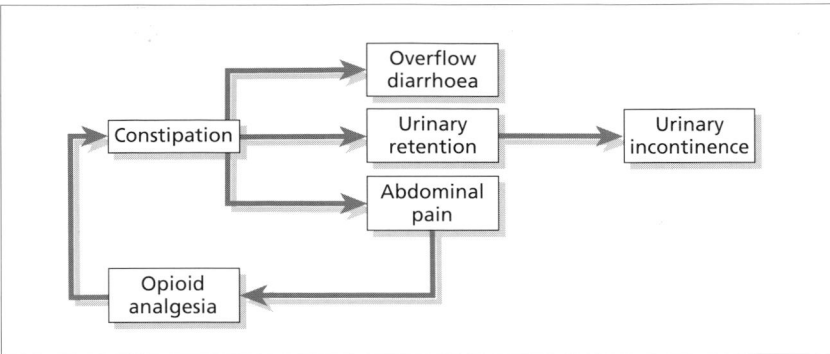

Fig. 10.2 The consequences of constipation-related pain treated inappropriately with opioids.

Management

Management will involve removing any underlying causes if possible, prescribing an appropriate oral laxative, and considering the use of per rectal/stomal measures (see Table 10.1). It should be remembered that one of the commonest reasons for failure of therapy is a prescription of a laxative which the patient dislikes.

Various types of laxative are available:

1   Stimulant oral laxatives (starting dose): bisacodyl (10 mg nocte) *or* senna (15 mg nocte). Latency of action 6–12 h.

2   Softening oral laxatives (starting dose): docusate sodium (100 mg t.d.s.);

Table 10.1 Treatment of constipation.

Examination finding	Treatment
Rectum full of hard faeces	Soften with glycerine suppositories +/– arachis oil enema. Commence combined stimulant and softening oral laxative.
Rectum full of soft faeces	Stimulate evacuation with bisacodyl suppository +/– stimulant enema. Commence stimulant oral laxative.
Empty distended rectum	Exclude obstruction. Stimulant suppository or enema will enhance colonic contraction. Commence oral laxative.

lactulose (15 ml b.d.). Latency of action 1–2 days. N.B. lactulose can cause flatulence, bloating, and increase discomfort.

3   Combined softening and stimulant oral laxatives (starting dose): Co-danthramer (two capsules nocte: 10 ml nocte); Co-danthrusate (one capsule or 10 ml nocte). Latency of action 6–12 h.

4   Rectal laxatives:

   Suppositories: glycerine (softening and mild stimulant); bisacodyl (stimulant);

   Enemas: arachis oil (130 ml) (softening); phosphate, sodium citrate (stimulant).

If the rectum is empty and stool is high in the colon, enemas should be administered through a rubber Foley catheter. Oil enemas should be warmed before use.

Bulk-forming laxatives have a very limited place in the management of constipation in patients with advanced disease, since they are generally burdensome to take, rely on a high oral fluid intake, and are not appropriate for the management of opioid-induced constipation.

All laxative doses should be titrated according to response.

Stoma care

Patients with stomas require both physical and psychological support. Good preparation before stoma formation and adequate time spent with the patient after stoma formation by a specialist (stoma care) nurse help in the transition and continued successful management. Patients vary in the time needed to adapt to and manage their stoma.

The most common physical difficulties are:
- when a bowel stoma becomes overactive, often with a more fluid faecal output;
- when constipation occurs;
- when patients are less able to manage their own stoma care because of the effects of their treatment or their disease.

Evaluation and management of these problems will involve examination of the stoma and effluent, including a digital examination of the stoma. There must also be a review of skin protectives/adhesives and bag size, together with a review of laxatives and antidiarrhoeal agents along with all other drugs.

If a stoma is impacted, suppositories and enemas can be given as for rectal impaction; however, a stoma has no sphincter. Suppositories should be gently pushed through the stoma as far as possible and gauze held over the stoma for a few minutes. If an enema, either oil or phosphate, is used it should be administered via a medium-size Foley catheter. This should be passed well into the stoma (identify direction of the bowel by digital examination beforehand). Inflate the balloon to 5 ml for 10 minutes while instilling the enema.

Control of fluid loss from an overactive ileostomy can be troublesome and specialist advice may need to be sought. Various treatments are available. The administration of opioids can reduce bowel motility; for example loperamide 4–8 mg b.d. *or* codeine phosphate 30–60 mg q.d.s. If the patient is already taking morphine for pain relief an increase in this may reduce bowel motility further but will also increase sedation and other central effects, and is not the preferred option unless it is also useful to improve pain control. A reduction of bowel motility and secretions may be achieved by use of anticholinergics, for example hyoscine butylbromide s.c. 60–180 mg/24 h, while H_2 antagonists or proton pump inhibitors can reduce gastric secretion.

Ispaghula (1–2 sachets t.d.s.) aids thickening of the motions, as does the use of isotonic and avoidance of hypotonic oral fluids. A subcutaneous infusion of octreotide can reduce small bowel secretions (see p. 141 'Obstruction'). However, doses required can be much greater than in treating obstruction.

The principles of management of a stoma and stoma care equipment can also be used to contain the output from faecal fistulae and protect the skin. Subcutaneous octreotide has been used to decrease the volume of fistula effluent and in some cases has aided healing.

Hiccup

This is a pathological respiratory reflex characterized by spasm of one or both sides of the diaphragm, causing sudden inspiration with associated closure of the vocal cords. The afferent arm of the reflex arc consists of the phrenic nerve, vagus nerve, and thoracic sympathetic fibres, which pass to the brainstem. There is central association of brainstem centres: involving the respiratory, phrenic, reticular formation, and hypothalamus, and the efferent arm to diaphragm is via the phrenic nerve. An inhibitory afferent pathway via the pharyngeal and glossopharyngeal nerves is apparent, but poorly understood.

Causes

The pathophysiology of hiccup is varied and there are many pathologies that lead to the symptom. Identification of cause may sometimes enable a logical and successful approach to treatment.

Irritation of branches of the vagus nerve in the abdomen can be due to gastric distension, peritonitis, or tumour, while similar irritation in the thorax may follow oesophageal obstruction or pneumonia. Vagal irritation can also stem from the larynx, pharynx, ear, or meninges.

Irritation of the phrenic nerve may be caused by diaphragmatic tumour, mediastinal tumour, or tumours in the neck.

Hiccup may also be caused by central nervous system pathology, including: intracranial tumours; brainstem lesions; toxic irritation (e.g. uraemia); or meningitis.

Management

Stimulation of the pharynx may be successful in reducing hiccup. This can be achieved in various ways, including: holding iced water in the oropharynx, soft palate massage, oropharyngeal or nasopharyngeal catheter placement, and agitation.

Additional management will be led by an understanding of individual aetiology but in practice it is often empirical. Common treatments are:
- a defoaming antiflatulent before and after meals and at bedtime (e.g. Asilone 10–20 ml);
- domperidone 10–20 mg t.d.s.; or metoclopramide 10 mg t.d.s. half an hour before meals if delayed gastric emptying; or cisapride 10 mg b.d.;
- nifedipine 10–20 mg b.d.–t.d.s.(assess effect on blood pressure);
- baclofen 5–10 mg b.d. (higher doses can be used with caution);
- chlorpromazine—use with care and only if simpler measures fail: 10–25 mg p.o. t.d.s. (it has a diffuse depressant effect on the reticular formation);
- sodium valproate—for hiccup of central origin.

Phrenic nerve stimulation or ablation are only occasionally an appropriate treatment in patients with advanced disease.

Mouth care

Saliva functions to maintain the optimum pH (6–7), reduce friction when chewing, aids talking, and helps form the food bolus. It contains bactericidal elements, proteolytic enzymes, and amylase, and therefore protects against infection and begins digestion of food. In total, about 1–1.5 l are produced per day in the healthy individual.

A dry mouth (xerostomia) is a common and major problem for many patients with advanced disease. Drugs such as opioids, antihistamines, anticholinergics, diuretics, beta blockers and anticonvulsants may produce xerostomia. Dehydration, anxiety, and mouth breathing also result in a dry mouth. Radiotherapy and chemotherapy can cause particular oral problems, which are discussed further in Chapter 12.

The aims of mouth care are to:
- keep the oral mucosa clean, soft, moist, and intact in order to prevent infection;
- keep the lips clean, soft, moist, and intact;
- remove food debris/dental plaque without damaging the gingival membrane;
- alleviate pain and discomfort thus enabling greater oral intake;
- prevent halitosis;
- promote taste, appetite, and speech;
- prevent a potential source of psychological distress.

The frequency of mouth care is of greater importance than the agent used. Mouth care every two hours prevents infection more effectively than sporadic mouth care [16].

Management of xerostomia

Simply taking frequent sips of water, sucking ice poles, or using glycerine (which tends to make the mouth sticky) and chewing gum may be helpful. Lemon may stimulate saliva flow but if there are mucosal breaks it will cause pain. An enzyme in pineapple helps clean the mouth, particularly when the tongue is coated. Effervescent vitamin C held on the tongue may also be useful to clean a coated tongue.

For very sick patients sucking on moist cotton swabs (e.g. Moistir) or sponge swabs on sticks dipped in water will be helpful.

The salivary substitutes, which contain either carboxymethycellulose or mucin, are useful. The latter may have marginal advantages in terms of longer duration of action. They should be sprayed beneath the tongue and between the buccal mucosa and the teeth (i.e. mimic the pooling of saliva) and not in the back of the throat.

The cholinergic agonist pilocarpine (5 mg t.d.s. with or after food) has been shown to increase saliva production, especially post-irradiation. This is contraindicated in obstructive airways disease and asthma, and is often poorly tolerated because of sweating, gastrointestinal, and other side-effects.

Prevention and management of oral infections

For patients with reduced saliva meticulous care of the oral cavity, teeth, and dentures will reduce infection and maintain function and comfort. Sodium bicarbonate mouthwashes repeated regularly (2-hourly) coupled with gentle brushing of the teeth (or cleaning dentures) twice per day is a simple but effective technique. The aim is to keep the pH alkaline—*Candida* prefers an acid environment [17].

Candidal infections are treated with nystatin, miconazole, or amphotericin administered orally. Dentures should be cleaned in Sterident or Milton with or without nystatin. If the patient is severely affected, has symptoms suggestive of oesophageal infection, or is taking antibiotics and steroids a systemic antifungal is indicated; for example, fluconazole 50 mg o.d. for 7–14 days, or itraconazole 100 mg o.d for 10–15 days.

Herpes simplex infections present as very painful, vesicular, and ulcerating lesions. Oral aciclovir 200 mg five times daily, or valaciclovir 500 mg b.d. for 5 days is indicated. Bacterial infection will usually respond to antibiotics.

A sore mouth, from whatever cause, may be helped by sucking anaesthetic lozenges or using local anaesthetic mouthwashes or sprays. A cocaine-based mouthwash may sometimes be helpful.

References

1 Grond S, Zech D, Diefenbach C, Bishcoff A. Prevalence and pattern of symptoms in patients with cancer pain: a prospective evaluation of 1635 patients referred to a pain clinic. *J Pain Symptom Manage* 1994; 9: 372–382.
2 Dunlop GM. A study of the relative frequency and importance of gastrointestinal symptoms, and weakness in patients with far advanced cancer. *Palliat Med* 1989; 4: 37–43.
3 Ashby MA, Game PA, Devitt P *et al*. Percutaneous gastrostomy as a venting procedure in palliative care. *Palliat Med* 1991; 5: 147–150.
4 Taylor RH. Laparotomy for obstruction with recurrent tumour. *Br J Surgery* 1985; 72: 327.
5 Krebs H, Goplerud DR. Surgical management of bowel obstruction in advanced ovarian cancer. *Obstet Gynaecol* 1983; 61: 327–330.
6 DeConno F, Caraceni A, Zecca E, Spondi E, Ventafridda V. Continuous subcutaneous infusion of hyoscine butylbromide reduces secretions in patients with gastrointestinal obstruction. *J Pain Symptom Manage* 1991; 6: 484–486.
7 Fallon MT. The physiology of somatostatin and its synthetic analogue, octreotide. *Euro J Palliat Care* 1994; 1: 20–22.
8 Riley J, Fallon MT. Octreotide in terminal malignant obstruction of the gastrointestinal tract. *Euro J Palliat Care* 1994; 1: 23–25.
9 Blazeby JM, Williams MH, Brooks ST, Alderson D, Farndon JR. Quality of life measurement in patients with oesophageal cancer. *Gut* 1995; 37: 505–508.
10 Blazeby JM, Alderson D. The modern management of patients with oesophageal cancer. *Prog Palliat Care* 1995; 3: 215–218.

11 Rey JF, Romanczyk T, Graff M. Metal stents for palliation of rectal carcinoma: a preliminary report on 12 patients. *Endoscopy* 1995; 27(7): 501–504.

12 McElligot E, Quigley C, Hanks GW. Tranexamic acic and rectal bleeding. *Lancet* 1991; 29: 37–39.

13 Regnard CFB. Control of bleeding in advanced cancer *Lancet* 1991; 337: 974.

14 Sykes NP. Constipation and diarrhoea. In: Doyle D, Hanks, MacDonald N, eds. *Oxford Textbook of Palliative Medicine*. Oxford: Oxford University Press, 1993: 299–309.

15 Fallon MT, Hanks GW. Is morphine-induced constipation dose elated? *Palliat Med*, in press.

16 Jobbins J, Bogg J, Finlay I, Addy M, Newcombe RG. Oral and dental disease in terminally ill cancer patients. *BMJ* 1992; 304: 1612.

17 Ventafridda V, Ripamonti C, Sbanotto A, DeConno F. Mouthcare. In: Doyle D, Hanks, MacDonald N, eds. *Oxford Textbook of Palliative Medicine*. Oxford: Oxford University Press, 1993: 434–435.

11: The Management of Respiratory Symptoms

ANDREW WILCOCK

Introduction

Respiratory symptoms are a common problem for patients with advanced illness. As many as 70% of patients with cancer will experience significant breathlessness in the last six weeks of life. In patients with end-stage congestive cardiac failure (CCF) or chronic obstructive pulmonary disease (COPD) the prevalence may be even greater. This chapter will discuss the management of the three commonest respiratory symptoms: cough, breathlessness and haemoptysis.

The evidence base for the symptomatic management of these problems is limited. Particular caution and close, objective evaluation should therefore be used when extrapolating from experience in patients with cancer to the needs of patients with more chronic, non-malignant disease. There may, however, be few, if any, other options available to improve the clinical picture.

Cough

Cough is a physiological reflex (Fig. 11.1) that clears the central airways of foreign material and secretions. It becomes pathological when excessive, ineffective, or persistent, affecting the patient's sleep, rest, eating, and social functioning. It may lead to muscular strain and discomfort, rib or vertebral fracture, syncope, headache, or retinal haemorrhage. In patients with cancer the prevalence of cough varies between 50% and 80%, being highest in patients with lung cancer.

The commonest cause of acute cough is respiratory tract infection. The commoner causes of chronic cough are summarized in Table 11.1.

Management of the cough

The cause can be established in 80% of patients by a careful history alone. Investigations appropriate to the clinical condition of the patient may include chest X-ray, sputum culture, spirometry (pre- and post-bronchodilator), sinus X-rays, or barium swallow. Stimuli that exacerbate coughing such

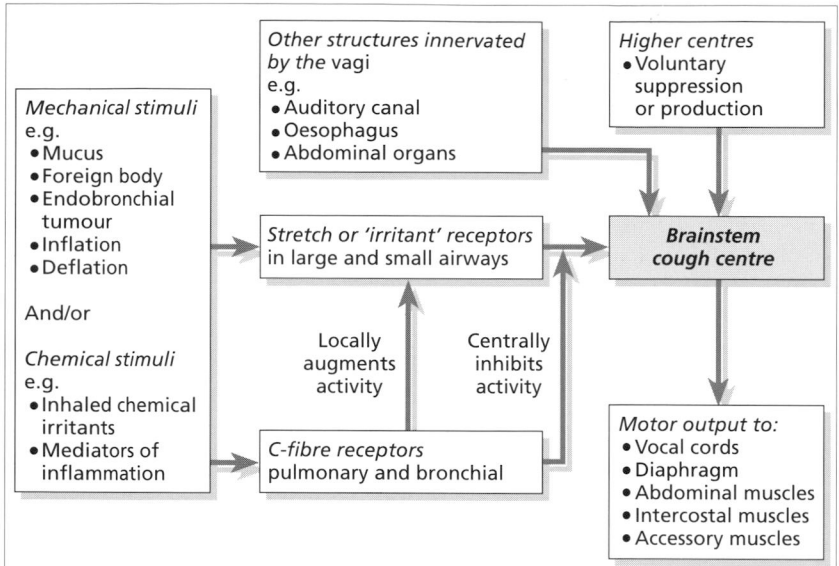

Fig. 11.1 The pathophysiology of the cough reflex.

as smoke, cold air, and exercise should be established for the individual patient and avoidance measures taken.

In a patient with cancer ask the following questions.
• Is the cough due to the cancer? It is easy to attribute all symptoms to the cancer. Other non-cancer-related causes must be considered and appropriate treatment given or existing therapies maximized (e.g. for asthma/COPD). If there is any doubt then consult appropriate colleagues for advice.
• Can the cancer be modified? This may include radiotherapy, chemotherapy, hormone therapy, or surgery. Obtain advice from your local oncology team.
• Can the effects that the cancer produces be modified? This includes, for example, the insertion of stents or the drainage of pleural effusions.

TREATMENT STRATEGY

It is useful to divide cough into 'wet' or 'dry'. A wet cough serves a physiological purpose and expectoration should be encouraged and facilitated. Conversely, a dry cough serves no purpose and should be suppressed. A wet cough that is distressing a dying patient who is too weak to expectorate should also be suppressed (Fig. 11.2).

Table 11.1 Causes of chronic cough.

Cancer related
Primary or secondary cancer causing airway:
  infiltration
  compression
  distortion
  obstruction, leading to collapse +/– infection.
Pulmonary infiltration
Pleural infiltration
Tracheo-oesophageal fistula
Mucus secretion and retention
Ineffective cough due to:
  generalized weakness
  vocal cord palsy
  pain on coughing.

Treatment related
Cancer treatment:
  pulmonary infiltration/fibrosis related to chemotherapy, e.g. bleomycin,
  methotrexate, cyclophosphamide, busulphan and radiotherapy.
Non-cancer treatments:
  nitrofurantoin–pulmonary infiltration/fibrosis
  ACE inhibitors–increase cough reflex
  beta-blockers–induce bronchoconstriction.

Other causes
Infection, 'smoker's cough', COPD, asthma, post-infection increased cough reflex,
lung abscess, bronchiectasis, post nasal drip syndrome due to (due to sinusitis,
rhinitis), gastro-oesophageal reflux, pulmonary oedema, pulmonary infarction,
recurrent aspiration, pleural effusion.

There is no evidence to support the routine use of expectorants to increase the volume of secretions (e.g. ipecacuanha and squill) or mucolytics to reduce the viscosity of secretions (e.g. carbocisteine and methyl cysteine hydrochloride) [1]. However, some individual patients do benefit from mucolytics and a therapeutic trial could be considered if all other approaches have failed (e.g. carbocisteine 750 mg t.i.d.). Nebulized acetylcysteine appears sometimes to be more effective than nebulized 0.9% saline [2]. However, it has an unpleasant sulphurous odour and can cause bronchoconstriction, nausea, or vomiting. It is inactivated by oxygen and the nebulizer must be driven by compressed air.

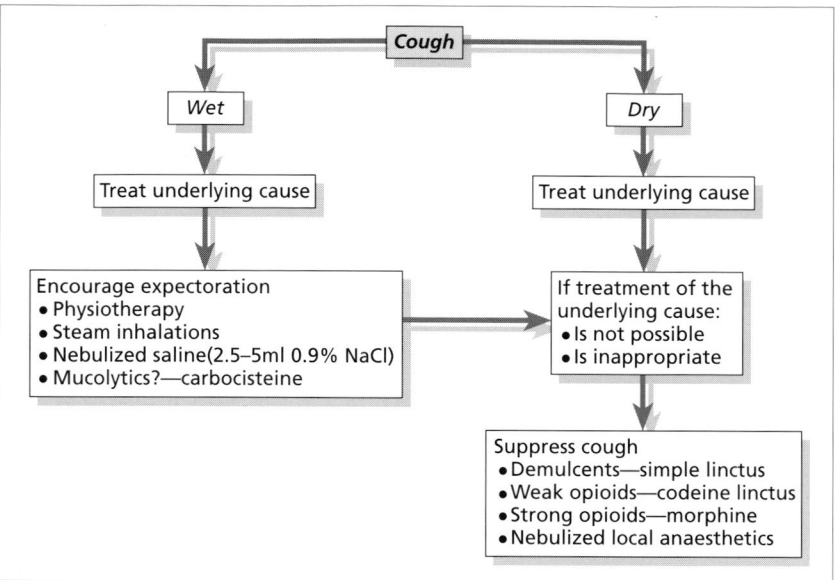

Fig. 11.2 The management of cough in patients with cancer.

COUGH SUPPRESSION

Demulcents

Demulcents contain soothing substances such as syrup or glycerol. Their high sugar content stimulates saliva production and swallowing which may inhibit the cough reflex. Their effect is short lived and there is no evidence to suggest that compound preparations offer any advantage over simple linctus (5 ml t.–q.i.d.).

Opioids

Opioids primarily work by suppressing the cough reflex centre in the brainstem. A peripheral action to reduce mucus production and cough may be of little clinical relevance as nebulized opioids do not suppress cough in humans [3]. Patients will require concomitant prescription for a stimulant laxative and perhaps initially an antiemetic.

Codeine. Codeine, pholcodine, and dextromethorphan are common ingredients in compound cough preparations. Evidence supports the use of codeine and dextromethorphan, but not pholcodine [1]. However, the effective dose of codeine or dextromethorphan is greater than that usually delivered by compound preparations, where the sugar content may in fact be the main effective ingredient. Therefore codeine linctus 5–10 ml (15–30 mg t.–q.i.d.) should be used.

Similar to its analgesic effect, the antitussive effect of codeine may rely partly on its conversion to morphine, an enzymatic process deficient in 5–10% of the population, who may fail to benefit from its use [4].

If codeine is ineffective a strong opioid such as morphine should be used. If a patient is already receiving a strong opioid for pain relief there is no logic in adding codeine, or another opioid as a separate cough suppressant.

In this situation check with the patient if a 'prn' dose helps relieve the cough. If so, use as required or consider increasing the regular dose. If not, there is little point in further dose increments or advantage in adding another strong opioid.

Morphine. The prescription of morphine (2.5–10 mg every 4 hours (q4h) initially) often raises issues for the patient and family, and time is required to listen, clarify, explain, and reassure them about these. The dose can be titrated upwards as allowed by side-effects and then converted to a modified-release preparation.

Methadone. Methadone has no clear advantage over morphine for the treatment of cough. There is a wide variation in its pharmacokinetics between individuals, and a risk of accumulation with repeated use.

Nebulized local anaesthetics

These inhibit afferent nerve endings. Their use in patients with cough due to cancer or other disease has not been fully evaluated and cannot be routinely recommended. They should be considered only when other avenues have failed. Their use is limited by their unpleasant taste, oropharyngeal numbness, risk of aspiration and bronchoconstriction and a short duration of action (10–30 minutes) [5].

Suggested doses are 2% lignocaine (5 ml) or 0.25% bupivacaine (5 ml) t.–q.i.d. [6]. A test dose should always be given under close observation to ensure bronchospasm or other adverse effects are rapidly treated.

Breathlessness

Breathlessness on exertion (dyspnoea) is a normal 'physiological' experience. It becomes pathological when it limits normal activity or is associated with disabling anxiety. Breathlessness can be difficult to describe and vary qualitatively depending on the underlying cause [7,8]. The experience of breathlessness includes the perception of difficulty in breathing and the physical, behavioural, and emotional responses to it. It should not be confused with an increase in respiratory rate (tachypnoea) or ventilation (hyperpnoea).

Chronic breathlessness is common in patients with cardiorespiratory disease and it is a likely symptom in the 25 000 patients who die from COPD each year in England and Wales and in the 250 000 living with CCF in the UK.

Breathlessness occurs in 70% of patients with cancer in the last six weeks of life. It is more likely in patients with primary or secondary lung cancer, pleural disease and pre-existing cardiopulmonary disease. In 25% of breathless patients, however, generalized muscle weakness (which will include the respiratory muscles) resulting from cancer cachexia may be the only apparent factor. Both the prevalence and the severity of breathlessness increase as death approaches, with 25% of patients describing their breathlessness as 'severe' or 'horrible' in the last week of life [9,10].

Breathlessness, in cancer at least, is a strong, independent predictor of survival second only to performance status [11].

Pathophysiology

How the sensation of breathlessness is generated remains unclear but it appears related to the degree of activation of brainstem structures concerned with the automatic control of breathing. Inputs from cortical and other higher centres are important and help explain why the threshold and tolerance to breathlessness appears to vary between individuals and is influenced by mood, anxiety [12], and encouragement [13] and can occur in several psychiatric disorders in patients who are otherwise healthy.

A model of chronic breathlessness identifying the antecedents, mediators, reactions, and consequences of breathlessness is illustrated in Fig. 11.3. This model attempts to encompass the complex integration between the physical and emotional dimensions of breathlessness.

The behavioural and practical responses to breathlessness can vary between patients, and include changes in position, moving more slowly, adjusting medication, and using breathing strategies. The most common adaptive strategies include reducing functional performance, obtaining assistance with activities of daily living, and altering, reducing, or discontinuing work [15]. The psychological responses may include anxiety,

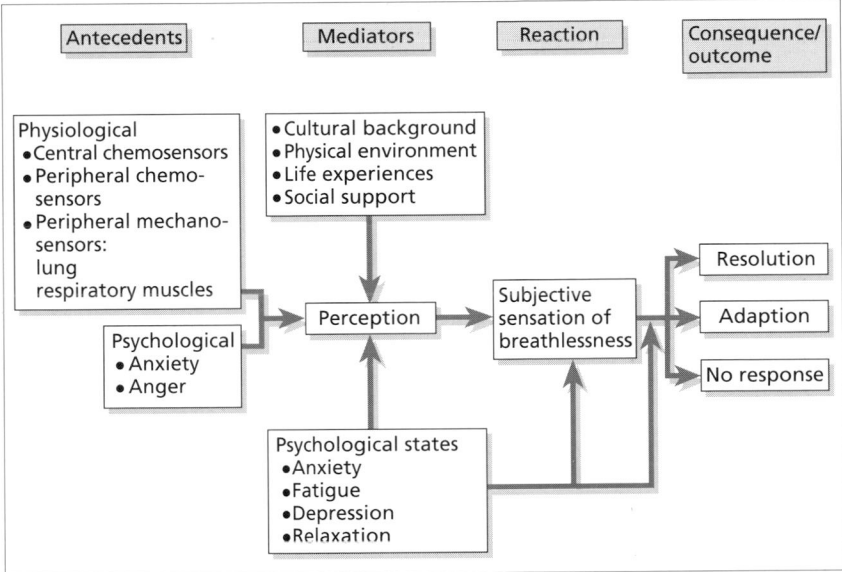

Fig. 11.3 A model of breathlessness after McCord and Cronin-Stubbs [14].

fear, panic and depression. Adaptive strategies may include breathing exercises and relaxation.

Assessment of breathless patients

Breathlessness is difficult to treat and so it is vital to identify any of the causes that may be partially or fully reversible (Table 11.2). Diagnosing the cause of breathlessness requires a thorough history and examination combined with appropriate investigation (see Box 11.1). A chest X-ray is often valuable as clinical examination of the chest may reveal few signs even in the presence of significant disease.

Assessment should also identify any symptoms of anxiety and depression, the impact of the breathlessness on the patient's lifestyle, the patient's (and family's) coping strategies, and the meaning of the breathlessness for the patient.

Increasingly severe breathlessness is accompanied by increased levels of anxiety and depression in patients with COPD. In patients with cancer, anxiety is more common and more severe in those with breathlessness compared to those with other symptoms. Reduction in anxiety or depression can lead to an improvement in breathlessness.

Table 11.2 Causes of breathlessness.

Cancer related
Primary and secondary lung cancer causing:
  airway obstruction (+/– collapse)
  mass effect
  lung infiltration
  tumour emboli
  lymphangitis carcinomatosis.
Generalized weakness causing:
  loss of 'fitness'
  respiratory muscle weakness.
Pleural effusion
Superior vena cava obstruction
Pericardial effusion
Phrenic nerve palsy
Splinting of the diaphragm caused by:
  ascities
  hepatomegaly.
Chest wall infiltration
Chest wall pain
Anaemia; of chronic disease due to marrow infiltration

Treatment related
Cancer treatments
  Surgery
  lobectomy, pneumonectomy
  Radiotherapy
  pneumonitis leading to fibrosis (usually with higher doses)
  Chemotherapy
  bleomycin, methotrexate–pneumonitis
  cyclophosphamide, busulphan–fibrosis
Non-cancer treatments
  Drugs precipitating fluid retention,
  e.g. corticosteroids
  Drugs precipitating bronchospasm,
  e.g. beta-blockers

Other causes
Infection
  bacterial, viral, fungal
Chronic respiratory disease,
  e.g. COPD, asthma
Chronic cardiac disease,
  e.g. ischaemic heart disease, CCF
Pulmonary oedema
Pneumothorax
Pulmonary embolism
Cardiac arrhythmia
Psychological factors,
  e.g. anxiety, fear, anger, frustration, isolation, depression

Box 11.1 The assessment of the breathless patient with cancer

History
Important things to note are:
- Speed of onset
- Associated symptoms, e.g. pain, cough, haemoptysis, sputum, stridor, wheeze
- Exacerbating and relieving factors
- Symptoms suggestive of hyperventilation:
    poor relationship of dyspnoea to exertion
    presence of hyperventilation attacks
    breathlessness at rest
    rapid fluctuations in breathlessness within minutes
    fear of sudden death during an attack
    breathlessness varying with social situations.
- Past medical history, e.g. history of cardiovascular disease
- Drug history, e.g. drugs precipitating fluid retention or bronchospasm
- Symptoms of anxiety or depression
- Social circumstances—support networks
- Level of independence:
    ability to care for themselves
    identify coping strategies.
- What the breathlessness means to the patient
- How do they feel when they are breathless

Examination
- Very useful to observe the patient walking a set distance or carrying out a specific task
- Does hyperventilation reproduce symptoms?

Investigations
Commonly performed:
- Chest X-ray
- Haemoglobin

Less commonly performed:
- Ultrasound scan—useful for differentiating between pleural effusion and solid tumour
- Oxygen saturation—may be useful if assessing value of oxygen
- Peak flow/simple spirometry—assessing response to bronchodilators or corticosteroids

Continued on p. 166

Box 11.1 *Continued*

- Electrocardiogram
- Echocardiography
- Ventilation / perfusion scan

Hyperventilation is a common accompaniment in patients with breathlessness 'disproportionate' to the severity of their pulmonary disease [16]. It occurs in up to 28% of patients with cancer who are breathless. If hyperventilation is suspected then ask the patient to take up to 20 deep breaths and monitor if this reproduces the patient's symptoms. This is also therapeutic as it helps to demonstrate the cause of the symptoms and allows the introduction of breathing control/relaxation exercises that aim to give the patient a greater feeling of control over their breathing.

The impact of breathlessness on the patient can be observed by asking the patient to carry out a set task. This may reveal hyperventilation, which can be highlighted to the patient. Alternatively, beneficial coping strategies that the patient uses can be reinforced. It also provides a baseline against which to monitor progress.

It is important to explore what the patient and their carers understand about breathlessness. It is a common belief that the heart or lungs are being further damaged by becoming breathless and many fear that they might die suddenly during an episode of breathlessness. Activities are subsequently curtailed or avoided and many become socially isolated. It is important to stress that becoming breathless in itself is not dangerous, and to encourage patients to remain as active as possible.

An exploration of the patient's emotional reactions to breathlessness is also important. Patients with lung cancer describe emotions such as anger, helplessness, depression, loss of strength, agitation, anxiety, fear of suffocating and nervousness during episodes of breathlessness [17].

Management of breathlessness in patients with cancer

First, consider the following questions.

Is the breathlessness due to the cancer?

It is easy to attribute the breathlessness to the cancer and fail to consider other causes. For example, a survey of patients with lung cancer attending a chest clinic found that half had airflow obstruction which was associated with more severe breathlessness. Of these, only 14% were taking bronchodilator therapy. A trial of bronchodilator therapy improved breathlessness in 60% of the previously untreated patients [18]. Patients should receive the most appropriate treatment or have any existing treatment optimized.

Can the cancer be modified?

Consider if radiotherapy, chemotherapy, hormone therapy, or surgery have any place. Endobronchial tumour causing large airway obstruction may be treated by surgical resection, brachy-, cryo-, or laser therapy.

Can the effects the cancer produces be modified?

This may involve the drainage of pleural and pericardial effusions or ascites and the insertion of endobronchial [19] or superior vena cava stents. Corticosteroids are used for their anti-inflammatory effect (thereby reducing peri-tumour oedema) to treat the symptoms of superior vena cava obstruction, tracheal compression/stridor or carcinomatosis lymphangitis. As there is little evidence to support their use, corticosteroids should not be a substitute for or delay the use of more definitive therapies when appropriate.

An overall strategy for the treatment of breathlessness

It is useful to consider the treatment of breathlessness in three clinical settings that relate to the prognosis of the patient:
• breathlessness on exertion (months to years);
• breathlessness at rest (weeks to months);
• terminal breathlessness (last days of life).
    Pharmacological or non-pharmacological treatments are both important but the relative contributions made by these two approaches varies according to the patient's prognosis. Pharmacological treatments predominate in the terminal phase and non-pharmacological methods in patients who are breathless on exertion (Fig. 11.4).

BREATHLESSNESS ON EXERTION (MONTHS TO YEARS)

This is common in patients with COPD, CCF, and cancer (especially those with coexisting cardio disease). The treatment of any underlying

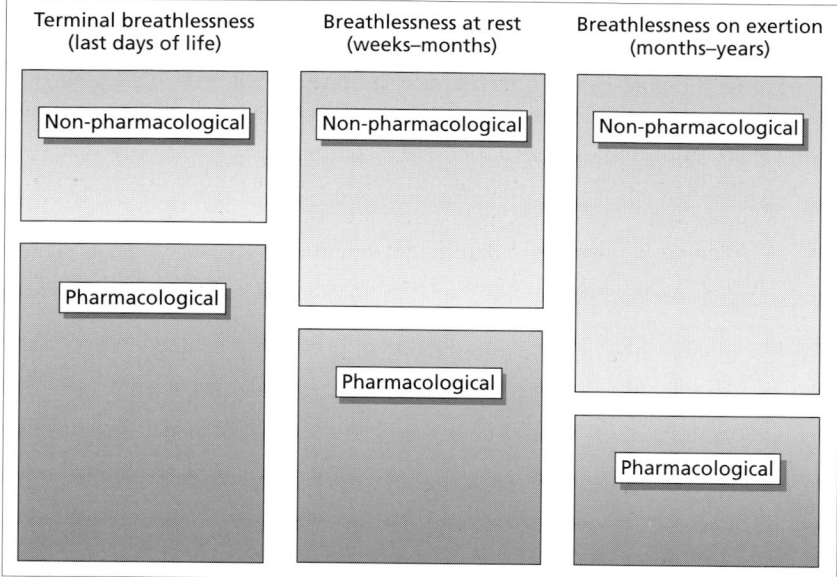

| Terminal breathlessness (last days of life) | Breathlessness at rest (weeks–months) | Breathlessness on exertion (months–years) |

Fig. 11.4 The relative contributions of pharmacological and non-pharmacological approaches to the management of breathlessness in patients with cancer according to the severity of the breathlessness and the patient's prognosis. *Note:* episodes of hyperventilation (panic attacks) are most appropriately managed by a predominantly non-pharmacological approach.

cardiorespiratory disease should be optimized. In the author's experience pharmacological therapies such as opioids are usually of little benefit and can be poorly tolerated in this setting.

Non-pharmacological approaches in managing breathlessness are therefore particularly important in this group of patients. This strategy requires the input of the whole multidisciplinary team in what is the palliative care equivalent of pulmonary rehabilitation. This is outlined in Box 11.2 [19].

BREATHLESSNESS AT REST (WEEKS TO MONTHS)

Opioids

Morphine acts centrally to diminish ventilatory drive stimulated by hypercapnia, hypoxia, and exercise. Depression of ventilation occurs in a dose-dependent manner largely by a reduction in tidal volume. The reduction in respiratory rate can be more variable, making it a less reliable

---

Box 11.2 Non-pharmacological approaches to breathlessness

Exploring the perception of the patient and carers
- Exploration of anxieties—especially fear of sudden death when breathless
- Explanation of symptoms and meaning
- Informing patient and carers that breathlessness in itself is not dangerous
- What is/is not likely to happen—'you won't choke or suffocate to death'
- Help come to terms with deteriorating condition
- Help to cope with and adjust to 'losses' (of role, abilities, etc.)

Maximizing the feeling of control over breathlessness
- Breathing control advice
- Relaxation techniques
- Plan of action for acute episodes:
  simple written instructions—step-by-step plan
  increase confidence in coping with acute episodes.
- Use of an electric fan
- Complementary therapies may benefit some patients

Maximizing functional ability and support
- Encourage exertion to breathlessness to increase tolerance to breathlessness and maintain fitness
- Assessment by the district nurse, occupational therapist, physiotherapist and social worker may all be necessary to identify where additional support is required.

Reduce feelings of personal and social isolation
- Meet others in similar situation
- Attendance at a day centre
- Respite admissions

---

index of respiratory depression. The respiratory and analgesic effects of morphine appear to be mediated by different receptors.

In patients with COPD or cancer the efficacy and tolerability of opioids for the relief of breathlessness varies widely (Table 11.3). In patients with COPD opioids are not seen as a useful routine therapy [20]; conversely in patients with cancer they are recommended and widely used [6].

Clinical aspects. For opiate-naive patients use small doses initially (e.g. 2.5 mg oral morphine q4h–q.i.d.) and titrate the dose and dose interval according to response and side-effects. For patients already receiving

Table 11.3 A summary of research into the efficacy and tolerability of opioids for breathlessness in patients with COPD and cancer (see text for clinical recommendations).

Effective and tolerated	Effective but poorly tolerated	Ineffective and poorly tolerated
Patients with COPD		
Dihydrocodeine 1 mg/kg p.o. single dose [21]	Morphine 0.8 mg/kg p.o. single dose [24]	Codeine 30 mg p.o. q.i.d. 4 weeks (worsening of pulmonary function, urinary retention) [26]
Dihydrocodeine 15 mg p.o. prior to exercise up to t.i.d. [22]	Dihydrocodeine 30–60 mg p.o. q.i.d. 2 weeks (nausea, vomiting, constipation, drowsiness) [25]	Dextromethorphan 60 mg p.o. single dose (nausea) [27]
Hydromorphone 3 mg p.r. q.i.d. [23]		Diamorphine 2.5–5 mg p.o. q.i.d. 2 weeks and 7.5 mg p.o. single dose (itching, constipation, vomiting) [28]
Patients with cancer		
Morphine 2.5 times the regular q4h dose s.c. or 5 mg s.c. if opiate naive Then as a single dose All patients on oxygen None had COPD (nausea and sedation only in the opiate naive patients) [29]		Morphine 10 mg b.i.d. (MST continues) or equivalent q4h dose opiate niave or 30% increase in dose p.o. none on oxygen 25% of patients had COPD (drowsiness, dizziness, falls) [31]
Morphine 1.5 times the regular q4h dose s.c. Then as a single dose All patients on oxygen None had COPD [30]		

p.o. = by mouth; p.r. = by rectum; s.c. = subcutaneously; b.i.d. = twice a day; t.i.d. = three times a day; q.i.d. = four times a day; q4h = four hourly.

opiates, observe whether there is benefit from an additional dose. If so, increase the regular opiate in steps of 30–50%. If there is no improvement or side-effects occur then reduce the dose.

A continuous subcutaneous infusion of opiate may be better tolerated and be more effective for some patients—possibly by avoiding the peaks (with side-effects) and troughs (with loss of effect) of oral medication.

Nebulized opioids

Evidence suggests that nebulized opioids act through a central [32,33] as opposed to a local pulmonary mechanism [34]. However, if this is the case then the nebulized route is a relatively inefficient way of administering morphine. Further studies are required to clarify the role of nebulized opioids and they should not be seen as a routine therapy for the relief of breathlessness in patients.

Oxygen

Supplemental oxygen has been shown to improve exercise tolerance and prolong life in patients with COPD who are severely hypoxic ($Pao_2 < 9 kPa$). The role of oxygen in less hypoxic patients is more difficult to determine as there is great variability between individuals in subjective response to oxygen. In addition the oxygen saturation level does not predict benefit from oxygen. Improvement with oxygen is therefore often considered to be a placebo effect due to the emotive connotations of its use. Alternatively, the cooling flow of oxygen against the face or through the nose may be reducing breathlessness (as does a stream of air) by stimulating facial and nasal receptors of the trigeminal nerve. This finding also supports the use of an electric fan to help relieve breathlessness. In patients with cancer the benefit of oxygen is also variable [35,36].

Clinical aspects. Oxygen therapy should be available to severely hypoxic patients. In those less hypoxic a trial of oxygen therapy can be given via nasal prongs for an agreed fixed period of time. A pulse oximeter will help identify those patients whose oxygen saturation is objectively improved by oxygen therapy (although initial saturation can be a poor predictor of who will benefit). If on review the patient has found it useful it can be continued. If the patient has any doubts concerning its efficacy then it should be discontinued.

Oxygen can be delivered at home via cylinders or an oxygen concentrator. The latter is more convenient but can be limited by its maximal flow rate

(4 l/min). If necessary tubing from two machines can be joined by a T-piece to deliver higher flow rates.

The use of an electric fan or portable hand fan may be beneficial.

Benzodiazepines, phenothiazines, and other anxiolytics

The use of benzodiazepines in patients with pulmonary disease requires caution following reports of ventilatory depression [37] although this has not been a universal finding [38]. They appear to reduce breathlessness by relieving coexistent anxiety rather than by any specific effect on breathlessness. Drowsiness is a common side-effect.

In patients with cancer, benefit from benzodiazepines is reported anecdotally but there have been no studies. Benzodiazepines should not be prescribed routinely as a treatment for breathlessness in patients without coexistent anxiety.

Clinical aspects. The oral benzodiazepine of choice is diazepam initially 2–5 mg t.i.d., reducing over several days as levels of active metabolites rise, to a maintenance dose of 2–5 mg at night. Chlorpromazine has been used for the relief of terminal breathlessness in patients with cancer [39]. Buspirone is an anxiolytic acting predominantly via serotonin receptors ($5HT_{1A}$). It is as effective as diazepam in the relief of anxiety and is free of sedative or respiratory depressant effects. In patients with COPD, buspirone improve anxiety levels along with breathlessness and exercise tolerance [40]. Further evaluation is necessary but buspirone appears to be a useful alternative to diazepam.

TERMINAL BREATHLESSNESS

Patients often fear suffocating to death, and it is important that there is a positive approach to the patient, their family, and to colleagues about the potential to relieve terminal breathlessness.
- No patient should die with distressing breathlessness.
- Failure to control is a failure to utilize drug therapy correctly.
- Combination of a parenteral opioid with a sedative anxiolytic such as midazolam is effective (Table 11.4).
- If the patient becomes agitated or confused (sometimes aggravated by midazolam), haloperidol or methotrimeprazine should be added.

Usually, due to distress, inability to sleep, and exhaustion, patients (and their carers) accept the risk of increasing drowsiness in order that they may be made more comfortable. Sedation is not the primary aim of

Table 11.4 Drugs used in treatment of terminal breathlessness.

Drug	Starting dose	Upper dose range	Route
Diamorphine	10 mg/24 h (opioid naive)	Titrate according to symptoms	s.c. infusion
Midazolam	10–30 mg/24 h	200–260 mg/24 h	s.c. infusion
Chlorpromazine	12.5 mg i.v. q4 h 25 mg p.r. b–t.i.d.	300–900 mg/24 h	i.v. rectal
Methotrimeprazine	12.5–50 mg/24 h	200–300 mg/24 h	s.c. infusion

i.v. = intravenous; s.c. = subcutaneous; q4h = four hourly; b.i.d. = twelve hourly; t.i.d. = eight hourly.

therapy (unless there is overwhelming distress) and some patients often become 'brighter' with improvement in their symptoms. However, as increasing drowsiness is usually a feature of their deteriorating clinical condition it is important to explain clearly to the relatives the aims of treatment and the gravity of the situation.

Haemoptysis in patients with cancer

The expectoration of blood is frightening and will lead most people to seek medical attention. In the majority of cases the amount of blood expectorated is small but large bleeds can occur with little or no warning. The management of massive, fatal haemoptysis is discussed in Chapter 12.

One-third of patients with bronchogenic carcinoma experience haemoptysis, with an incidence of acute fatal bleeds of 3%. Of these, 20% occur without prior warning. Haemoptysis from bronchogenic carcinoma can occur with any histological type although massive fatal haemoptysis is most likely to be due to squamous cell tumours (83%) that are located centrally or causing cavitation (48%).

In patients with metastatic lung disease from solid malignancies, haemoptysis is usually due to endobronchial disease. Oesophageal carcinoma may extend directly into the tracheobronchial tree to cause massive haemoptysis. Infection (bacterial and fungal), low platelets, and abnormal clotting increase the risk of haemoptysis.

Management of haemoptysis

Is the haemoptysis due to the cancer?

The history will help determine if the haemoptysis is related to the cancer, to its treatment, or to the common differential diagnoses of infection or pulmonary embolism. Investigations appropriate to the clinical condition of the patient depend upon the causes being considered and the severity of the haemoptysis.

Can the cancer be modified?

Radiotherapy is the treatment of choice for haemoptysis, leading to prolonged relief in 85% of patients. The dose given is palliative and the treatment can usually be repeated if the symptom recurs. For patients with unrelieved or recurrent haemoptysis, in whom further external beam irradiation is not possible, brachytherapy, laser therapy or cryotherapy may be considered depending on local access to specialist services.

Can factors increasing the risk of bleeding be modified?

It may help to discontinue drugs with antiplatelet effects (e.g. aspirin, NSAIDs). If this is not possible the NSAID could be substituted by a non-acetylated salicylate NSAID (e.g. diflunisal) or paracetamol, which do not interfere with platelet function.

Can the bleeding be prevented medically?

Tranexamic acid (500 mg q.i.d.) is an antifibrinolytic agent and ethamsylate (500 mg q.i.d.) is a haemostatic agent that inhibits the synthesis of prostaglandins that cause platelet disaggregation. Both appear effective in reducing blood loss in a number of conditions.

References

1 Irwin RS, Curley FJ, Bennett FM. Appropriate use of antitussives and protussives. A practical review. *Drugs* 1993; 46 (1): 80–91.
2 Gallan AM. Evaluation of nebulised acetylcysteine and normal saline in the treatment of sputum retention following thoracotomy. *Thorax* 1996; 51: 429–432.
3 Fuller RW, Karlsson JA, Choudry NB, Pride NB. Effect of inhaled and systemic

opiates on responses to inhaled capsaicin in humans. *J Appl Physiol* 1988; 65 (3): 1125–1130.

4 Twycross RG. Weak opioids. In: *Pain Relief in Advanced Cancer*. Edinburgh: Churchill Livingstone, 1994: 233–254.

5 Karlsson JA. Airway anaesthesia and the cough reflex. *Bull Eur Physiopathol Respir* 1987; 23 (Suppl. 10): 29–36.

6 Ahmedzai S. Palliation of respiratory symptoms. In: Doyle D, Hanks GWC, Macdonald N, eds. *Oxford Textbook of Palliative Medicine*. Oxford: Oxford Medical Publications, 1993: 349–378.

7 Simon PM, Schwartzstein RM, Weiss JW, Fencl V, Teghtsoonian M, Weinberger SE. Distinguishable types of dyspnea in patients with shortness of breath. *Am Rev Respir Dis* 1990; 142: 1009–1014.

8 Elliot MW, Adams L, Cockcroft A, MacRae KD, Murphy K, Guz A. The language of breathlessness: use of verbal descriptors by patients with cardiopulmonary disease. *Am Rev Respir Dis* 1991; 144: 826–832.

9 Reubin DB, Mor V. Dyspnea in terminally ill cancer patients. *Chest* 1986; 89: 234–236.

10 Groud S, Zech D, Diefenbach C, Bischoff A. Prevalence and pattern of symptoms in patients with cancer pain: a prospective evaluation of 1635 cancer patients referred to a pain clinic. *J Pain Symptom Manage* 1994; 9: 372–382.

11 Reubin DB, Mor V, Hiris J. Clinical symptoms and length of survival in patients with terminal cancer. *Arch Intern Med* 1988; 148: 1586–1591.

12 Morgan AD, Peck DF, Buchanan DR, McHardy GJR. Effect of attitudes and beliefs on exercise tolerance in chronic bronchitis. *BMJ* 1983; 286: 171–173.

13 Guyatt GH, Pugsley SO, Sullivan MJ *et al*. Effect of encouragement on walking test performance. *Thorax* 1984; 39: 818–822.

14 McCord M, Cronin-Stubbs C. Operationalizing dyspnoea: focus on measurement. *Heart Lung* 1992; 21: 167–179.

15 Carrieri VK, Janson-Bjerklie S. Strategies patients use to manage the sensation of dyspnea. *West J Nurs Res* 1986; 8: 284–305.

16 Heyse-Moore LH. On dyspnoea in advanced cancer. MD thesis; University of Southampton, 1993.

17 Brown ML, Carrieri V, Janson-Bjerklie Dodd MJ. Lung cancer and dyspnea: the patient's perception. *Oncol Nurs For* 1986; 13: 19–24.

18 Congelton J, Meurs MF. The incidence of airflow obstruction in bronchial carcinoma, its relation to breathlessness and response to bronchodilator therapy. *Respir Med* 1995; 89: 291–296.

19 Corner J, Plant H, Warner L. Developing a nursing approach to managing dyspnoea in lung cancer. *Int J Palliat Nurs* 1995; 1 (1): 5–11.

20 Shee CD. Palliation in chronic respiratory disease. *Palliat Med* 1995; 9 (1): 3–12.

21 Woodcock AA, Gross ER, Gellert A, Shah S, Johnson M, Geddes DM. Effects of dihydrocodeine, alcohol and caffeine on breathlessness and exercise tolerance in patients with chronic obstructive lung disease and normal blood gases. *N Engl J Med* 1981; 305: 1611–1616.

22 Johnson MA, Woodcock AA, Geddes DM. Dihydrocodeine for breathlessness in pink puffers. *BMJ* 1983; 2: 675–677.

23 Robin ED, Burke CM. Single-patient randomized clinical trial. Opiates for intractable dyspnea. *Chest* 1986; 90: 888–892.

24 Light RW, Muro JR, Sato RI, Stansbury DW, Fischer CE, Brown SE. Effects of oral morphine on breathlessness and exercise tolerance in patients with chronic obstructive airways disease. *Am Rev Respir Dis* 1989; 139: 126–133.

25 Woodcock AA, Johnson MA, Geddes DM. Breathlessness, alcohol and opiates (letter). *N Engl J Med* 1982; 306: 1363–1364.

26 Rice KL, Kronenberg RS, Hedemark LL, Niewoehner DE. Effects of chronic administration of codeine and promethazine on breathlessness and exercise tolerance in patients with chronic airflow obstruction. *Br J Dis Chest* 1987; 81: 287–292.

27 Giron AE, Stansbury DW, Fischer CE, Light RW. Lack of effect of dextromethorphan on breathlessness and exercise performance in patients with chronic obstructive pulmonary disease (COPD). *Eur Respir J* 1991; 4: 532–535.

28 Eiser N, Denman WT, West C, Luce P. Oral diamorphine: lack of effect on dyspnoea and exercise tolerance in the "pink puffer" syndrome. *Eur Respir J* 1991; 4: 926–931.

29 Bruera E, Macmillan K, Pither J, MacDonald RN. Effects of morphine on the dyspnea of terminal cancer patients. *J Pain Symptom Manage* 1990; 5: 341–344.

30 Bruera E, Maceachern T, Ripamonti C, Hanson J. Subcutaneous morphine for dyspnoea in cancer patients. *Ann Int Med* 1993; 119: 906–907.

31 Boyd K, Kelly M. Oral morphine for dyspnoea in cancer patients? [abstract]. *Prog in Pall Care* 1994; 210.

32 Leung R, Hill P, Burdon J. Effect of inhaled morphine on the development of breathlessness during exercise in patients with chronic lung disease. *Thorax* 1996; 51: 596–600.

33 Davis CL, Penn K, A'Hern R, Daniels J, Slevin M. Single dose randomised controlled trial of nebulised morphine in patients with cancer related breathlessness [abstract]. *Palliat Med* 1996; 10 (1): 64–65.

34 Young IH, Daviskas E, Keena VA. Effect of low dose nebulised morphine on exercise endurance in patients with chronic lung disease. *Thorax* 1989; 44: 387–390.

35 Bruera E, de Stoutz N, Velasco-Leiva A, Schoeller T, Hanson J. Effects of oxygen on dyspnoea in hypoxaemic terminal cancer patients. *Lancet* 1993; 342: 13–14.

36 Booth S, Kelly MJ, Cox NP, Adams L, Guz A. Does oxygen help dyspnea in patients with cancer? *Am J Respir Crit Care Med* 1996; 153: 1515–1518.

37 Clark TJH, Collins JV, Tong D. Respiratory depression caused by nitrazepam in patients with respiratory failure. *Lancet* 1971; 2: 737–738.

38 Kronenberg RS. Tranquilizers can be used safely in severe obstructive lung disease. *Clin Res* 1973; 21: 891.

39 McIver B, Walsh D, Nelson K. The use of chlorpromazine for symptom control in dying cancer patients. *J Pain Symptom Manage* 1994; 9 (5): 341–345.

40 Argyropoulou P, Patakas D, Koukou A, Vasi liadis P, Georgopoulos D. Buspirone effect on breathlessness and exercise performance in patients with chronic obstructive pulmonary disease. *Respiration* 1993; 60 (4): 216–20.

12: Managing Complications of Cancer

CHRISTINA FAULL AND RACHAEL BARTON

Introduction

Metastatic or advanced cancer may cause complications which require urgent intervention to palliate symptoms and either restore function or prevent deterioration. Although common, these complications are rarely seen by those working outside the field of oncology. Such complications often have a profound effect on a patient's functional ability and quality of life. It is important to identify early those who may benefit from specific treatment since a prompt referral allows the rapid palliation of symptoms and may prevent loss of function and independence. It is equally important to identify those patients who are in the terminal stage of their disease, and who may be helped more by symptomatic measures alone.

This chapter outlines the clinical problems most frequently encountered and gives management guidelines so the non-specialist may have confidence in dealing with what is often a frightening situation for both patient and carer.

Spinal cord compression

This requires early recognition and prompt referral. Restoration of sphincter and motor function is rarely possible for those who have lost it by the time they start treatment. Despite the development of cord compression being a poor prognostic sign, active management is indicated in all but very terminally ill patients.

Epidemiology

Spinal cord compression is common, affecting 5% of all cancer patients. In 8–47% it is the first presentation of cancer. It is particularly frequent in myeloma and lymphoma and in those cancers which metastasize readily to bone, i.e. breast, prostate, lung, and renal carcinomas, affecting up to 10% of all patients with these diseases. In children spinal cord compression is very rare but may occur with Ewing's sarcoma,

177

neuroblastoma, Hodgkin's disease, germ cell tumours, and soft tissue sarcomas [1].

Pathophysiology

Neurological dysfunction is caused by a combination of spinal cord oedema, ischaemia, and direct pressure. Of the total, 85–90% are due to compression of the cord by vertebral metastases, while 10% are due to compression from growth of a paraspinal mass into the spinal canal (commonly lymphoma). A small proportion are due to meningeal carcinomatosis in vertebral sites:
- thoracic: 70%;
- lumbar: 20%;
- cervical: 10%;
- multiple sites: 20%.

Metastatic disease is present in more than one vertebra in >70% of patients.

Diagnosis and early suspicion

Any patient with known vertebral metastases is at risk of spinal cord compression. A history of increasing back pain is the presenting symptom in 60–95% of patients. This may be localized axial pain but often a radicular pain develops. The pain may be worsened by coughing, sneezing, straining, movement, lying supine (patient may prefer to sleep sitting up), percussion over the vertebrae, or neck and hip flexion.

Muscle weakness generally occurs symmetrically in the proximal leg groups. Sensory loss may be in any modality, symmetrical in pattern or of Brown-Séquard type. Sphincter dysfunction occurs late except in compression of the cauda equina, with painless urinary retention and overflow and faecal incontinence.

The cardinal features of spinal cord compression are:
- pain;
- muscle weakness;
- sensory loss;
- abnormal reflexes;
- sphincter dysfunction.

Likewise, the cauda equina syndrome produces the following:
- sciatic pain;
- saddle anaesthesia;
- urine retention;

- loss of anal tone.

Once mobility or sphincter function are lost they are unlikely to be regained. More than 25% of patients develop paraplegia within 48 h of presentation and 50–65% develop paraplegia by 7 days; 10–20% develop paraplegia more slowly. Unfortunately 50% of people are already paraplegic by the time they are referred for treatment.

Treatment

IMMEDIATE TREATMENT

The patient diagnosed as suffering from spinal cord compression should be prescribed dexamethasone 8 mg immediately and 4 mg q.d.s. Suitable analgesia is instigated (see Chapter 9), using NSAIDs, opioids, and antispasmodics. Urgent referral to an oncologist or neurosurgeon for investigation and further management is vital.

SUBSEQUENT TREATMENT OPTIONS

Radiotherapy. Radiotherapy (RT) is the mainstay of treatment. It relieves pain, may prevent deterioration but will not restore function that is lost.

Surgery. Surgery may be indicated when the histology of the primary cancer is unknown; when there is limited disease with a good prognosis; when there is spinal instability causing pain; or when the tumour is radioresistant. An anterior (transabdominal) approach may provide better results than laminectomy [2].

Chemotherapy. Chemotherapy (CT) may be indicated for very chemo-sensitive tumours.

Rehabilitation and discharge planning

Many patients have a dramatic change in their functional ability and independence. The physiotherapist and occupational therapist play a key role in achieving maximum potential in function and independence. Patients may need to adapt to catheterization and faecal incontinence.

Patients and their carers may need:
- special equipment;
- adaptations to home or perhaps a new place of care;

- a large 'package' of social and health care including respite care;
- support in psychological adaptation to the life change and poor prognosis.

It is vital that the hospital team, primary health care team, social workers, community health professionals (occupational and physiotherapy), and community palliative care services are in close contact to plan and achieve optimum results.

Outcomes

FUNCTION

Functional outcome is influenced by several factors [3]. These include: the degree of neurological impairment at diagnosis, the tumour histology, the extent of myelographic block, the rapidity of development of neural compression and structural changes in the spine itself. Overall, 40% will walk again. However, 25% of patients relapse at the same site within 6 months and 50% relapse within a year.

SURVIVAL

Overall median survival is 7–10 months; 10% die within 1 month and 18–30% live for more than 1 year. Lung cancer carries a particularly poor prognosis, with a median survival of 2–3 months.

PLACE OF CARE

Many people who are paretic or paraplegic will be unable to be cared for at home and may require further care in a nursing home. If the prognosis is very short (i.e. short life expectancy) or there are particular physical, psychological or other problems then in-patient care in a palliative care unit may be appropriate.

Follow-up

These patients are at increased risk of further spinal cord compression since >70% will have other vertebral sites affected by metastatic disease. To continue to optimize function, pain control, and quality of life, regular follow-up in the community is vital.

Superior vena cava obstruction (SVCO)

In 50% of cases, SVCO is the first manifestation of disease so it is important to make the underlying diagnosis to determine treatment. Patients require urgent referral to a specialist centre. Although the symptoms are often uncomfortable, they are rarely life-threatening. Active treatment of SVCO may give good relief from distressing symptoms and is indicated in all but the frail, terminally ill patient who may be helped more by simple symptomatic measures alone.

Lung cancer causes 70% of cases of SVCO; lymphoma causes 8% of cases; and 10% are caused by other malignancies; 12% of cases have a non-malignant cause.

Pathophysiology

Malignant obstruction to blood flow usually results from extrinsic compression by tumour or lymph nodes although intracaval thrombus may complicate the extrinsic compression. Swelling of the face and arms results from elevation of venous pressure above the obstruction.

Diagnosis and early suspicion

Any patient known to have a primary lung tumour, especially right-sided, is at risk. The onset is usually insidious allowing collaterals to develop, visible as engorged subcutaneous veins. Two-thirds of patients complain of breathlessness and half of facial swelling or a feeling of fullness in the head. All symptoms and signs (see Box 12.1) may be exacerbated by bending forwards or lying down.

Management

The slow rate of onset usually allows collateral circulation to develop and unless oxygenation is severely compromised, the syndrome is rarely life-threatening. Urgent telephone referral should be made to a chest physician if there is no prior diagnosis, or to an oncologist if the patient has known malignant disease.

IMMEDIATE MEASURES

The patient is prescribed bed rest. Elevation of the bed head is helpful. Oxygen should be given a therapeutic trial and continued only if it gives

> **Box 12.1 Symptoms and signs of superior vena cava obstruction**
>
> *Symptoms*
> - Dyspnoea
> - Facial/arm swelling
> - Head fullness
> - Headache
> - Cough
> - Chest pain
> - Dysphagia
>
> *Physical signs*
> - Neck vein distension
> - Chest vein distension
> - Breathlessness
> - Plethora
> - Facial +/or conjunctival oedema
> - Central +/or peripheral cyanosis

symptomatic relief. Hypoxia, if present, is usually due to the underlying tumour.

The role of steroids is unproven. Dexamethasone 4 mg q.d.s. may help but should not be given 'blind' if the underlying diagnosis is not known. Rarely, high-grade mediastinal lymphoma may present as SVCO, in which case steroids may induce tumour lysis, threatening renal function and obscuring a histological diagnosis. Anticoagulants are not indicated routinely.

SUBSEQUENT TREATMENT

The aim of treatment is to relieve symptoms and, if possible, to cure the underlying process. Patients with SVCO who are otherwise well can be treated as out-patients.

Radiotherapy is the mainstay of treatment and can usually be completed in one to two weeks. Chemotherapy may be useful for some tumours. Radiological intervention with thrombolysis and/or stenting is occasionally indicated.

Symptomatic measures alone may provide some relief for terminally ill patients who are too unwell for active treatment. These include: steroids; raising the head of the bed; analgesia; antitussives; soft/liquid diet or trial of home oxygen.

Outcome

The average survival of a patient diagnosed with a malignant cause of SVCO is 8 months, but the prognosis depends on the underlying histology and stage of their disease [4]. Radiotherapy results in symptomatic improvement in up to 70% of patients within two weeks of starting treatment. Correction of venous pressure with stenting gives rapid relief in selected patients.

With chemotherapy, rapid resolution of symptoms within 7–10 days is seen in over 75% of patients with small cell lung cancer (SCLC) and in almost all patients with lymphoma.

In those patients with bronchial carcinoma who respond to treatment, 20% will relapse with SVCO. Those who do not respond have a short life expectancy.

Follow-up

During active treatment and until toxicity has settled, care should be centred on the specialist unit providing the treatment. Patients with incurable lung cancer are best followed by infrequent routine hospital visits with an 'SOS' option. Other effects of lung cancer are common, such as haemoptysis, pain, effusions, cough, cachexia, and metastases to bone or brain. The patient, family, palliative care and primary health care teams should all be made aware of likely symptoms and who to contact should they arise.

Brain metastases

In most cases brain metastases indicate a poor prognosis, but prompt diagnosis and treatment will often relieve symptoms and may restore function.

Metastases to the brain are a common problem in oncology, affecting 17–25% of the cancer population. They are common in cancers of the lung (26% of patients), breast (16%), kidney (13%), colon/rectum (5%), and in melanoma (4%).

Diagnosis and early suspicion

Patients with the sites of cancers given above are at particular risk but the diagnosis should be considered in all those with advanced cancer presenting any of the symptoms or signs listed in Table 12.1 [5].

Table 12.1 Frequencies of symptoms and signs associated with brain metastases.

Symptom	Frequency (%)	Sign	Frequency (%)
Headache	53	Cognitive impairment	77
Focal weakness	40	Hemiparesis	66
Confusion	30	Sensory loss	27
Ataxia	20	Papilloedema	26
Seizures	15	Ataxia	24
Visual disturbance	12	Aphasia	19
Speech abnormality	10		

Management

In some patients, the presence of cerebral metastases is a component of widely disseminated disease with consequent poor performance status and prognosis. The focus of management for this group of patients is general symptomatic care and consideration of psychosocial needs and place of care. For less unwell patients, more intrusive treatment is appropriate.

GENERAL SYMPTOMATIC MEASURES

Cerebral oedema and raised intracranial pressure is treated acutely with high-dose steroids: dexamethasone 8 mg immediately and 4 mg q.d.s. The first dose should be given parenterally if there is any chance that absorption will be poor. Occasionally steroids can induce distressing side effects (e.g. agitation). Intravenous mannitol may be needed rarely to reduce the intracranial pressure in a patient whose condition is worsening rapidly.

Seizures are often controlled once the intracranial pressure is reduced but some patients require anticonvulsant drugs. The terminally ill patient with cerebral metastases and uncontrolled fitting may require rectal or infusional benzodiazepines (see Chapter 20). The nausea and vomiting of raised intracranial pressure respond best to measures which reduce pressure, but antiemetics (e.g. cyclizine 50 mg t.d.s.) may be required and may need to be given parenterally or rectally at first.

Headache is very common and may be helped by steroids and analgesics. An NSAID and/or codeine phosphate given regularly is often helpful but occasionally stronger analgesia may be required. Confused, agitated, or psychotic patients may require sedative medications.

SPECIFIC TREATMENT OPTIONS

Radiotherapy

This is the most commonly used treatment. Treatment is usually given over 2 or 5 days to the whole brain [6]. No complex planning is needed and the treatment is well tolerated. Steroids are continued throughout the treatment but are tailed off once it is complete, typically reducing the dose by 25% every 3–5 days. If the clinical condition deteriorates when steroids are withdrawn, they should be restarted and tailed more slowly.

In selected patients with a good prognosis, stereotactically guided radiotherapy may be used for solitary brain metastases not amenable to surgery [7].

Toxicity. Various side-effects may follow radiotherapy. Total scalp alopecia is usual. The hair regrows although it often remains thin. Headache may occur during treatment and often responds to simple analgesia or to an increase in steroid dose. Radiotherapy may induce some increase in cerebral oedema and symptoms may transiently worsen, requiring an increase in steroid administration. This may be particularly apparent in neurologically compact areas such as the brainstem. Rarely, dementia develops in long-term survivors and necrosis of treated brain may occur, presenting with similar features to relapsed disease.

Chemotherapy

Chemotherapy is useful for some tumours which are chemosensitive, such as SCLC.

Surgery

Surgery is most commonly carried out where there is diagnostic uncertainty. It may be considered appropriate in highly selected patients with known metastatic cancer, a solitary brain metastasis, and a good prognosis. Surgery may also be considered if symptoms persist from a metastasis which has proved resistant to other treatment.

Rehabilitation and discharge planning

Many patients with brain metastases have a dramatic change in their functional ability, independence, and personality. Many of their rehabilitation needs are similar to those outlined for patients with spinal cord compression. In addition some patients will need the help of speech therapy and communication experts, while others may need advice on feeding and may require nasogastric or gastrostomy feeding. There is a need for psychological support for the patient and their carers, particularly for patients with personality change and cognitive impairment.

Outcomes

FUNCTION

Following radiotherapy, 60–80% of patients will show functional and sensory improvement and reduction in headache and confusion [8]. A complete response (i.e. a complete resolution of symptoms and signs of brain metastases) will occur in 35–55% of patients, but many have significant residual disability.

SURVIVAL

The median survival for various treatments is shown in Table 12.2. Twenty percent of patients will fail to complete a course of radiotherapy because of deterioration. The benefit of radiotherapy is relatively short lived: up to 50% of those surviving for 6 months will relapse in the brain. Box 12.2 summarizes the factors that may improve or reduce survival.

PLACE OF CARE

Many patients will be unable to be cared for at home because of loss of independence in activities of daily living, nursing care needs, and cognitive impairment. Changes in cognitive function in particular make care at home problematic and distressing to relatives.

Table 12.2 Effect of treatment on median survival in patients with brain metastases.

Treatment	Median survival
None	1–2 months
Steroids	10 weeks
Steroids and radiotherapy	3–6 months
Re-irradiation	5 months
Surgery	8–9 months

Box 12.2 Factors affecting survival in patients with brain metastases

Factors that improve survival
• Brain as first site of relapse of disease
• Long disease-free interval prior to relapse
• Primary site breast
• Early response to radiation

Factors that reduce survival
• Multiple lobes involved
• Meningeal disease

The short life expectancy, complex physical and psychological needs, and carer distress often make in-patient palliative care more appropriate than nursing home placement, but patient and carer preference and geographical factors, as well as needs, will influence this.

Follow-up

Relapse of brain metastases is common and close follow-up in the community is essential. Patients with a good prognosis and limited disease may be helped by further specific treatment. Those with a poor outlook and progressive systemic disease without a valid treatment option will be helped more by symptomatic measures alone.

Metabolic emergencies

Hypercalcaemia

Hypercalcaemia is the commonest metabolic emergency associated with cancer and is usually but not always associated with widespread bone involvement (80%). The outlook for patients with tumour-induced hypercalcaemia is poor, but prompt active treatment may relieve symptoms rapidly with minimal toxicity. Specific therapy with rehydration and bisphosphonates should be offered in all but the very frail, terminally ill patient in whom hypercalcaemia is a terminal event and who may be helped more by simple symptomatic measures.

Hypercalcaemia is common in breast cancer and myeloma, affecting up to 50% of patients with these diseases. It is also common in carcinoma of the lung, kidney, cervix, and head and neck [9].

PATHOPHYSIOLOGY

Tumour-induced hypercalcaemia results from the action of various factors released from, or induced by the tumour. This is most commonly parathyroid hormone-related protein (PTH-RP), which acts to increase both the reabsorption of calcium from bone and its renal tubular reabsorption. Other substances which may act locally on bone to increase the mobilization of calcium include prostaglandins and cytokines.

Hypercalcaemia induces vomiting and an osmotic diuresis leading to polyuria and dehydration. The resultant hypovolaemia compromises renal function, which further escalates calcium levels. The action of a raised serum calcium concentration on smooth muscle and the CNS leads to the characteristic symptoms of constipation and confusion and nausea.

DIAGNOSIS AND EARLY SUSPICION

The diagnosis should be considered in any patient with advanced cancer who becomes unwell. Bony metastases are usually but not always associated. Onset is often gradual and the symptoms are non-specific, often mimicking the general debility of a patient with advanced cancer (see Box 12.3).

Investigations

Serum calcium, renal function, and albumin should be checked. The serum calcium should be corrected for the serum albumin concentration (the precise formula will depend on the units in which the calcium and albumin are measured; details should be sought from the local biochemistry laboratory):

corrected calcium (mmol/l) = measured calcium (mmol/l) + [40 − albumin (g/l)] × 0.02

Uncontrolled diabetes mellitus should be excluded concurrently as the clinical features are similar.

MANAGEMENT

The urgency of treatment is dictated by symptoms rather than serum calcium concentration. For patients at home with mild symptoms suggestive of hypercalcaemia the results of blood tests should be established within 48h. Definitive treatment should be started as soon as possible

---

Box 12.3 Clinical features of hypercalcaemia

General
- Thirst
- Polyuria
- Polydipsia
- Dehydration
- Weight loss
- Anorexia
- Lethargy
- Fatigue

Neurological
- Confusion
- Psychosis
- Coma

Gastrointestinal
- Nausea/vomiting
- Constipation
- Peptic ulceration
- Pruritus

Cardiac
- Bradycardia
- Arrhythmias

---

as the metabolic disturbance may worsen rapidly. Patients with serum calcium >3.5 mmol/l, even if well should be admitted within 24 h.

A patient with cancer who becomes unwell with suspected hypercalcaemia should be admitted urgently under the oncology or medical team for investigation and treatment. Many hospices will have facilities for treatment of patients who have more advanced disease and recurrent hypercalcaemia. The admission should be discussed with palliative care and oncology teams and with the patient to ensure the most appropriate place of treatment.

Immediate treatment

Rehydration is the first requirement. Oral fluids are encouraged and intravenous normal saline is infused at a rate determined by the clinical condition. Drugs that inhibit urinary calcium excretion or decrease renal blood flow should be stopped (e.g. thiazide diuretics, NSAIDs).

High-dose steroids are of limited use and should be used with caution in elderly patients undergoing vigorous rehydration who are at risk of heart failure. Steroids should not be used 'blind' if the underlying diagnosis is unknown. High-grade lymphomas may rarely present with hyper-calcaemia and treatment with steroids may cause tumour lysis precipitating renal failure and obscuring the histological diagnosis.

Symptom control

Rehydration alone may be sufficient to relieve many of the symptoms. Analgesia may be required for the pain of bony metastases or abdominal symptoms. The constipation and nausea associated with hypercalcaemia are often severe and should be treated vigorously (see Chapter 10).

Specific treatment of hypercalcaemia

Intravenous bisphosphonates are the mainstay of the treatment of cancer-induced hypercalcaemia [10]. The serum calcium concentration begins to fall within 24 h, with nadir after 3–4 days. Symptom improvement may lag behind biochemical improvement.

Oral formulations of the bisphosphonate clodronate are licensed for the maintenance of normocalcaemia after the correction of hypercalcaemia. It has been shown to reduce the incidence of subsequent episodes of hypercalcaemia in myeloma and breast cancer.

Specific treatment of the underlying cancer

Unless treatment is directed at the underlying problem, hypercalcaemia will recur. In patients for whom there is a therapeutic option, specific anticancer treatment such as chemotherapy or hormonal therapy should be started as soon as the clinical condition allows. Rarely tamoxifen may induce hypercalcaemia in patients with bony metastases from breast cancer.

OUTCOME

With the exception of myeloma the prognosis for most patients with cancer-induced hypercalcaemia is very poor. If an anticancer treatment is available the median survival is 3 months, otherwise it is only 1 month.

Similarly, if the patient becomes normocalcaemic with the administration of bisphosphonates the median survival is 7–8 weeks; if not, it is less than 3 weeks.

Hypercalcaemia in patients with myeloma indicates stage III disease, which has a median survival of up to 2 years.

Follow-up

Expectant, close follow-up at home is vital as hypercalcaemia commonly recurs. It is often a preterminal or terminal event and further admission to a hospice or hospital oncology unit should be discussed with the teams involved. The symptoms of patients not treated with bisphosphonates can be managed at home if the carers are well supported by community nurses.

Obstructive nephropathy

Pelvic malignancies predispose to the development of ureteric obstruction. If left untreated, progressive disease will lead to acute or chronic renal failure, which will ultimately prove fatal. Relief of the ureteric obstruction by nephrostomy or stenting is a relatively simple procedure with good resolution of symptoms in most patients. However, if renal failure is relieved, many patients must continue to bear the burden of suffering arising from the disease processes leading to death. This gives rise to a dilemma commonly encountered in palliative care: *is relief of the obstruction, and therefore prolongation of life, in the patient's best interests?* Consequently, discussion with the patient and their informed consent are crucial but this is often very difficult if this issue is only raised when the need for treatment has become urgent.

Of patients presenting with acute renal failure secondary to bilateral ureteric obstruction, two-thirds will have underlying malignant disease. For half of these it will be their first manifestation of disease [11]. This is particularly common in cancers of the cervix and bladder.

DIAGNOSIS AND EARLY SUSPICION

Obstruction of a single kidney is often not noticed unless imaging of the abdomen takes place. Once the second kidney becomes involved, the clinical features of obstructive nephropathy become evident (see Box 12.4). As with hypercalcaemia, the features are non-specific unless anuria occurs and may mimic the general debility of a patient with advanced cancer.

Box 12.4 Clinical features of obstructive nephropathy

- Anorexia
- Anuria/oliguria
- Bleeding tendency
- Cardiac arrhythmias
- Confusion
- Drug toxicity
- Hypertension
- Myoclonic jerks
- Nausea
- Oedema
- Susceptibility to infection
- Vomiting

Investigations

Both blood urea and creatinine are usually raised in obstructive nephropathy and potassium may also be raised. Ultrasound and/or computed tomography (CT) scan examination of the renal tracts and pelvis will usually be able to confirm obstruction to renal outflow with dilation of the renal pelvis and may be able to demonstrate the cause of the obstruction.

MANAGEMENT

If appropriate, the obstruction needs to be relieved promptly before irreversible damage is caused to the kidneys. Acute management of the associated hyperkalaemia, metabolic acidosis, and fluid overload may be necessary if the deterioration in renal function has been rapid.

Symptomatic measures

Hydration should aim to replace losses and prevent thirst while avoiding fluid overload and the distressing features of pulmonary oedema. All drugs should be used with caution in renal failure (see *British National Formulary*, Appendix 3). Haloperidol 1.5–5 mg o.d.–t.d.s. orally or 5–20 mg/24 h by subcutaneous infusion will help control nausea, myoclonic jerks, confusion, and agitation.

Pain from hydronephrosis and other aspects of the malignant disease may require strong opioids. Morphine and many other opioids accumulate in renal failure and should be used with longer dosing intervals and daily review. Fentanyl has little renal excretion and accumulates less in renal failure than other opioids.

Haemorrhage

There are several reasons why a patient with cancer may haemorrhage including:
- bleeding directly from tumour or metastases;
- invasion of tumour into blood vessels;
- bleeding tendency:
  thrombocytopenia (sometimes as a result of anticancer treatment);
  disseminated intravascular coagulation;
  uraemia;
  anticoagulants.
- bleeding from post-radiotherapy telangiectasia (especially bladder and gastrointestinal tract).

The management of massive, terminal haemorrhage is discussed in Chapter 20.

Management of bleeding directly from tumour

RADIOTHERAPY

Palliative radiotherapy to control bleeding is usually restricted to a short course of treatment with few planning stages. A typical course lasts 1–3 weeks. Radiotherapy is useful for bleeding skin metastases but locally recurrent breast cancer usually occurs in skin which has already received radiotherapy to tolerance doses. Advice should be sought from the treating radiotherapist.

Haemoptysis responds well to radiotherapy (see Chapter 11).

Previous radical radiotherapy to the pelvis usually rules out further treatment to a bleeding central pelvic lesion but this is not always so and the advice of a radiotherapist should be sought in individual cases.

Symptomatic measures

Drugs which decrease the tendency to bleed may be helpful: for example, tranexamic acid 500 mg q.d.s. or ethamsylate 500 mg q.d.s. Mucosal bleeding may be reduced by using 1% alum as a bladder irrigation or enema. Tranexamic [acid] enema (5 g in 50 ml water twice daily or 1–2 g mixed with KY jelly) may reduce bleeding from rectal tumours. The application of adrenaline-soaked swabs (1 : 1000), alginate dressings, and sucralfate paste (in KY jelly) may reduce capillary bleeding. Oral or rectal sucralfate (1 g b.d.–q.d.s.) may stop bleeding from oesophageal, gastric, or rectal tumours, respectively.

Itch

Itching, or a sensation that produces a desire to scratch and is a problem for many patients with cancer. It can cause profound debility as it prevents sleep and leads to painful excoriation of skin. It is associated with various conditions.
• Blood disorders: lymphoma (itch may be the presenting feature of Hodgkin's disease); leukaemia; polycythaemia rubra vera.
• Iron deficiency.
• Cholestatic jaundice.
• Uraemia.
• Allergens causing eczema and contact dermatitis.
• Drugs: opioids (histamine release); chlorpromazine (cholestasis).
• Skin infections and infestations:
  scabies;
  fungal infection.
• Advanced cancer.

Pathophysiology

Irritant substances in the skin stimulate receptors of unmyelinated nerve fibres (C fibres). The chemical irritant may be histamine, tissue proteinases, prostaglandins, or bile acids.

Management

If possible the underlying cause should be addressed. There are no specific antipruritic drugs.

GENERAL MEASURES

Various simple measures can be taken to reduce itching. For example, the patient should, as far as possible, avoid: friction from rough clothing and bed linen, overheating, vasodilators and soap which drys the skin. Scratching only exacerbates the itchiness.

Cooling and moistening the skin with moisturizers and emollients is helpful, for example menthol 0.25–1% in aqueous cream. Cucumber is soothing but may be impractical if the itch is generalized. Calamine lotion may overdry the skin.

Oral antihistamine in the form of a sedative preparation may be useful at night (e.g. chlorpheniramine 4 mg). A less sedative preparation is used in the day (e.g. terfenadine 120 mg daily).

A trial of oral corticosteroids may be of value in some patients, particularly those with lymphoma or with bile duct obstruction due to tumour or lymph node. NSAIDs are helpful in some patients, presumably where prostaglandins play a role in the pathophysiology. They are particularly helpful for the itch of cutaneous tumour infiltration.

A hypnotic may be helpful.

OTHER MEASURES

Various treatments can reduce itch in certain conditions. For instance, cimetidine may be helpful in Hodgkin's disease, whereas erythropoietin is very helpful for the itch of chronic uraemia, although its place in treating itch of other aetiology is, as yet, unknown.

Cholestyramine if tolerated (4–8 g daily), colestipol (5–10 g daily), stanozolol (5–10 mg daily), and rifampicin (300–600 mg daily) may all be useful for the itch associated with cholestasis.

$5HT_3$ antagonists such as ondansetron and granisetron have been found to be effective for itch associated with cholestatic jaundice of advanced cancer and of non-malignant origin. Acupuncture may also be helpful in treating itch.

Fever and sweating

Patients with cancer and other serious illnesses are vulnerable to the troublesome symptoms of fever and sweating. The two are related but sweating may occur without fever. These symptoms are generally distressing to patients and can result in fatigue, drowsiness, and confusion. The aetiology can be related directly to the tumour (neoplastic fever) or secondary to co-morbidity (e.g. infective process). Neoplastic fever is experienced by 0.7–60% of patients [12]. Both fever and sweating are more common in patients with Hodgkin's disease, leukaemia, and tumours with liver metastases.

Management

Although it is inappropriate within a palliative care setting exhaustively to investigate patients with fever and sweats, it is important to consider the differential diagnoses which may aid appropriate treatment.
- Infection. Look for common foci of infection (e.g. chest, urine, upper respiratory tract, pressure sores, tumour site). Be especially cautious in patients who are susceptible to neutropenia (e.g. chemotherapy, marrow invasion). Fever may not occur if patients are on steroids.
- Neoplastic fever.
- Treatment related. Certain chemotherapeutic agents produce fever (e.g. bleomycin), as can blood transfusion.
- Hormonal (e.g. thyrotoxicosis and menopause).
- Anxiety.
- Physiological (secondary to environmental conditions).

In many cases it is necessary to resort to general measures to provide relief. Paramount among these is a high standard of nursing care, including: the provision of a fan, sponging and regular washing and encouraging oral fluids. The effectiveness of paracetamol may be reduced in neoplastic fever. Other options include aspirin, NSAIDs [13] and thioridazine [14]. High-dose steroids have a role in chronic lymphatic leukaemia.

Side-effects of palliative oncology treatments

Severe side-effects of chemotherapy and radiotherapy weigh heavily in the cost-benefit analysis of palliative interventions. It is important for the patient, the health care teams, and the carers to know what effects are likely, how long they may last and what can be done to alleviate them. Late side-effects of palliative treatments are rarely a concern.

Gastrointestinal system

PROBLEMS OF THE MOUTH, OROPHARYNX, AND OESOPHAGUS

Oral mucositis is most common with radiotherapy to head and neck tumours, whereas oesophageal mucositis is seen with radiotherapy to the mediastinum or neck. Reactions begin 1–2 weeks after the start of treatment and continue for the same period after completion. Chemotherapy often temporarily affects taste and may give a mild to moderate mucositis.

Management of dry or sore mouth

Several steps can be taken to ease the discomfort of a dry or sore mouth. The first is for the patient to avoid agents that exacerbate the problem, such as smoking, spicy foods, and undiluted spirits. The second is the observance of basic oral hygiene: rinse and gargle with 0.9% saline after each meal; clean the teeth thoroughly with a soft brush; use a mouthwash (e.g. thymol or chlorhexidine) two to four times a day.

For analgesia use the following: benzydamine oral rinse 15 ml 3–6 hourly; plus soluble aspirin 300 mg in 5 ml mucilage q.d.s.; rinse and swallow (if not contraindicated) before meals. Dry or sore lip scan be soothed with soft yellow paraffin (avoid before radiotherapy if lips in field).

Management of ulceration, severe pain and difficulty in swallowing

These distressing symptoms can be treated in several ways. The patient should observe basic oral hygiene, as outlined above and consume soft foods. Typical medication could consist of: dilute benzydamine mouthwash (1 : 2) 1–3 hourly; mucaine 10 ml before meals; sucralfate suspension 1 g before meals (coats raw mucosa). Consider the use of an antifungal, for example nystatin suspension 1 ml q.d.s. or fluconazole 50 mg o.d. Also consider oral acyclovir if the ulcers are very painful—herpes simplex sometimes becomes activated in these cases.

To determine the most appropriate oral analgesics consult the WHO analgesic ladder (see Chapter 9). Assess the patient's nutritional state and consider temporary tube feeding (see Chapter 15).

NAUSEA AND VOMITING (see also Chapter 10)

Nausea and vomiting are worsened by anxiety about cancer, the treatment, and its side-effects so reassurance is important.

Highly emetogenic chemotherapy

Nausea and vomiting usually occur in the first 24–72 hours post-chemotherapy. They can be managed by administering a $5HT_3$ antagonist plus dexamethasone intravenously pre-chemotherapy, followed by metoclopramide 10 mg p.o. q.d.s. (domperidone if extrapyramidal side-effects) plus dexamethasone 2 mg p.o. t.d.s. for 3 days afterwards.

Less emetogenic chemotherapy

In situations where chemotherapy is likely to cause less severe nausea and vomiting, management employs oral or rectal antiemetics, for example cyclizine 50 mg t.d.s. or metoclopramide 10 mg t.d.s. Rarely, 5HT$_3$ antagonists are required.

Radiotherapy

Nausea and vomiting can follow radiotherapy, especially if the stomach or liver is in the treatment field. The symptoms usually occur acutely after each treatment and remit once treatment is complete. Vomiting may be a side-effect of radiotherapy to the brain.

For managing the symptoms, oral antiemetics usually suffice, for example cyclizine 50 mg t.d.s. or haloperidol 1.5 mg b.d.

PROBLEMS OF THE LOWER BOWEL

Diarrhoea

Diarrhoea is common with pelvic or abdominal radiotherapy. It often begins in the second week of radiotherapy and lasts 1–2 weeks after completion.

Management involves: a low-fibre diet (special advice is required for vegetarians); loperamide titrated to effect (suggested maximum 16 mg/day); codeine phosphate 30–60 mg b.d.–q.d.s. (if the patient is not already receiving a strong opioid). Oral rehydration usually suffices.

Proctitis

Proctitis is common with pelvic radiotherapy. The timing of occurrence is the same as for diarrhoea (see above). Rectal bleeding may occur.

Management involves the use of Anusol or other soothing suppositories p.r.n., or suppositories with steroid and/or local anaesthetic. If symptoms are more severe, steroid foam enemas may be used. Rarely, surgery may be needed for the prolonged (>6 months) side-effect of rectal bleeding, but this is hazardous as healing is poor.

Skin

Skin reactions are common with high-dose radiotherapy [15]. Moist regions with opposed skin surfaces, such as the perineum or inframammary fold, are particularly affected. Reactions occur 1–2 weeks after the start of radiotherapy and take approximately the same time to heal.

The skin is less commonly affected by chemotherapy. Discoloration, erythema, and peeling of the palms and soles are sometimes seen.

ERYTHEMA, SORENESS, AND ITCHING

Several steps can be taken to reduce erythema, soreness, and itching.
• Protect from friction, e.g. from tight clothing, straps, etc.
• Avoid strong sunlight, hot baths, wet shaving or brisk towelling, cosmetics, deodorants, adhesive plasters, and perfumed soaps or creams.
• Wash with warm water and pat dry with a soft towel; air dry if possible.
• Skin may be soothed with Unguentum Merck, E45, or 1% hydrocortisone cream applied sparingly. Avoid hydrocortisone cream in the genital area.
• Baby talc or sodium bicarbonate solution (1 teaspoon in a cup of warm water) applied to the skin may help itching.

DESQUAMATION

Dry desquamation is the dry, flaking skin seen with radiotherapy. The management is as for erythema. Moist desquamation is painful ulceration with exposed dermis and oozing of serum. It is seen after three or more weeks of radiotherapy where there has not been healing of the basal layer of the epidermis. It is most common in moist skin folds. Re-epithelialization usually occurs within 2–3 weeks of completing radiotherapy. Management consists of easing pain, reducing exudate, and preventing infection while healing takes place. Crystal violet paint can be used on all moist areas, including the genitals, where it dries skin and eases pain while acting as a local antiseptic. Proflavine lotion or cream is preferred by some as crystal violet stains clothes heavily. Silver sulphadiazine cream may be helpful. Occlusive dressings should be avoided.

Other side-effects

HAIR LOSS

Temporary hair loss is a variable feature of many chemotherapy regimes. Radiotherapy will also provoke patchy hair loss. The psychological impact should not be underestimated, and wigs and camouflage should be introduced pretreatment.

MARROW SUPPRESSION

Patients with advanced cancer may have reduced bone marrow reserve making further radiotherapy and chemotherapy more toxic with consequent anaemia, thrombocytopenia, and neutropenia. Symptoms of anaemia and bleeding may be managed by transfusion. Neutropenia predisposes to overwhelming bacterial sepsis, particularly when the absolute neutrophil count is less than $1 \times 10^9/l$.

Neutropenic sepsis requires urgent specialist in-patient treatment with intravenous antibiotics. Urgent admission to the treating oncology unit should be arranged for assessment of any patient on chemotherapy who develops symptoms or signs of sepsis, particularly: sore throat, fever >38°C, rigors, cough productive of purulent sputum, or shock.

References

1 Klein SL, Sandford RA, Muhlbower MS. Paediatric spinal epidural metastases. *J Neurosurg* 1991; 74: 70–75.
2 Kramer JA. Spinal cord compression in malignancy. *Palliat Med* 1992; 6: 202–211.
3 Findlay GFG. Adverse effects of the management of malignant spinal cord compression. *J Neurol Neurosurg Psych* 1984; 47: 761–768.
4 Yahalom J. Superior vena cava syndrome. In: DeVita VT Jr, Hellman S, Rosenberg SA, eds. *Cancer Principles and Practice of Oncology*, 4th edn. Philadelphia: J.B. Lippincott, 1993: 2111–2118.
5 Wright DC, Delaney TF, Buckner JC. Treatment of metastatic cancer to the brain. In: DeVita VT Jr, Hellman S, Rosenberg SA, eds. *Cancer Principles and Practice of Oncology*, 4th edn. Philadelphia: J.B. Lippincott, 1993: 2170–2186.
6 Priestman T, Brada M, Dunn J, Rampling R. Final results of the Royal College of Radiologists trial comparing 2 different radiotherapy schedules in the treatment of cerebral metastases. *Br J Cancer* 1996; 74 (S28): 19.
7 Wurm RE, Warrington A, Shepherd S, Sardell S, Hines F, Brada M. Stereotaxic radiation-therapy for solitary brain metastases as an alternative to surgery. *Radiology* 1995; 197 (SS): 264.
8 Borgelt B, Gelber R, Kramer S *et al.* The palliation of brain metastases: final results of the first two studies by the Radiation Therapy Oncology Group. *Int J Radiother Oncol Biol Phys* 1980; 6: 1–9.
9 Ling PJ, A'Hern RP, Hardy JR. Analysis of survival following treatment of tumour-induced hypercalcaemia with intravenous pamidronate (APD). *Br J Cancer* 1995; 72: 206–209.
10 Ralston SH, Gallacher SJ, Patel U *et al.* Comparison of three intravenous bisphosphonates in cancer-associated hypercalcaemia. *Lancet* 1989; ii: 1180–1182.

11 Watkinson AF, A'Hern RP, Jones A, King DM, Moskovic EC. The role of percutaneous nephrostomy in malignant urinary tract obstruction. *Clin Radiol* 1993; 47: 32–35.

12 Johnson M. Neoplastic fever. *Palliat Med* 1996; 10: 217–224.

13 Tsvaris N, Zinelis A, Karabelis A. A randomised trial of the effect of three non-steroidal anti-inflammatory agents in ameliorating cancer induced fever. *J Intern Med* 1990; 228: 451–455.

14 Regnard C. Use of low dose thioridazine to control sweating in advanced cancer. *Palliat Med* 1996; 10: 78–79.

15 Sitton E. Early and late radiation-induced skin alterations. Part 1: mechanisms of skin changes. *Oncol Nurs For* 1992; 19 (5): 801–807.

13: Palliative Care for People with Acquired Immune Deficiency Syndrome (AIDS)

GWYNETH JONES, CHRISTINA FAULL
AND YVONNE CARTER

Introduction

There are many issues in the management of patients dying with AIDS-related illness that concern not only the disease but also society's attitudes to the illness, and moral perceptions of risk factors for infection. Since 1981 more than 1.3 million cases of AIDS have been reported from 193 countries. By the turn of the millennium it is estimated there will be 26 million men, women, and children infected with the human immuno-deficiency virus (HIV) most of whom will be living in developing countries. Whilst there is hope that new combinations of antiretroviral therapies will transform HIV from a lethal pandemic to a chronic, manageable illness, for many patients these will come too late or only delay death, while millions of others can never hope to have access to such expensive treatments. The provision of good palliative care is, and will remain, a major facet of care for the majority of patients.

Many patients with HIV and AIDS choose to receive much of their care from hospitals, and the primary care team may have very little involvement with the patient until the end of their illness. Issues about safety and control of infection are included in the Appendix (see p. 223).

Prognosis and the transition to palliative care

Life expectancy for patients with AIDS in the developed world has improved over the last decade from a median survival time of 6 months to over 2 years. The clinical course is very variable but is influenced by the nature of the AIDS-defining illness and tolerance of different treatment regimens as medical complications accumulate.

It is perhaps more difficult in AIDS than in other terminal illness to determine when the emphasis of care should turn towards palliating symptoms rather than pursuing investigations and curative treatment regimens. The average age of the patient is much younger than for most malignant conditions. Many can battle through numerous opportunistic infections, each potentially life threatening, before the cumulated toll leads to progressive cachexia, development of HIV-related malignancy, or features of dementia. Undoubtedly, the best control of many physical symptoms is often achieved by drugs specific for an underlying infective agent (Table 13.1). Boosting the immune status with new antiretroviral regimens may reduce the development of further opportunistic infections and other AIDS-defining events and can also improve chronic but distressing conditions. Thus even in very advanced disease patients continue to take many, often unusual medications (Table 13.1). Frank discussion with the patient will often clarify the most appropriate course but they must be guided in their expectations, particularly in situations when significant improvement is unlikely. Certain conditions are associated with a particularly poor prognosis (Table 13.2) and likelihood of death in less than six months. This should prompt a change in focus with more consideration of quality of life, palliating symptoms, and anticipating the individual's and carer's terminal care needs.

Epidemiology

The global epidemiology of HIV has been changing over the last 15 years, with rates of infection stabilizing or falling in 'high-risk' groups but with an explosion into the heterosexual population in Africa and more recently Asia.

England, Wales, and Scotland

In England and Wales in 1995 the largest proportional increase in new cases occurred in the heterosexual population, and experience from Africa and the USA would suggest that this trend will continue.

The place of death of people with AIDS is not nationally collated. It is probable that the majority of patients die in hospital or a hospice.

General palliative care issues

Following progression to AIDS patients may benefit from greater practical and emotional support at home as mobility, strength, and often vision deteriorate making activities of daily living more difficult. A great number of agencies may be involved with this including the specialist palliative care services (see 'Useful Addresses', pp. 377–381).

Table 13.1 Antimicrobial drugs which are commonly used for symptom control in advanced AIDS.

Target organism	Drug	Prescribing order	Target symptom
HIV	Antiretrovirals		
	RTI zidovudine (AZT)	200 mg t.d.s oral	Dementia, neuropathy
	RTI didanosine (ddI)	125–200 mg b.d.s oral	Immune status
	RTI zalcitabine (ddc)	0.75 mg t.d.s oral	Immune status
	RTI lamuvidine (3TC)	150 mg b.d.s oral	Immune status
	RTI stavudine (d4T)	20 mg b.d.s oral	Immune statue
	PI ritonavir	600 mg b.d.s oral	Immune status
	PI saquinavir	600 mg t.d.s oral	Immune status
	PI indinavir	800 mg t.d.s oral	Immune status
Pneumocystis carinii	co-trimoxazole	960 mg o.d oral	Dyspnoea, fever
	or pentamidine	300 mg monthly nebulized	
	or dapsone	50–100 mg o.d oral	
Toxoplasma	pyrimethamine	25 mg o.d oral	Headache, features of space
	folinic acid	15 mg o.d oral	occupying lesion
	and clindamycin	450 mg t.d.s oral	
	or sulphadiazine	1 g t.d.s oral	

CMV	ganciclovir or foscarnet	5 mg/kg 5 days/week i.v. 900 mg/kg daily i.v.	Blindness, fever, headache
Herpes	aciclovir	400 mg b.d.s oral	Recurrent lesions, pain
Candida	fluconazole or itraconazole	50–200 mg o.d oral 100–200 mg o.d oral	Sore mouth, dysphagia
Atypical mycobacteria (*numerous regimens*) (*combining 3–4 drugs*)	rifabutin clarithromycin azithromycin ethambutol ciprofloxacin clofazimine	300–450 mg o.d oral 500 mg b.d.s oral 1 g weekly oral 15 mg/kg o.d oral 750 mg b.d.s oral 100 mg o.d oral	Fever, sweats, diarrhoea, weight loss, anaemia, abdominal pain, fatigue

* Multiple drug regimens increase likelihood of serious interactions.

Table 13.2 AIDS related conditions associated with a prognosis of less than six months.

Advanced AIDS dementia
Blindness from bilateral retinitis
Extensive pulmonary Kaposi sarcoma
Refractory wasting syndrome
Multiple concurrent opportunistic infections
Relapsed refractory HIV-related lymphoma

Management of common physical symptoms

Many of the symptoms in advanced AIDS are similar to those of advanced cancer and other terminal illnesses (Table 13.3). The principles of symptom control are identical to other diseases. Understanding the likely pathophysiology allows selection of the most appropriate management. Ideally, treatment should be holistic, tailored to the individual with frequent review of benefits, side-effects, and patient's wishes.

Many treatments have been extrapolated from their use in patients with advanced cancer and have been found to be effective. Unfortunately

Table 13.3 Common physical symptoms in AIDS [1].

Symptom	Patients (%)
Pain	60
Neuropathic	22
Pressure sore	12
Visceral	10
Headaches	8
Epigastric/retrosternal	7
Joint	7
Myopathic	5
Ano-rectal	4
General debility	61
Anorexia	41
Nausea	21
Confusion	29
Diarrhoea	18
Dyspnoea	11

studies continue to show that pain is considerably underestimated by clinicians, and consequently undertreated [2,3]. The management of pain and other symptoms is discussed in depth in other chapters of this book.

Psychosocial issues specific to AIDS

Many patients with HIV are greatly concerned that their diagnosis may become public knowledge and often fear the repercussions that this may have for them, their family members, and friends. Professional staff should enquire who has been informed of the diagnosis and make no assumptions. Written and verbal communications with the patient, family, friends, and other professionals should be sensitive and discreet. For some patients there is additional concern that their family should not be aware of their sexuality.

Homosexual men and drug users have often cared for friends or partners who have died from HIV-related illnesses and suffer anticipatory grief and fear as their own health declines. The families of haemophiliacs may have lost more than one son in quick succession or be living with that expectation. People from Africa may have experienced family and community decimation from AIDS and may have particular immigration and care issues.

Homosexual couples may need particular legal advice to ensure the financial security of the surviving partner who will not be regarded legally as 'next of kin' and will have no automatic right of inheritance.

Some drug users come from families in which substance abuse is common, and times of stress, such as a relative dying, may precipitate excesses of drugs and/or alcohol with unpredictable behaviour during visits. Setting clear guidelines on visiting (both in the home and in the hospital/hospice) and giving frequent and clear explanations about the patient's treatment plans and condition are crucial to avoid unpleasant confrontations around the dying patient.

The association with drug use has inevitably led to many patients with HIV spending time in prison. Whilst release on compassionate grounds may be considered appropriate for some terminally ill patients, others will be transferred to hospital/hospice under custodial supervision in the final stages of their illness. This can lead to additional stress for all involved and demands careful and considerate organization to preserve patient dignity yet fulfil Home Office supervision requirements.

The use of body bags can cause much distress to carers, so early discussion of this topic is helpful. Viewing of the body should still be possible but some undertakers request prior warning if this is likely.

Patients may be buried or cremated, and in many cities certain undertakers have established a good reputation for sensitivity in handling HIV-related deaths. Patient support groups or local HIV units should be able to advise families.

It should be remembered that death certificates are public documents. The HIV status need not be included on the form but the doctor should indicate that further information would be available for statistical records.

Controversies in prescribing

ANTIRETROVIRAL AGENTS

In 1987 zidovudine (ZDV or AZT) was the first antiretroviral agent shown to improve survival in patients with AIDS. Now there are eight antiretroviral agents (see Table 13.1) licensed for prescription in the UK: five reverse transcriptase inhibitors (RTIs) and three protease inhibitors (PIs). Clear benefit of dual RTI regimens over monotherapy has been reported [4]. Even in late-stage disease a change in combination of RTIs or addition of a PI can achieve both immunological and clinical benefit with dramatic decline in HIV viral load. However, the long-term benefits of such new combination regimes are set to be determined.

For the many individuals who have participated in clinical drug trials stopping treatment can feel like giving up and raises fear that the virus will immediately run rampant.

CORTICOSTEROIDS

Practitioners are often reluctant to prescribe steroids to patients with HIV because of fears that this will accelerate disease and predispose them to opportunistic infections. In particular the incidence of CMV (cytomegalovirus) retinitis, oropharyngeal candidiasis, and *Pneumocystis carinii* pneumonia (PCP) are increased and lesions of Kaposi's sarcoma may enlarge. The benefits of steroids in certain situations such as raised intracranial pressure or severe PCP are clearly established but they may also be helpful in palliating non-specific symptoms by:
- lifting mood;
- reducing fatigue;
- improving anorexia resistant to anabolic steroids;
- acting as an adjuvant antiemetic for nausea or vomiting;
- promoting weight gain with improved body image;
- modulating fever associated with HIV *per se,* lymphoma, or *Mycobacterium avium-intercellulare* complex (MAC) infection;

- reducing the oedema and pain from visceral Kaposi's sarcoma (KS);
- acting as an adjuvant to analgesia for patients with painful neuropathy or myopathy.

Short courses at a higher dose probably give more benefit than prolonged low-dose treatment. Patients need to be aware of the potential side-effects, and offered an initial trial of treatment.

OPIOIDS

There is some resistance and fear of prescribing opioids for pain for patients with a current or previous history of drug abuse (but not for other patients with HIV-related pain). In late-stage HIV the control of pain must be a priority. In addition, patients who have been on maintenance methadone for many years are sometimes fearful of changing to an alternative opioid. For such a patient in pain the choices are:

1   To continue same dose of methadone and *add* morphine or other opioid as an analgesic.
2   To increase methadone: using it for both 'maintenance' and analgesia.
3   To convert methadone to morphine (or diamorphine if not able to swallow) and increase the dose.

There is little evidence about the comparative efficacy of these methods but probably choice 1 is the most satisfactory method.

The two uses of opioids and the doctors' roles should be kept as clear and separate as possible. However, the doctor prescribing for addiction could also provide a separate prescription of the opioid for analgesia with advice from the GP or palliative care physician. This simplifies collection of prescription for patients and minimizes the potential for abuse.

For patients who cannot take oral medication diamorphine should be prescribed for analgesia *and* replacement of maintenance methadone. Close liaison with the drug addiction team is vital to avoid problems.

The appropriate dose of additional or alternative opioids should be calculated taking into account the chronic methadone use (see Box 13.1). In chronic use, oral methadone 10 mg = 20–40 mg oral morphine = 7.5–15 mg s.c. diamorphine.

The use of the additional opioid for *analgesia* should be fully discussed and clear guidelines, boundaries, and a plan for review unambiguously drawn up with the patient and their carers and other professionals involved in the patient's care in order to prevent abuse. Many of these patients exhibit remarkable opioid tolerance and sometimes pain control may be achieved and maintained only with what may appear to be an alarmingly high opioid dose. Appropriate antiemetic and laxative agents should always be prescribed and, if needed, sedative agents.

**Box 13.1 Examples of opioid dosage regimens for the
management of pain for AIDS patients who
are already taking methadone**

Example 1
A patient with nociceptive pain usually takes 60 mg methadone daily for
maintenance. They wish to continue methadone but have oral morphine
for analgesia.
    To calculate an initial dose of oral morphine to take in addition to
methadone 60 mg daily:
• 60 mg methadone = 120–240 mg oral morphine (mean 180 mg).
• To achieve analgesia a 30% increase in opioid dose is required = 60 mg
morphine/24 h.
• Divide into 4-hourly doses = 60 mg/6 = 10 mg oral morphine 4-hourly.
Therefore the patient will take methadone 60 mg o.d. and oral morphine
10 mg 4-hourly.
• Dose for breakthrough pain = 10 mg oral morphine.
    Review daily and titrate as usual to analgesic efficacy with 30–50%
dose increments.

Example 2
The same patient wishes to stop methadone and take only oral morphine
for pain relief.
    To calculate an initial analgesic dose of oral morphine:
• Total methadone dose in 24 h = 60 mg.
• Convert to equivalent morphine dose in 24 h = 120–240 mg (mean
180 mg).
• Analgesia will require a 30% increase in dose = 180 mg + 60 mg =
240 mg/24 h.
• Divide into 4-hourly doses = 240 mg/6 = 40 mg oral morphine 4-hourly.
• Dose for breakthrough = 40 mg oral morphine.
    Review daily and titrate as usual to analgesic efficacy with 30–50%
dose increments.

Example 3
A patient on 100 mg methadone is in pain and very unwell and you would
like to start a syringe driver with diamorphine.
    To calculate an initial analgesic dose of diamorphine:
• Total methadone in 24 h = 100 mg.
• Convert to equivalent s.c. diamorphine = 75–150 mg (mean 120 mg)/
24 h.

Continued

Box 13.1 *Continued*

- Analgesia will require a 30% increase in dose = 120 mg + 40 mg = 160 mg/24 h.
- Dose for breakthrough = 25 mg diamorphine.
  Review daily and titrate as usual to analgesic efficacy with 30–50% dose increments.

Complementary therapy

Many patients report a feeling of well-being following massage, aromatherapy, or reflexology (see Chapter 21). The human contact involved is particularly important in patients whose illness, sexuality, or chaotic lifestyle may have led to social isolation. It may also reassure those who have developed disfiguring skin conditions and fear rejection by partners or family members.

Specific AIDS-related physical problems

These are described in some detail in order that the clinician may feel confident in dealing with patients with these problems even though investigation and treatment is usually undertaken by specialist teams.

Oral problems

Painful oral lesions can cause disproportionate discomfort as patients become reluctant to eat or drink and the effects of dehydration compound their symptoms.

ANGULAR STOMATITIS

Angular stomatitis may be fungal or herpetic in origin. It is common in denture wearers. Swabs for viral culture are useful in persistent lesions and prior to commencing aciclovir.

ORAL CANDIDIASIS

Florid oral candidiasis (white plaques) is easy to diagnose but the earlier stage of erythematous candidiasis may be overlooked although patients will often describe discomfort, particularly when drinking hot liquids, halitosis, or altered taste.

The first line of treatment is the use of antiseptic/anti-inflammatory mouthwashes (chlorhexidine/benzydamine), coupled with topical nystatin and/or amphotericin; the latter require frequent dosing (alternating 2-hourly).

Extensive oral and oesophageal disease requires oral azoles (ketoconazole, fluconazole, or itraconazole). A liquid preparation of itraconazole is useful particularly with dysphagia in oesophageal disease. Interactions with H_2 blockers or rifampicin may render drug levels suboptimal.

In patients with persisting plaques the additional use of miconazole troches (or pessary slowly chewed) can avoid the need for intravenous amphotericin B, which is associated with significant toxicity and the need for additional blood monitoring.

Following widespread use of azoles resistant strains of *Candida albicans* have emerged as an increasing problem along with other candidal species (*C. tropicalis*, *C. glabrata*) that have intrinsic resistance to ketoconazole and fluconazole. Cultures and sensitivity profiles can be helpful, if available, in choosing the most appropriate agent.

ORAL HAIRY LEUKOPLAKIA (OHL)

Oral hairy leukoplakia (OHL) is a white, striped lesion on the lateral border of the tongue. It is common but rarely painful and will naturally remit and then reappear. If distressing, OHL responds to treatment with aciclovir.

ORAL ULCERATION

The treatment of mouth ulcers depends on their nature. Lesions should be swabbed for herpes and treated accordingly. Sterile, aphthous ulcers may respond to topical steroids (triamcinolone in orobase) or oral steroids (hydrocortisone pellets) although prolonged courses inevitably increase the susceptibility to oral candidiasis.

Persistent and painful lesions often respond dramatically to thalidomide, which must be prescribed on a 'named patient' basis with advice regarding safe storage and contraceptive precautions in sexually active women.

Biopsy of non-responding lesions may less commonly reveal underlying malignancy, especially lymphomas. Such lesions should also be examined for atypical mycobacterial organisms.

Oesophageal problems

Oesophageal disease is suggested by dysphagia, retrosternal pain or vomiting.

Candidiasis is the most frequent diagnosis and an empirical course of oral azole treatment is prescribed for 2 weeks. If symptoms persist diagnostic endoscopy should be considered, when it is crucial to biopsy and culture as well as visualize lesions.

Ulceration may be due to herpes or CMV infection, and superficial candidiasis can mask underlying pathologies such as lymphoma.

Treatment is directed to the underlying cause. Symptomatic relief may be achieved with mucaine 20 ml (4–6-hourly); steroids or thalidomide could also be considered.

When eating/swallowing becomes increasingly difficult PEG tubes may be considered (see Chapter 15) although delayed wound healing in a cachectic patient can make this problematic with leakage and recurrent stoma infections.

Lung problems

PNEUMOCYSTIS CARINII PNEUMONIA (PCP)

Mortality from acute *Pneumocystis carinii* pneumonia (PCP) has decreased dramatically over the last decade but breakthrough episodes on prophylactic treatment can be expected as immune function declines. Infection is also more likely in a patient receiving corticosteroids. It is useful to continue PCP prophylaxis in the final stages of terminal care. The condition is associated with an increased risk of pneumothorax.

BACTERIAL INFECTIONS

Drug users in particular are prone to recurrent bacterial chest infections (*S. pneumoniae, H. influenzae*), which should respond to appropriate antibiotics.

Mycobacterial tuberculosis infections

Mycobacterial infections, including tuberculosis, are common in patients with AIDS (see also 'Gastrointestinal problems', p. 215) and the emergence of multidrug resistant tuberculosis (MDR-TB) in association with HIV has highlighted the importance of infection control measures and the need for continued bacteriological surveillance.

Tuberculosis (TB) should be considered in any respiratory illness with cough, and the patient isolated until diagnosis is excluded by smear examination of sputum. Cough-inducing procedures should never be performed in an open area. Directly observed treatment facilitates compliance at all stages of the disease but particularly in those with chaotic lifestyles, visual impairment, or dementia.

KAPOSI'S SARCOMA (KS)

Extensive pulmonary Kaposi's sarcoma (KS) is often diagnosed on bronchoscopy in dyspnoeic patients who have failed to respond to antibiotic therapy. It carries a poor prognosis. Chemotherapy (see below) has not been clearly shown to improve survival but it may palliate symptoms. Oxygen delivered by nasal cannulae can maintain mobility in patients who rapidly desaturate on exertion.

Endobronchial lesions can cause coughing, which is relieved by antitussives, opioids, and nebulized local anaesthetics (see Chapter 11) or corticosteroids. Profuse bleeding and massive haemoptysis may occur although it is rare.

Cardiac problems

Features of HIV-related cardiomyopathy include increasing dyspnoea, fatigue, and ankle oedema. Conventional treatment of cardiac failure with loop diuretics and an angiotensin-converting enzyme (ACE) inhibitor to improve ventricular function may relieve symptoms. Median survival is around 3 months.

Gastrointestinal problems

DIARRHOEA

Diarrhoea is distressing, often painful, and associated with rapid weight loss. It is socially inhibiting and demoralizing, ruining attempts to maintain a normal lifestyle. It is helpful in all but those patients very near death to treat any infective cause. Stool samples should be sent for microscopy, culture, and sensitivity including *Clostridium difficile* toxin and culture.

General symptomatic management of diarrhoea may include:
• agents to reduce gut motility and stool frequency, e.g. loperamide 4–8 mg q.d.s.;
• relief of colic and other pain, e.g. hyoscine butylbromide 20 mg q.d.s. p.o. or 60–120 mg/24 h s.c.;
• relief of nausea, e.g. cyclizine 50 mg t.d.s.;
• stronger opioids may be needed and drugs given parenterally particularly if there is vomiting or evidence of malabsorption;

- stool thickeners, e.g. ispaghula husk (Fybogel one sachet t.d.s.);
- maintenance of hydration;
- practical support with commodes, toilet rails, incontinence pads, and help with washing and laundry.

Infective causes

Infective diarrhoea is usually associated with fever or sweats. Patients with HIV are more susceptible to food poisoning organisms and should receive dietary and cooking advice.

Invasive salmonellosis is an AIDS-defining condition and can cause recurrent symptoms. A quinolone such as ciprofloxacin (500 mg b.d.s.) is the treatment of choice.

Cryptosporidiosis is commonly a water-borne infection leading to profuse diarrhoea associated with marked weight loss and low-grade fever. Response to antibiotic therapy is poor and rarely sustained. Octreotide has been used in an effort to reduce the volume in apparently secretory diarrhoea with variable success. Questran may be helpful to diminish bile acid volume. Occasionally parenteral nutrition is useful for patients with profound weight loss but otherwise 'limited' HIV disease.

Microsporidiosis is difficult to diagnose, requiring duodenal aspirate or biopsy, but diarrhoea may be associated with features of ascending cholangitis including abnormal liver function tests and right upper quadrant pain. Albendazole is often an effective treatment.

Atypical mycobacteria infection is probably acquired through the gut, and diarrhoea may be associated with anaemia, raised alkaline phosphatase, abdominal pain with lymphadenopathy, and intermittent high fever. Organisms are typically resistant to many drugs but symptoms may improve on a variety of regimens incorporating two or more of the second-line antimycobacterial drugs, usually with ethambutol.

Giardiasis should be considered, particularly in patients who have been abroad.

Cytomegalovirus (CMV) gut disease including cholecystitis can occur earlier in the natural history of HIV disease than eye disease (see below) and often responds well to a three-week course of parenteral ganciclovir without any need for long-term prophylaxis.

Non-infective causes

Diarrhoea may also be non-infective in origin. Drug-related diarrhoea is particularly common with agents with low bioavailability such as oral ganciclovir, saquinavir, and didanosine (ddI). These are often prescribed in late-stage disease with numerous other medications (see Table 13.1). Overflow diarrhoea may relate to analgesic opioid use or occur in patients with a history of drug abuse. Abdominal X-ray is helpful in diagnosing these conditions.

Neurological disease such as spastic paraparesis and autonomic neuropathy can lead to diarrhoea with loss of sphincter control, often coinciding with poor mobility, causing particular distress and difficulties for carers.

Diarrhoea may also accompany malabsorption due to small bowel partial villous atrophy. Elemental nutritional supplements may be of value in these cases.

CONSTIPATION

This is a chronic problem in patients receiving maintenance methadone for opiate addiction. It often becomes worse with progressive weight loss and diminished muscle tone (see Chapter 10 for details of management).

New or persisting constipation should prompt investigation for obstructing lesions if the patient is likely to benefit from interventional treatment. Intestinal KS may initially respond well to chemotherapy, and resection of discrete lymphomas or other tumours offers good palliation.

Ophthalmic problems

The incidence of eye disease increases during the course of HIV, with as many as 75% of patients experiencing problems.

EYELIDS

Herpes zoster ophthalmicus is associated with conjunctivitis and dendriform keratitis. Persistent problems with neuralgic pain may occur.

For details of KS pathology affecting the eyes, see below.

CONJUNCTIVAE

Around 10% of patients with AIDS develop non-specific, culture-negative conjunctivitis. Discomfort may be relieved by cool compresses and careful lid hygiene. Dry-eye syndrome can be relieved with substitute tears. Topical antibiotics are used for superadded bacterial infections.

CORNEA

Herpes simplex keratitis presents with visual blurring and should be treated promptly with oral aciclovir (400 mg five times daily for 7 days) to avoid corneal scarring.

ANTERIOR UVEITIS

A red, painful, photophobic eye suggests uveitis and should prompt formal ophthalmic review. It has been reported most commonly in patients receiving treatment for atypical mycobacteria.

RETINAL PROBLEMS

More than 50% of patients with AIDS have fluffy, retinal cotton wool spots (CWS) which do not cause visual disturbance and require no intervention although their presence may indicate a greater risk of CMV retinitis. Retinitis occurs in about 25% of patients and is most commonly due to CMV; other causes include *Toxoplasma*, *Candida*, syphilis, herpes simplex, or herpes zoster.

CMV retinitis

The initial lesions of CMV retinitis are similar to CWS. The lesions typically spread along the retinal vessels with perivascular exudates, followed by haemorrhages and necrotic lesions with the appearance of 'cottage cheese and tomato sauce'. Papillitis and retinal detachment can also occur.

The risk of contralateral eye disease is 85% and immediate treatment is indicated even in late disease to avoid blindness (see Table 13.1). Treatment with intravenous ganciclovir or foscarnet is associated with significant side-effects and patients require careful monitoring. Many patients learn to administer their own intravenous treatment and this may be facilitated by devices such as portacaths and Hickman lines.

BLINDNESS

Becoming blind during the final stages of a progressive disease which impairs many other bodily functions is extremely disabling. Involvement of the visual impairments services at an early stage can facilitate the learning of new skills and set in place practical help (e.g. simple kitchen stabilizing devices, textural colour coding for clothes) as well as providing emotional support as sight deteriorates. Teaching a partner or friend how to guide safely can avoid patients becoming housebound and help maintain their independence.

Dermatological problems

Skin diseases can cause distress from itching, pain, and social embarrassment. Many conditions progress as immune function deteriorates.

FUNGAL INFECTIONS

Seborrhoeic dermatitis caused by *Pityrosporum orbiculare* is characterized by erythema and scaling of the nasolabial folds, eyebrows, beard area, scalp, and chest wall. Topical antifungal agents (including shampoos) combined with a low-dose corticosteroid are effective. Patches of tinea elsewhere on the body can be treated similarly or with oral antifungals.

MOLLUSCUM CONTAGIOSUM

Lesions are commonly found on the face and numbers increase as immunocompetence declines. They may be itchy, and squeezing can lead to local spread or superadded bacterial infection. Once lesions start to coalesce they are difficult to eradicate. Cryotherapy is safe and simple but needs to be applied on a weekly basis to be effective. Atypical lesions should be biopsied since cutaneous lesions due to cryptoccocal infection or atypical mycobacteria can be easily confused.

BACTERIAL INFECTIONS

Staphylococcal infections are more common in patients with symptomatic HIV and AIDS and may present as folliculitis, impetigo, abscesses, or cellulitis. Syphilis and mycobacterial infections may present as ulcers, plaques, or cold abscesses and biopsy is recommended in painful or growing lesions. Bacillary angiomatosis caused by *Rochalimaea henselae* can present with a few or hundreds of lesions that mimic KS. It responds to tetracycline.

SCABIES

Generalized itching should always prompt consideration of infection with *Sarcoptes scabiei*. The usual manifestations may be absent, particularly in

Norwegian scabies when hyperkeratotic skin plaques may be teeming with mites. Treatment with conventional agents (malathion 0.5% or permethrin 5%) is appropriate but more frequent applications may be necessary. Calamine lotion and oral antihistamines may help itching that persists after effective antiparasitic treatment.

PSORIASIS

The incidence of psoriasis does not appear to be increased in patients with HIV but it is often more aggressive/extensive and arthritis is more common. Topical agents and the retinoids are used but methotrexate and ultraviolet (UV) treatment are avoided because of their immunosuppressive effect.

PRESSURE SORES

The profound weight loss experienced in late-stage HIV, often in association with neurological impairment, creates an ideal scenario for the development of pressure sores (see Chapter 18).

Tumour-related problems

HIV infection predisposes individuals to early development of several neoplastic conditions including Kaposi's sarcoma, non-Hodgkin's lymphoma, invasive cervical cancer, and probably anal tumours.

KAPOSI'S SARCOMA

In western countries HIV-associated Kaposi's sarcoma (KS) is seen predominantly in homosexual men or women who have had sexual partners with KS; it is rare in drug users. KS appears as nodular, purplish lesions commonly affecting the face and trunk. Skin lesions are usually present when visceral disease develops. Lesions frequently occur in the oropharynx but can develop in the bronchial tree, lungs, and lower gastrointestinal tract. Cutaneous disease may regress spontaneously but patients may require advice on cosmetic masking techniques if it is noticeable or unsightly. For large single lesions or sites of lymph node obstruction, radiotherapy is the most effective treatment. Active treatment of associated lymphoedema is important (see Chapter 19).

Other treatment options include subcutaneous alpha interferon, which is associated with shrinkage of lesions but has significant side-effects.

Systemic or aggressive cutaneous disease requires combination chemo-therapy with a response rate of around 50% using vincristine and bleomycin. Addition of an anthracycline improves response rates, and liposomal preparations of daunorubicin may result in 90% of patients initially responding although it is not clear whether longer remissions can be maintained. Bone-marrow toxicity may necessitate blood transfusions during treatment.

NON-HODGKIN'S LYMPHOMA (NHL)

Some 3–10% of patients with AIDS will develop NHL, which most frequently involves extranodal sites or the central nervous system (CNS). Most are large B-cell lymphomas (60%) although Burkitt's lymphoma (30%) is commonly seen in younger patients. Symptoms relate to the site of the tumour, and localized disease is best treated by surgical resection. Cerebral or disseminated disease poses a difficult therapeutic problem, when the benefits of treatment may be marginal compared to the toxicity of the drugs. Radiotherapy may provide good palliation but most patients relapse after cytotoxic regimens, with a median survival of 5–8 months.

Problems of the nervous system

HEADACHE

Headaches are often multifactorial, with stress, anxiety, and drug side-effects probably the most common causes. Space-occupying lesions may be associated with headache and features of raised intracranial pressure. A meningeal headache may relate to aseptic meningitis due to HIV *per se* and usually develops as CD4 counts decline. Tuberculous and cryptococcal meningitis often present with non-specific symptoms but usually in association with fever.

PERIPHERAL NEUROPATHY

The commonest neuropathy is a distal, axonal and predominantly sensory polyneuropathy that presents with painful dysaesthesias of the feet that are usually worse at night and may prevent walking. Power and proprioception are usually relatively preserved. It may be due to late-stage HIV infection or drugs, including zalcitabine, didanosine and stavudine. Drug-related symptoms are dose related and usually reversible on discontinuing treatment.

HIV-related symptoms may be improved by commencing an antiretroviral agent.

Symptomatic control is often difficult. This is neuropathic pain and may be partially opioid responsive, but treatment will often require adjuvant analgesics such as carbamezepine, amitriptyline, or mexiletene (see Chapter 9). Occupational therapy assessment is important due to the progressive debility.

CMV can cause a subacute progressive polyradiculopathy or mononeuritis multiplex. Treatment can arrest and partly reverse the condition.

A vacuolar myelopathy is often associated with AIDS dementia complex (see below) and presents with difficulty in walking, with spastic-ataxic gait and brisk reflexes with clonus. Anal and bladder sphincters are commonly affected, which creates great difficulties in maintaining continence when mobility is so poor.

MYOPATHY

Myopathic pain may relate to HIV *per se* but can also be caused by the toxic effects of zidovudine on muscle mitochondrial DNA polymerase. Aspirin may be surprisingly effective.

FOCAL CEREBRAL DEFICIT

Hemispheric dysfunction is most commonly due to toxoplasmosis or primary CNS lymphoma. Both will show a mass effect on computed tomography (CT) with surrounding oedema but are difficult to distinguish radiologically. Whilst the initial response to treatment in toxoplasmosis is usually good, the prognosis in cerebral lymphoma is very poor.

Progressive multifocal leukoencephalopathy has a more distinct radiological appearance with lesions confined to white matter with no mass effect or contrast enhancement. Whilst prognosis is very poor some improvement may be seen with high-dose zidovudine.

AIDS DEMENTIA COMPLEX

The HIV-associated cognitive/motor complex encompasses subcortical dementia with slowness and imprecision of cognition (initially manifested as poor concentration and forgetfulness) and impaired motor control. The mortality rate at 6 months has been reported to be as high as 67%.

In the early stages patients with a history of drug use can often become more chaotic, for example losing prescriptions and turning up late or on the wrong day for appointments. Important information should be conveyed in written as well as verbal form, and patients encouraged to keep lists and appointment diaries.

As the condition progresses motor abnormalities become more apparent, sometimes progressing to quadriparesis. Some patients may develop antisocial and aggressive behaviour and like other patients with dementia require constant supervision.

The demands on the carers of such patients are immense and regular respite admissions can provide a way for them to cope. The progressive decline in both mental and physical faculties makes home care extremely difficult. Provision of appropriate community and in-patient care for such patients is often a problem for the health, social, and voluntary services.

Decisions around the ending of life

Suicide is higher in populations with AIDS than other terminal illnesses and much greater in those with inadequately treated pain [5]. Advance directives or living wills are common in this group of patients [6] (see Chapter 6).

Bereavement in AIDS

Carers, family, friends, and professionals are particularly at risk of difficult and abnormal grief in relation to deaths from AIDS (Table 13.4). Chapter 7 discusses in detail the identification of risk factors and the prevention of problems.

Table 13.4 Risk factors for difficult bereavement in AIDS related deaths.

For homosexual men
Multiple loss experiences
History of alcohol and drug abuse
Bereaved are also ill
Denial of status as a lover/partner
Social isolation
Stigma of the disease
Stigma of their lifestyle

Continued

Table 13.4 *Continued*

Undisclosed diagnosis
Family rejection

For i.v. drug abusers
Multiple loss experiences
History of alcohol abuse
Bereaved are also ill
Social isolation
   Stigma of the disease
   Stigma of their lifestyle
Family rejection

For parents
Loss of children (multiple in haemophilia)
Social isolation
   Stigma of the disease
   Stigma of their lifestyle
   Undisclosed diagnosis
Anger

For health care professionals
Multiple losses
Powerlessness
Disenfranchised grief

Appendix

Control of infection and safety when caring for patients with AIDS

Contact	• There is no risk of HIV transmission from social contact such as hugging, kissing or sharing cutlery. Basic hygiene practices should always be followed • Wearing gloves should be normal practice when changing wound dressings, giving injections or handling body fluids. Broken skin should be covered with a waterproof dressing
Body fluids	• Body fluids can be discarded into a normal sluice or toilet • Baths and toilets should be cleaned as normal after use with Milton/bleach
Clinical waste	• Clinical waste should be divided from domestic waste for disposal in standard sacks

Continued on p. 224

Appendix *Continued*

Sharps	• Sharps should never be resheathed but put directly after use into a sharps bin, within the patient's room, to avoid corridor accidents
Facial masks	• Facial masks are incorporated into guidelines for care of patients with tuberculosis but must be of recommended standard to be effective. Disposable particulate respirators provide a better facial fit and filtration capacity (1 μg) and should be used
	• Masks and visors should be used for any procedure that may involve facial splashing with blood or body fluids
Clinical equipment	• Non-invasive clinical equipment (e.g. infusion pumps) that has been used for patients with HIV requires no special cleaning
	• Suction machines should be fitted with disposable liners and hydrophilic filters
	• Companies leasing Clinitron bead beds destroy the beads after use
Blood	• Blood spillage should be contained and can be mostly easily absorbed using granular sodium dichloroisocyanurate, e.g. Presept left for a few minutes then wiped with disposable paper. Alternatively a strong solution of sodium hypochlorite (equivalent to 1 part household bleach and 10 parts water) left for 20–30 minutes can be used. The area is then washed with hot, soapy water. Superficial contamination is wiped with a weak (1 in 100 dilution) solution of hypochlorite
Use of body bags	• Following death from certain infections a body bag is required prior to transport. Conditions classified as high risk include hepatitis B and C and medium risk HIV/AIDS [7]. Details of risk category are put on the patient identifier card and inner and outer bag
Needlestick injuries	• Many patients with HIV have also acquired hepatitis C and/or B which must be considered in the event of a needlestick injury. Medical, nursing staff and appropriate lay carers should be immunized for hepatitis B and have antibody levels checked to ensure that protective titres are maintained.
	• Every team caring for patients with HIV should have an incident plan that enables needlestick injuries to be dealt with in a calm but supportive manner. The risk for HIV infection through percutaneous injury is around 0.3% and is lower for mucous membrane (0.1%) and skin (<0.1%) exposure. There is now evidence to suggest that post exposure prophylaxis (PEP) zidovudine (ZDV/AZT),

Appendix *Continued*

significantly (79%) [8] reduces chance of seroconversion to HIV following percutaneous exposure. A starting pack of drugs should be immediately available either on site or through liaison with a designated occupational health service or infectious diseases unit with 24 hour access. Carers in the community should also be aware of who to contact and what action to take

- Most accidents occur because safe practices have not been followed. Particular care should be taken with disposal of 'butterfly' needles which may spring back.
- The area should be washed in warm water with Hibiscrub with gentle downward pressure to encourage bleeding
- Prior to commencing treatment blood should be taken for storage. Protocols vary but it is usual to offer HIV and hepatitis B and C testing 3 and 6 months post injury. Later seroconversions have been reported but are unusual. Safer sex guidelines should be followed until sero-status is known
- Non-immune individuals should receive hepatitis B immunoglobulin and vaccine if the patient was an infectious carrier
- PEP should ideally be commenced within 1–2 hours of exposure and zidovudine 500 mg – 1 g stat should be given if there is likely to be any delay obtaining other drugs or further advice
- Because of concerns about viral resistance new guidelines in 1996 advised dual or triple antiviral therapy to be continued for a 4 week course [8].
- Close follow-up is essential since antiretroviral therapies have significant side effects, particularly marrow toxicity

References

1 Sims R, Moss VA. *Palliative Care for People with AIDS*, 2nd edn. London: Arnold, 1995.
2 Larue F, Fontaine A, Colleau SM. Underestimation and undertreatment of pain in HIV disease: multicentre study. *BMJ* 1997; 314: 23–28.
3 Breithcart W, Rosenfeld BD, Passik SD, McDonald MV, Thaler H, Portenoy RK. The undertreatment of pain in ambulatory AIDS patients. *Pain* 1996; 65: 243–249.
4 Gazzard BG, Moyk GJ, Weber J *et al.* British HIV Association Guidelines for Antiretroviral Treatment of HIV seropositive individuals. *Lancet* 1997; 349: 1086–1092.

5 Marzuk P, Tierney H, Tardiff K *et al.* Increased risk of suicide in persons with AIDS. *J Am Med Assoc* 1988; 259: 1333–1337.
6 Richardson A. Living wills. In: Sherr L, ed. *Grief and AIDS.* Chichester: Wiley, 1995: 129–143.
7 Healing TD, Hoffman PN, Young SEJ. The Infection Hazards of Human Cadavers. *Communicable Disease Report* 1995; 5:
8 CDC. Update: Provisional Public Health Service Recommendations For Chemoprophylaxis After Occupational Exposure to HIV. *MMWR* 1996; **Vol.45/ No.22:**

Further reading

Brettle RP, Bisset K, Burns S *et al.* Human immunodeficiency virus and drug abuse: the Edinburgh experience. *BMJ* 1987; 294: 421–424.
Pizzo PA, Wilfert CM. *Pediatric AIDS: The Challenge of HIV Infection in Infants, Children and Adolescents,* 2nd edn. Baltimore: Williams & Wilkins, 1994.
Pratt R. *HIV & AIDS—A Strategy for Nursing Care,* 4th edn. London: Edward Arnold, 1995.
Quinn TC. Global burden of the HIV pandemic. *Lancet* 1996; 348: 99–106.
Sherr L, ed. *Grief and AIDS.* Chichester: Wiley, 1995.
UK Department of Health. *Guidance for Clinical and Health Care Workers: Protection Against Infection with HIV and Hepatitis Viruses.* London: HMSO, 1990.

14: Palliative Care for People with Motor Neurone Disease

FIONA HICKS

Introduction

Motor neurone disease (MND) was first described in the mid-19th century, and is a progressive, degenerative disease of motor neurones of unknown cause (Table 14.1). All treatment for patients with MND is palliative.

Although there is no cure for MND, much can be achieved to maximize a patient's function and comfort within the confines of the disease. Caring for patients with MND will be a rare experience for the primary health care team. This chapter will help the team to understand the issues facing patients and their carers, and to feel confident in the management of specific problems.

What is MND?

In MND there is a progressive loss of motor neurones. Muscles are not directly affected, but show denervation atrophy and irritability, leading to cramps and fasciculation. Some people with MND may have episodes of paroxysmal laughing or crying which do not represent true emotion; this can be difficult for both patients and carers. The mechanism behind this is not clear.

Unlike other progressive neurological conditions such as multiple sclerosis, there are no occasions in MND where function improves. However, periods of stabilization of the disease may occur but are of unpredictable duration.

Epidemiology

MND is a relatively rare condition. It has an incidence of approximately 2 per 100 000. A general practitioner with an average list size might expect to see one new patient with MND every 25 years. Affected individuals have a median survival of 3 years, leading to an overall prevalence of about 6 per 100 000.

Table 14.1 Clinical variants of MND.

Areas affected	Functions spared

Motor neurones in the:
  Cerebral cortex
  Brainstem motor nuclei
  Anterior horn of the spinal cord.
	Intellect and memory
	Cranial nerves controlling eye movements
	Sacral nerves supplying sphincters
	Sexual function
	Sensory nerves

MND is largely a disease of middle to late life. Males are more commonly affected than females. A rare, hereditary form may have an onset in childhood or adolescence.

Variants of MND

Three clinical variants of MND have been described (Table 14.2). These may present differently in their early stages but there is inevitably some overlap between them as the disease progresses.

Organization/co-ordination of care

Poor organization of care is a common feature for patients with MND and contributes to a sense of loss of control and poor quality of life for

Table 14.2 Summary of the variants of MND.

Variant of MND	Clinical findings	Prognosis
Amyotrophic lateral sclerosis (ALS); 66% of patients	Lesions of lower motor neurones, combined with involvement of the corticospinal tracts	Median survival in this group is around 3 years.
Progressive muscular atrophy (PMA); 8% of patients	Largely affects lower motor neurones in the first instance	The most favourable prognosis, with some patients surviving more than 15 years.
Progressive bulbar palsy (PBP); 26% of patients	Involvement of the brainstem motor nuclei predominates	The most sinister prognosis with death often occurring within a year.

patients and families. As MND is a comparatively rare condition, the primary health care team will have little experience of the disease. However, the majority of the work will fall to them. MND is a complex disorder requiring the skills of many professionals at different times. The number of people involved can be bewildering for patients and professionals alike and may lead to a breakdown in communication. It is essential that each patient is nominated a *key worker* from diagnosis, whose name and contact number is known to both the patient and the caring team.

The role of the key worker

The key worker may be drawn from any discipline, and should have an interest in the disease, a good relationship with the patient, and the ability to communicate well with all those involved in the patient's care.

Coping with disability

Occupational therapists, speech and language therapists, and physiotherapists can be of great help to patients with MND facing progressive disability (see Chapter 2).

Treatment against the disease process

In the 1990s, the first compound shown to have efficacy against the course of MND was discovered—Riluzole. In practice, Riluzole should be given early in the course of the disease where possible, as it appears to slow the rate of loss of motor neurone function but does not restore function. It is unclear how well Riluzole preserves functional ability, although it certainly does appear to have a modest effect on survival. Riluzole 50 mg b.d. is well tolerated by patients but should only be initiated by specialist physicians with experience in the management of MND.

Common physical symptoms in people with MND

The common physical problems encountered by patients with MND are listed in Table 14.3 [1].As outlined in Chapter 1, good symptom control requires:
- a thorough history of each symptom;
- a careful physical examination;
- conducting relevant investigations;
- discussing the problem with the patient (and carers where appropriate)

Table 14.3 Common physical problems in patients with MND.

	Percentage of affected patients with MND (*n* = 124) [1]
Constipation	65
Pain	57
Dyspnoea	47
Dribbling saliva	38
Cough	53
Insomnia	48

including the therapeutic options and their potential advantages and disadvantages.

Constipation

Constipation is the most common symptom found among MND patients. Possible causes include a low-residue diet, immobility, drug side-effects (e.g. anticholinergics, opioids), and reduced power of the abdominal muscles used to aid evacuation.

MANAGEMENT

Remove the cause of the constipation if possible, especially if drug-related. It is possible to give dietary advice even in patients with swallowing difficulties. If aperients are needed, ensure that they can be swallowed easily by patients with dysphagia. Oral aperients are usually preferable to suppositories. A combination of a stimulant laxative and a softener is usually required, for example:
• Co-danthramer, initially 5–10 ml b.d. (dose may be increased or given as Co-danthramer forte as necessary);
• senna syrup 5 ml b.d. with lactulose 5–10 ml b.d. (dose titrated as required). Flatulence may limit the dose of lactose that can be tolerated.

Pain

MUSCULOSKELETAL PAIN

There are two main factors which contribute to the development of musculoskeletal pain: (i) restricted movement leading to stiff joints; and (ii) reduced muscle tone around joints leading to loss of the normal positioning (shoulder joints are most commonly affected).

Pain should be prevented wherever possible by careful positioning. Physiotherapy, including passive movements, helps to maintain joint mobility. Once musculoskeletal pain has become established, joint positioning and exercise remain critical but pharmacological treatment will also be necessary.

- Non-steroidal anti-inflammatory drugs (NSAIDs) in tablet, suspension, or suppository form as required.
- NSAID gel applied to the affected areas may be of benefit.
- Intra-articular injections of local anaesthetic and steroid are worth considering, especially for shoulder pain.

MUSCLE CRAMPS

Muscle cramps can be a very troublesome problem and may respond to simple stretching exercises. However, if drugs are required, various muscle relaxants may be tried, for example: baclofen 5–20 mg q.d.s. (larger doses may be necessary for some patients); dantrolene 25–100 mg q.d.s.; diazepam 5 mg nocte increased as necessary to 10 mg q.d.s. or more, depending on side-effects; or quinine sulphate 200 mg nocte, increased to 600 mg as necessary.

These drugs should be titrated against the response of the patient until cramps are controlled or side-effects become troublesome. Some authors would advocate higher maximum doses than described here [2]. A combination of drugs may be used if necessary, although drowsiness is a common problem with higher doses. All these drugs may also be used for troublesome spasticity (e.g. adductor spasm) but it is important to remember that in ambulatory patients, some spasticity may be necessary to keep the patient mobile.

SKIN PRESSURE

Skin pressure causes pain in patients with advanced disease who are unable to move and change position. Attention to the care of pressure areas is very important both for patients in wheelchairs and for bed-bound patients (see also Chapter 18). Unfortunately some patients with established pressure sores often need a period of admission to a hospital or hospice unit for intensive nursing support. Pain may be relieved with NSAIDs as before, but analgesics may well have to be increased according to the WHO analgesic ladder (see Chapter 9).

Some patients with MND are most uncomfortable at night, and a dose of slow-release opioid only at night may be helpful to improve sleep.

Up to 60% of patients with advanced MND require regular opioids for non-specific pain.

Breathlessness (dyspnoea)

Breathlessness in MND patients can have several possible causes.
• Lower respiratory tract infection, often caused or compounded by aspiration pneumonia.
• Weakness of the muscles of ventilation, particularly the diaphragm and intercostal muscles, sometimes aggravated by poor nutrition.
• Coexistent cardiac or lung pathology (e.g. left ventricular failure (LVF), chronic obstructive pulmonary disease) in a largely elderly population.

MANAGEMENT

Infection

Management of infective causes should comprise appropriate antibiotics and consideration of alternative methods of feeding if aspiration is a problem.

Weakness of ventilatory muscles

Nocturnal ventilatory failure may precede daytime breathlessness. Precarious ventilatory reserve is exhausted by lying supine at night. Raising the head of the bed or sleeping in a reclining chair may be of benefit. In many patients breathlessness is a poor prognostic sign, and ventilatory failure sufficient to cause daytime breathlessness usually heralds the terminal phase of MND.

For a few patients who may be otherwise fit, non-invasive nocturnal ventilation may be considered and is possible in the home. It is important to have a full and frank discussion with patients before embarking on such treatment, as increasing dependence on the ventilator is likely and the limits of such treatment should be made clear [3]. Life can be prolonged indefinitely in this way, and this raises many ethical issues. It is not usual practice in the UK to use these measures.

For most patients treatment is purely symptomatic (see Chapter 11). Sitting upright with a stream of air passing across the face is helpful. Calm reassurance, company, relaxation, and breathing exercises have important therapeutic roles. Pharmacological treatment is aimed at reducing anxiety and decreasing the subjective experience of breathlessness. This may be done using diazepam 2–5 mg t.d.s. Lorazepam 0.5–1 mg may be given for acute attacks, as it is shorter acting. Another option is morphine sulphate 2.5–5 mg every 4 h. These drugs can be given together as required.

Salivary drooling

CAUSES

Bulbar palsies make it difficult for patients to manipulate saliva in the mouth and then swallow it. This may be compounded by weakness of facial and neck muscles, causing parting of the lips and a tendency for the head to fall forwards. This then leads to salivary drooling. Drooling is often a distressing symptom for patients, who may isolate themselves from company due to embarrassment.

MANAGEMENT

Explanation to the patient and carer and attention to posture may be all that is needed. Drug treatment may be used to dry up saliva, and in this case a compromise must be reached between drooling and a dry mouth. Anticholinergic drugs are the mainstay of treatment:
- hyoscine hydrobromide patches (500 μg over 72 h); 1 to 5+ patches may be needed, titrated according to response; or
- hyoscine hydrobromide 300–600 μg sublingually q.d.s.; or
- glycopyrronium bromide 1.2 mg s.c. over 24 h.

If a patient is also suffering from depression, amitriptyline may be used for both problems. Beta blockers may be useful, for example propranolol 10 mg t.d.s.

A few patients may tolerate having a dry mouth but dislike taking medication in the longer term. Radiotherapy to the salivary glands may then be considered. This is usually done unilaterally in the first instance to assess its acceptability to the patient.

Cough

A weak, ineffectual cough may be a troublesome symptom in MND. This is often compounded by a lower respiratory tract infection.

MANAGEMENT

If aspiration is a problem, consider alternative methods of feeding. Treat infection appropriately and consider physiotherapy and suction. If mucus is tenacious, this may compound the difficulties of a weak cough. Consider mucolytics such as: nebulized saline 5 ml prn., or carbocysteine 500–750 mg t.d.s. A distressing cough, particularly at night, may be helped by nebulized local anaesthetic.

Insomnia

CAUSES

Insomnia may have various causes, including: pain/discomfort, anxiety, and depression. The patient's sleep may be disturbed by a troublesome nocturnal cough due to increased secretions. Moreover, nocturnal ventilatory failure causes hypoxia resulting in frequent night-time wakening, morning headache (CO_2 retention), and daytime somnolence.

The management should be directed at the underlying causes of the insomnia, which have been discussed elsewhere in this chapter.

Introduction of aids and appliances

The introduction of new aids and appliances requires sensitive handling. The necessity for new equipment serves to remind patients of their deterioration. Equipment may be rejected or simply not used if it is introduced too early or with inadequate explanation. However, there is nothing more demoralizing than waiting so long for a much-needed piece of equipment that by the time it arrives the disability has progressed too far for it to be of use. For example, an electric wheelchair is of no use to a patient who has lost the function of their hands.

There is a large variety of equipment available for most conceivable needs. Equipment should be loaned wherever possible, as its usefulness may be short-lived if disability progresses rapidly. Various agencies may be of help (see Useful Addresses, pp. 377–381, for more details).

- The Motor Neurone Disease Association (MNDA).
- Disablement Resettlement Officers.
- Disablement Living Centres.
- The Disablement Living Foundation.
- REMAP (Rehabilitation Engineering Movement Advisory Panels).

Upper limb weakness

Many appliances are available to help with the common problems of upper limb weakness in MND, such as: weak grip; inability to raise the arms, necessitating forearm supports; carrying aids; dressing aids.

Lower limb weakness

There is a variety of equipment that may be used to maintain mobility where this is compromised by lower limb weakness. If continued home care is desired, consideration should be given to necessary alterations in the home, before mobility is lost.

Communication difficulties

Many patients with MND will develop difficulties with speech, ranging from quiet speech, to dysarthria and anarthria. It is vital that wherever possible, the caring team builds up a good relationship with the patient while speech is preserved. This may entail visiting the patient more often than is strictly necessary during the early part of their illness. During this time, attitudes to illness and treatment can be explored along with other issues and fears that are important to the patient. This will aid communication in the later phases of the disease when speech may be difficult or absent, although the patient's attitudes and fears may change. When a patient becomes anarthric, it is important to remember that their hearing and intellect are almost always preserved.

A speech and language therapist may be most useful in this instance. He/she will establish the cause of speech problems and give advice on maintaining intelligible speech where possible. Advice on the choice and use of communication aids will be given. These range from amplifiers for those with a weak voice to a keyboard operated by hand or by eye movements. Communication Aid Centres have been set up around the country, where aids can be tried out.

Feeding problems

Feeding difficulties may be due to upper limb weakness or difficulty in swallowing. These are often of great embarrassment to patients as feeding is often a social event. A speech and language therapist will help diagnose causes of swallowing problems and advise on how a patient may optimize their swallowing. Oral or oesophageal candidiasis should not be overlooked in patients with dysphagia; this can be treated with ketoconazole 200 mg o.d. for 5 days.

Food of uniform, semisolid consistency is the easiest to swallow in patients with bulbar palsies. Dieticians can advise on palatable, nutritious recipes.

If oral feeding becomes untenable, usually due to recurrent aspiration into the trachea, alternative methods of feeding may be considered with the patient. This may remove the stress of needing to maintain nutrition and will probably prolong survival. It should be remembered, however, that the risk of aspiration remains even when the patient only has the occasional cup of tea. The reason for considering alternative feeding methods should be weighed up carefully.

Nasogastric feeding has little place now for these patients. Percutaneous endoscopic gastrostomy (PEG) feeding is a much more satisfactory alternative.

Psychosocial problems commonly affecting people with MND

Difficulties for patients

ANXIETY

Anxiety affects many patients with MND, often becoming more manifest as the illness progresses. It is often most disabling at night. Management may include reassurance, and cognitive or behavioural techniques. A good therapeutic relationship and efficient management of coexisting symptoms are of great benefit. If medication is needed, a short-acting benzodiazepine, such as temazepam 10–20 mg at night is often sufficient. If daytime anxiety is also a problem, a longer-acting preparation such as diazepam 5–10 mg at night is preferable, although some people prefer to take 2–10 mg t.d.s.

DEPRESSION

A low mood may be expected in patients suffering from a progressive, ultimately fatal disorder such as MND, but a treatable, clinical depression should not be overlooked. The diagnosis of depression poses a particular challenge in those with severe speech difficulties alongside a severe physical illness. An all-pervading sense of hopelessness and loss of self-worth may point to the diagnosis. Treatment is with conventional antidepressants. If insomnia is a problem, amitriptyline 25 mg at night, increased as necessary to 150 mg, is the drug of choice. Alternatively a selective serotonin reuptake inhibitor (SSRI) such as paroxetine 20 mg o.d. may be used.

FEAR ABOUT THE MANNER OF DEATH

When MND is portrayed by the lay media, death by choking is often mentioned. The fear of choking combined with impending loss of speech and function in the arms and legs leads some patients to make advance directives requesting assisted suicide or euthanasia. Requests like this must be handled with great sensitivity and the underlying fears explored. An explanation about the likely mode of death, including signs that the terminal phase is approaching, can be of great benefit to some people. Reassurance about the drugs that are available to manage symptoms in the terminal phase can be helpful.

Difficulties for lay carers

The physical and emotional demands on the families and friends of people with MND can be enormous. These demands are compounded where speech problems hinder normal communication. The possibility of respite care should be explored and discussed with patients and their carers. Options include day care, a home sitting service, or periods of in-patient care in hospital, hospice, or nursing home. The advantage of admission to a hospice for respite care is that a thorough nursing and medical reassessment can take place by staff with experience in the care of patients with advanced MND [4]. This may make subsequent care at home more manageable.

Difficulties for professional carers

Many professionals find caring for patients with MND and their families very distressing. Managing patients with a relentlessly progressive and disabling condition with no cure may elicit feelings of hopelessness and

despondency among the caring team. Reactions may vary; typical ones include:
- keeping a distance, not getting too involved;
- referring the patient to someone else;
- being over-optimistic about the prognosis;
- being nihilistic about any interventions;
- being drawn towards physician-assisted suicide or euthanasia.

However, there is no substitute for getting involved, being honest and sensitive with the patient and family, and striving to address each problem as it arises. This will maximize physical function and comfort within the limits of the disease.

Terminal care

Terminal care for patients with MND follows the same principles as for other conditions (see Chapter 20). Ideally a decision about the place of death will have been made in advance by the patient and their carers. Every effort should be made to achieve those wishes where possible. Once respiratory complications become apparent, however, the terminal phase may be short. In one large series 40% of patients deteriorated suddenly and died within 12 h [1].

Common causes of death

The major cause of death in MND is respiratory failure. Patients often have a pronounced fear of choking to death, but this is rarely seen in practice.

Management

Medications given for symptomatic benefit should be continued in a convenient form during the terminal phase. This may be via a gastrostomy tube where present, or a subcutaneous syringe driver. Common drugs used subcutaneously in terminal care include:
- diamorphine for pain or breathlessness;
- midazolam 10–30 mg/24 h for sedation or anxiety. An alternative is methotrimeprazine 12.5–150 mg/24 h;
- hyoscine hydrobromide 1.2–2.4 mg/24 h. Glycopyrronium can be used as an alternative in this instance.

The Motor Neurone Disease Association (MNDA)

The MNDA is a national, voluntary organization and registered charity.

It has regional care advisors who have direct contact with patients and families and also have an educational role to health care professionals. They serve a wide area so the amount of direct patient contact they can provide is limited.

The MNDA also runs an information service, with a wide range of publications written for both the lay public and professionals involved in the care of people with MND. A comprehensive list of useful addresses and telephone numbers is provided in the MNDA booklets.

Conclusions

This chapter outlines various aspects of a strategy designed to help professionals work successfully with MND patients and their carers in order to achieve good palliative care.

- Get involved early, while the patient can still communicate.
- Nominate a key worker to educate the team, provide a focus for care, and ensure that appropriate actions are taken at appropriate times.
- Remember to pay attention to details, especially with aids and appliances and symptom control.
- Remember the psychosocial impact of MND, particularly for patients with communication difficulties.
- Be mindful of experts/agencies that can help.

References

1 O'Brien T, Kelly M, Saunders C. Motor neurone disease: a hospice perspective. *BMJ* 1992; 304: 471–473.
2 Norris F, Smith R, Denys E. Motor neurone disease: towards better care. *BMJ* 1985; 291: 259–262.
3 Shneerson J. Motor neurone disease, some hope at last for respiratory complications. *BMJ* 1996; 313: 244.
4 Hicks F, Corcoran G. Should hospices offer respite care to patients with MND? *Palliat Med* 1993; 7 (2): 145–151.

Further reading

Oliver D. *MND—A Family Affair*. Sheldon Press, 1995.
Walton J, ed. Motor neurone disease. In: *Brain's Diseases of the Nervous System*, 10th edn. Oxford: Oxford Medical Publications, 1993.
Motor Neurone Disease Association booklets for patients and professionals are available from the MNDA (see Useful Addresses, p. 377).

15: The Management of People with Head and Neck Cancers

NICKY RUDD AND JANE WORLDING

Introduction

The care of patients with relapsed head and neck cancer is rarely mentioned in medical literature. Yet this group pose a unique challenge as they often experience unpleasant local symptoms, difficulty in swallowing and speech, and gross disfigurement, leading to psychological distress and social isolation.

Fortunately head and neck tumours are rare and many are curable, but their rarity may disadvantage the patient, who does not have access to support systems and the self-help groups which are in place for patients with commoner cancers. The primary health care team may lack confidence in dealing with these patients as they are unlikely to see many in their professional life. Those patients whose heavy drinking and self-neglect have been an aetiological factor, are often socially isolated prior to diagnosis, living alone in poor circumstances with little help or social contact. Younger patients may have children who are frightened of their appearance, causing great distress to both parties.

Epidemiology of head and neck cancers

Head and neck cancers comprise 4% of all solid tumours, the majority of which are of squamous cell origin. They occur more frequently in the elderly than the young, and in the UK at least, have a higher incidence in the Asian population [1,2]. The main known aetiological factors in the UK are cigarette smoking and alcohol, particularly when combined and associated with poor nutrition. A known carcinogen in the Asian population is betel nut chewing. Nasopharyngeal cancer is also associated with Epstein–Barr virus [3].

Challenges of head and neck cancer

The natural history of the primary disease and its subsequent management depend largely on the stage at presentation. Those patients with early stage disease will be treated by surgery and/or radiotherapy. Surgical procedures are often major and may be disfiguring or leave residual disability; for example, partial glossectomy may cause residual speech impediment, while laryngectomy may entail the need for stoma care and communication aids. Radiotherapy requires careful planning, with moulding and wearing of a mask. Chemotherapy has, as yet, no proven long-term benefit and is generally used only in the context of large multicentre clinical trials.

Locally recurrent and advanced primary head and neck tumours can be most unpleasant, causing mainly localized symptoms. These include:

- pain;
- eating difficulties and dysphagia;
- difficulty in speaking (articulation and phonation);
- dribbling;
- an unpleasant taste;
- facial oedema;
- the disconcerting constant presence of a tumour within the oral cavity;
- fistulae, which are a common complication;
- highly visible, fungating offensive-smelling tumours.

Effective care of these patients demands a team approach, with different professionals intervening as the situation demands. The full team will comprise doctors, nurses, speech therapists, dieticians, physiotherapists, occupational therapists, social workers and chaplains (see also Chapter 2).

Body image counsellors and specialist nurses are invaluable in preparing for and supporting patients through their initial treatment and rehabilitation. They may visit patients in their homes, accompany them on clinic visits, and make regular contact when they are in hospital. They can help advise the primary health care team and other professionals on specific aspects of care such as the care of tracheostomies. The relationship which is forged is of great benefit if the patient relapses, and a good specialist nurse will remain an important psychological support to the patient and their family throughout the illness, and act as a source of professional support and advice to the primary health care team.

The management of symptoms and common procedures

Palliative radiotherapy and chemotherapy

In addition to its role as a primary curative treatment, radiotherapy is frequently employed for symptom control if the patient has not already received a maximum dose to the area of recurrence. It is an effective

Table 15.1 Side effects of radiotherapy to the head and neck.

Side effect	Treatment
Loss of taste	None
Xerostomia	Artificial saliva–water sprayer Room humidification Pilocarpine
Mucositis	Raspberry mucilage NSAID mouthwashes Local anaesthetic gel
Furred tongue	Half tablet effervescent vit C dissolved on tongue

Infection
  Odynophagia/dysphagia
  Osteoradionecrosis/soft
    tissue fibrosis
	Antifungal agents: antibiotics
	  Mucaine–10 ml q.d.s.
	  None

Patients who continue to smoke and drink whilst having radiotherapy may potentiate its side effects and compromise the success of treatment.

treatment for pain: by reducing tumour bulk radiotherapy reduces pain and improves secondary mechanical difficulties. It is also useful for controlling bleeding from a fungating wound, and for reducing odour.

Palliative radiotherapy aims to relieve symptoms whilst keeping side-effects to a minimum. Table 15.1 illustrates some of the typical and less frequently encountered side-effects and their subsequent treatment (see also Chapter 12).

The role of chemotherapy in head and neck cancer is controversial and currently the subject of clinical trials in combination with radiotherapy (it has no proven role as a monotherapy). Combined modality treatment may improve local disease control and symptom relief but has not yet been shown to alter prognosis.

Pain

Pain is seldom a feature of early disease but those who present with advanced disease may have considerable problems. A small number of disease-free patients experience chronic postoperative pain, but more commonly pain will be the first clue to relapsing disease (Table 15.2). It is important to exclude intraoral infections and abscesses as a cause for a

Table 15.2 Symptoms of diagnosis of recurrence in 24 consecutive patients with squamous carcinoma of the head and neck [4]. Disseminated disease is rare, the commonest site of distant metastases is the lungs.

New pain in the absence of palpable recurrence	9
Pain and palpable local or nodal disease	10
Painless local recurrence	4
Other symptoms	1

new pain or worsening of pre-existing pain and a trial of antibiotics is justified.

The principles of pain control, discussed in Chapter 9 should be followed in all patients. The head and face has a rich nerve supply and many patients will experience neuropathic pain. The following is a guide to the management of patients with pain.

• Elicit the cause and type of pain. Consider infections and abscesses.
• If recurrence, follow the WHO analgesic ladder when introducing opioids ('strong' opioids) for severe pain as appropriate.
• Non-steroidal anti-inflammatory drugs are often very effective because of bone involvement and general inflammation.
• Tricyclic antidepressants/anticonvulsants should be introduced early in neuropathic pain that is unresponsive to moderate doses of opioid analgesics.
• Flecainide and ketamine or other drugs for neuropathic pain may be appropriate but specialist advice should usually be sought.
• Nerve blocks may be helpful, but if permanent the associated anaesthesia or paralysis needs to be discussed with the patient.

It is important to consider routes of drug administration in this group of patients as treatment is commenced, bearing in mind that swallowing difficulties may develop as the tumour progresses. Most medicines can be given as liquids, but may taste unpleasant and be in large volumes. A gastrostomy or jejunostomy tube may be helpful (see Chapter 10). Transdermal, subcutaneous, and rectal routes are useful if acceptable to the patient.

Dysphagia, nutrition and feeding

Patients with advanced head and neck cancer will usually have altered anatomy as a consequence of previous surgery as well as their recurrent tumour. Neurological dysfunction and the side-effects of radiotherapy (e.g. mucositis or xerostomia) may further exacerbate dysphagia and interfere with the complex action of swallowing. Many patients are nutritionally disadvantaged prior to presentation as a result of high alcohol intake combined with a poor diet. Finally, malignancy itself causes cachexia via cytokines (see also Chapter 17).

The consequences of malnutrition are impairment of immune function and hence increased susceptibility to infection; decreased tolerance of chemotherapy or radiotherapy; reduced skin integrity leading to pressure sores and poor wound healing; and increased morbidity and mortality. The enormous psychological distress to both patient and carers should never be underestimated as weight loss continues and the patient has to alter eating habits or fails to participate in communal eating.

CRITERIA FOR IDENTIFYING THE NUTRITIONALLY
HIGH-RISK PATIENT

Various criteria can be used to help identify the patient who is at high risk of malnutrition. These include:
- recent loss >12% of body weight;
- alcoholism;
- no oral intake >10 days (on i.v. fluids only);
- protracted nutrient loss—fistula, fungating wounds;
- hypercatabolic state—infection, rapidly advancing tumour, protracted fever;
- drugs with antinutrient or catabolic properties, e.g. steroids, chemotherapy;
- severe mucositis secondary to radiotherapy.

NUTRITIONAL SUPPORT

Nutritional support should be provided in consultation with a dietician and considered before the patient at risk starts to lose a large amount of weight. High-calorie and high-protein drinks, liquidizing food, and eating and drinking little and often are helpful steps in maintaining an adequate daily intake. Helping to reduce family stress around meal times is also important. (See also Chapter 17).

More invasive support is appropriate in some patients but requires very careful consideration and fully informed consent. Many professionals will consider nasogastric or percutaneous endoscopic gastrostomy (PEG) feeding unnecessarily invasive. However, the patient may find contemplation of 'starving to death' worse than that of a protracted illness with worsening local symptoms. It is debatable whether supplementary feeding does prolong life. However, it does seem to improve quality of life, particularly if the procedure is carried out as dysphagia is developing.

A variety of routes are amenable to alimentation: nasogastric, gastrostomy, jejunostomy, peripheral or central venous access. Each of these routes has advantages and disadvantages which need to be assessed for an individual patient's comfort, nutritional needs, and the projected time span of feeding which is required. Parenteral nutrition is seldom appropriate or necessary if the gut is functional and can be accessed [5].

The timing of enteral feeding can be arranged to suit the patient's needs; it is usually done for 12–16h but can be interrupted. Overnight feeding is usually preferred but bottles may need to be changed during this period. Equipment is arranged via the community or hospital dietetic service.

Nasogastric feeding

Nasogastric feeding is useful for *short-term* use (weeks) or prior to surgery. Various difficulties can be encountered, including:
- accidental displacement of tube;
- aspiration;
- blockage;
- irritation of nasal tissue;
- narrow bore of tube necessitates prolonged feeding time;
- early satiety;
- diarrhoea;
- patient dislike.

Some patients have fewer problems with reflux symptoms if the feeding tube is placed in the jejunum.

Percutaneous endoscopic gastrostomy (PEG)

This technique allows fixed placement of a feeding catheter through the abdominal wall into the stomach under benzodiazepine sedation [6] (Fig. 15.1). The procedure is well tolerated by even quite sick patients. It can be performed as a day case but usually patients remain in hospital whilst learning about the enteral feeding apparatus and techniques.

If it is impossible to site a gastrostomy endoscopically it may be possible radiologically with ultrasound guidance.

PEG feeding is useful for long-term use (months to years) [8,9]. Box 15.1 outlines the indications and contraindications, and Box 15.2 describes the possible complications.

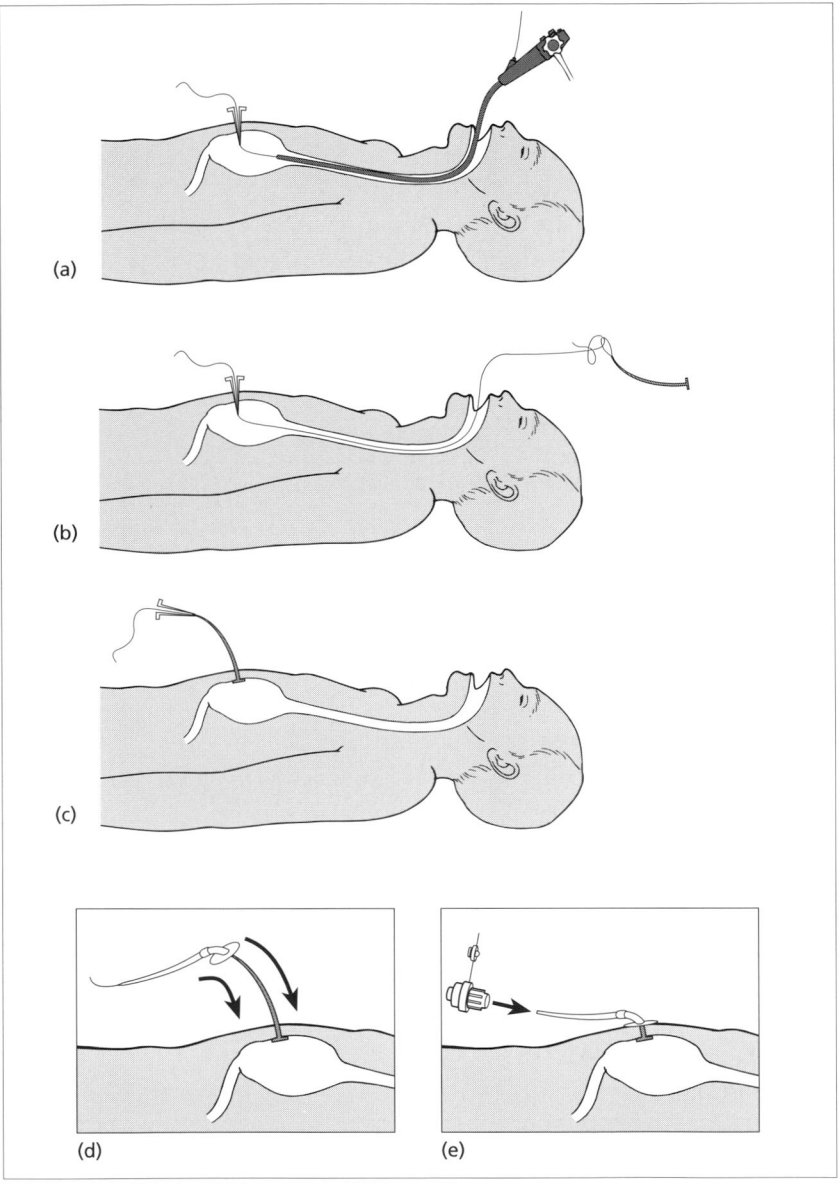

Fig. 15.1 Positioning a PEG tube. (a) Gastric puncture with a sheathed needle and introduction of a string or metal wire through the sheath after removal of the needle. While grasping the string or the metal wire, the endoscope is removed. (b) The loop of the gastrostomy tube is knotted at the string projecting from the mouth and by pulling at the abdominal end of the string the gastrostomy tube passes through the oesophagus and stomach and finally pierces the abdominal wall. (c) The retention disc of the gastrostomy tube is apposed against the gastric wall. (d) The outer retention disc, and (e) the feeding adaptor are put in place. Adapted from [7].

Box 15.1 PEG insertion in patients with head and neck cancer

Indications
- Tumour cachexia
- Oropharyngeal disease
- Inoperable obstruction—upper digestive tract
- Neurogenic dysphagia without risk of aspiration
- Major oral surgery
- Pre-radiotherapy

Contraindications
- Lack of diaphanoscopy
- Blood coagulation disorder
- Poor wound healing
- Ileus
- Ascites
- Sepsis
- Pancreatitis

Box 15.2 Complications of PEG

Major
- Gastric perforation
- Haemorrhage
- Haematoma

Minor
- Wound infection/stomal leak
- Regurgitation and aspiration
- Ileus, abdominal bloating, diarrhoea
- Tube migration/extubation
- Anorexia

PEG tube care. Certain routine measures and guidelines should be followed to minimize the risks associated with PEG feeding. Rinse the tube before and after each feeding or at least once daily using 30 ml cooled boiled water, or fennel or camomile tea. Always remember that any medicine administered via a PEG should be in liquid form or a dissolvable preparation. In the case of a blockage, never attempt to force flush the obstruction through, but replace the tube.

Good oral, dental, and pharyngeal hygiene is necessary, and the puncture site should be examined daily.

The risk of gastrointestinal infection can be reduced by discontinuing H_2 antagonists and antacids for 24 h prior to PEG and until PEG feeding has finished. Gastric prokinetic agents may be used if reflux or stasis is a problem.

Jejunal feeding

Some patients have considerable problems with enteral feeding into the stomach, with symptoms of: reflux, aspiration, hiccups, nausea, and vomiting. These may be particularly problematic in patients with gastric stasis or gastric emptying problems. Jejunal placement of the feeding tube may alleviate these symptoms.

A nasal feeding tube may be directed into the jejunum under fluoroscopic or endoscopic guidance. A jejunostomy tube may be placed by threading a fine feeding tube through the gastrostomy catheter and subsequent endoscopic manipulation into the upper small bowel. Patients with jejunal feeding tubes will be unlikely to tolerate bolus feeds since there is no gastric reservoir.

Airway patency and tracheostomies

A tracheostomy may be necessary to maintain airway patency and allow expectoration of secretions. The indications for tracheostomy include: bilateral vocal cord paralysis; laryngectomy, and a tumour occluding the airway.

A tracheostomy tube used in the palliative setting is usually a plastic single-lumen uncuffed tube suitable for long-term use. These tubes are lightweight and soften at body temperature, which reduces tracheal abrasion. They have an inner cannula which can be removed for cleaning or to allow suctioning, and can be periodically replaced. The outer housing and neck plate should not be replaced unless blocked, as re-siting in the presence of tumour may be difficult. Some inner cannulae are designed to allow speech, but more frequently (if the vocal cords are intact) the patient is taught to vocalize by temporary occlusion of the stoma with a finger. Occasionally a patient will have an 'electronic voicebox' or communicate by writing. This is often very frustrating and tiring for both patients and carers—patience is required!

COMPLICATIONS OF TRACHEOSTOMIES

The complications arising from a tracheostomy can be considered under three categories: immediate, early, and late.

- Immediate (0–24 h):
  anaesthetic complications;
  primary haemorrhage;
  damage to local structures, e.g. recurrent laryngeal nerve.
- Early (1–14 days):
  accidental decannulation;
  surgical emphysema;
  pneumothorax;
  tube obstruction;
  infection—wound, perichondritis, secondary haemorrhage;
  necrosis of the trachea leading to stenosis or fistulae;
  swallowing difficulty.
- Late (14+ days):
  subglottic or tracheal stenosis;
  fistulae—oesophageal, blood vessels, cutaneous;
  stomal recurrence tumour.

CARE OF A TRACHEOSTOMY

Many patients manage effective self-care and will wish to do so even in very advanced disease. They should be counselled to avoid polluted atmospheres, for example smoke or dust, and to avoid freezing temperatures. They should also wear a lint-free scarf or bib over the stoma to warm inspired air and trap foreign bodies. There are three basic aspects of care [10,11]: humidification of inspired air; mobilization of secretions; and suctioning.

Humidification

Due to the loss of air passing through the moist mouth and oropharynx, extra humidity is essential to keep secretions thin and easily removable in patients with tracheostomies. This can be provided by dampening the covering bib (not all varieties require this), by installing a room or bedside humidifier, or by using an ultrasonic nebulizer with specialized mask.

Mobilization and reduction of secretions

Regular deep-breathing exercises and chest physiotherapy will help move secretions and reduce pulmonary complications. If the patient is bed-bound, regular turning will aid drainage. Even a low level of activity, such as transferring from a bed to a chair, should be encouraged to help prevent basal atelectasis. Some patients will have coexistent chronic obstructive pulmonary disease: ipratropium bromide nebulizers, administered via the tracheostomy, may be useful in reducing secretions.

Suctioning

This is required if viscid secretions or mucous plugs develop and/or the cough reflex is ineffective. The catheter used for suctioning should be half the internal diameter of the tracheostomy tube. A sterile technique should be observed and the procedure explained to the patient.

Some patients may need preoxygenation. The catheter should be inserted 15 cm into the trachea. Suction should be applied as the tube is withdrawn, whilst being slowly rotated. Suctioning should not last longer than 15 s to enable the patient to breathe.

For patients with a lot of secretions

Special measures are required for patients who produce very high volumes of secretions. Cuffed tubes will prevent blood and secretions entering the airway. Inner tubes should be changed and cleaned (in sodium bicarbonate) frequently (2–6 times daily). Outer tubes may need specialist help in changing (1–2 times weekly).

Emergency care of acute tracheostomy obstruction

Tracheostomy tubes may become blocked acutely by bleeding from tracheostomal recurrence or severe crusting of secretions, often associated with tumour recurrence and poor humidification of inspired air.

When this happens, the following steps should be taken:
• remove the inner tube;
• suction through the outer tube (catheter < half diameter of the tube);
• Tilley's forceps (long fine prongs) may be introduced in the tube to relieve obstruction;
• If necessary instil 5 ml 0.9% saline into the tube and resuction, repeat as necessary.

If the obstruction persists the outer tube should be removed and cleaned and the stoma held open by tracheal dilators or immediate placement of a new tube. Tracheal dilators and a spare tube set must be available in case both inner and outer tubes are displaced and the stoma is closed.

Prosthesis

Some patients with advanced head and neck cancer may have facial prostheses to restore functional and cosmetic anatomy. For example, a maxillary bridge to facilitate swallowing and improve speech, or a false nose to support glasses and restore facial integrity. However, the process of facial reconstruction is time-consuming, requiring several long out-patient visits to a prostho-orthodontist as well as extensive laboratory work. Hence, many patients who have advanced disease would not be suitable for referral. Some patients who have relapsed following initial radical treatment and reconstruction may have a facial or dental prosthesis which requires revision.

Psychological problems

Contemporary society places great importance on physical attractiveness and the ability to communicate. It is therefore not surprising that head and neck cancer poses unique and distressing psychological problems. For example, when loss of speech is compounded by loss of facial expression, the powers of communication are doubly diminished. Facial deformity or functional changes, for example dysarthria, may draw unwanted attention to a patient already struggling to cope with loss of self-confidence, self-esteem, and sexuality.

Rapport *et al.* [12] suggest that patients with congenital abnormality cope better than those with acquired abnormality, as do longer-term survivors of facial injury who presumably have longer to come to terms with psychological problems. Clearly when the cause of the acquired abnormality is malignancy, there is a two-fold problem: the cancer itself as well as change in body image and self-concept.

Health professionals should be sensitive to the problems of depression and the social withdrawal which may arise. Consideration must also be given to the reaction of relatives and friends when faced with the altered appearance of a loved one. The patient and family may have a constant visual or audible reminder of their disease. Daily activities such as shaving, cleaning teeth, eating, and simply talking may become an ordeal. Each time the patients looks in a mirror, they may be confronted by their cancer or consequences of treatment, such as surgical scarring or radiation damage in the skin. Most cancer patients are able to assume a relatively 'normal' lifestyle in between symptomatic episodes, but this may not be the case for a patient with head and neck disease [13–15].

Cultural difficulties in dealing with cancer may also pose challenging difficulties in patient care. Disease may be viewed as a 'shame' or punishment which has been visited on an individual and/or his or her family. Frequent reassurance and clear communication must aim to dispel such beliefs and minimize social isolation and guilt.

Terminal care

The management of the last phase of life for patients with locally advanced disease may present some challenges. Many patients will become very weak and malnourished, while those with PEG feeding may remain systemically well, but may experience particular complications specific to local tumour growth. These complications may include:
- local infections;
- respiratory infections;
- tracheal obstruction/stridor;
- oesophageal obstruction;
- tracheo-oesophageal fistulae;
- pathological, compound fracture of mandible;
- arterial bleeds.

Local infections

A large proportion of fungating and recurrent tumours may become locally infected. It is usually worthwhile treating these aggressively as they ease unpleasant additional symptoms including pain, foul-smelling discharge, and a constant distressing unpleasant taste in the mouth. Superadded infection may rapidly worsen swallowing in the dysphagic patient.

Treatment involves culturing the organism and commencing appropriate antibiotics, including cover for anaerobic organisms.

Intra-oral infections

Candida and herpes simplex infections are the commonest infections and require prompt treatment to avoid needless distress. *Candida* usually produces white plaques but also may be present in the sore red mouth. Herpes may cause ulcers, mucositis, and plaques. A diagnosis of herpes should be suspected in the presence of any painful oral lesions, and rapidly treated (see Chapter 10).

Respiratory infections

Respiratory infections are the predominate infections in this group, often precipitated by fistulae and aspiration. Treatment decisions depend on the individual case, but antibiotics may alleviate cough and sputum production.

Large airway compression: stridor

The onset of tracheal compression may be slow, due to tumour growth, or rapid, precipitated by haemorrhage or infection (it may occur earlier in the disease and then requires urgent management by referral to the ear, nose and throat (ENT) or other relevant specialist team). Most patients will have previously received radical radiotherapy and treatment is therefore supportive.
- High-dose dexamethasone: start at 16 mg daily, either dissolved or subcutaneously.
- Benzodiazepines may reduce the sensation of panic: e.g. diazepam 5–10 mg orally or titrated i.v., or midazolam 2.5–5 mg titrated s.c. or i.v.
- Nebulized 0.9% saline + 2% lignocaine (5 ml volume).
- Oxygen: high flow (28% or more if possible).
- If there is no response to dexamethasone it may be appropriate to offer sedation. This may be via the PEG tube or subcutaneous infusion via a syringe driver.

Arterial bleeding

The possibility of arterial bleedings causes great anxiety to patients, carers, and health professionals. Many patients will have fungating, eroding tumours close to their carotid arteries but despite this arterial bleeding is a rare occurrence. Patients at risk may have a small warning bleed. However, unconsciousness and death may be too rapid to allow sedation (see Chapter 20). A green, red, or dark cloth is helpful in camouflaging blood.

Patients who are told about this possibility are often fearful and loath to leave the hospital. This should be considered when balancing the need for information with the likely ensuing anxiety. Discussion of such a possibility with the patient and carer is helpful. If a patient asks or is reported to be (or appears to be) worrying about such an event facilitating discussion may allow a more realistic scenario to be portrayed, with the opportunity to reassure the patient and the carer that suffering would be transitory as unconsciousness develops quickly. It is also an opportunity to inform many patients that such events are, in fact, very rare. Following this, a plan of care can be formulated together.

When there is a serious risk of such a terminal event many carers find it much less distressing to be forewarned despite the difficulty and distress of such a discussion. The discussion must be handled therefore with great sensitivity and followed-up with repeated support and review of the situation. The aims of such a discussion are threefold.

•   To give an opportunity for the carer to voice their own suspicions and fears and discuss them in realistic terms.

•   To help the carer plan what they might do so that they can feel less helpless and fearful.

•   To ensure that the carer understands the optimum sources of professional support and how to contact them. For example not necessarily to telephone the emergency services, but to have the telephone numbers of the GP and emergency hospice/palliative care services beside the telephone.

References

1   Peckham, Pinedo, Veronesi, Boyle, eds. In: *Oxford Textbook of Oncology,* Vol. 1. Oxford: Oxford University Press, 1995: 200–206.

2   Hifsa Haroon-Iqbal. *Palliative Care Service Use by Black and Minority Ethnic Groups in Leicester.* Fosse Health Trust and Coping with Cancer, 1994.

3   Souhami R, Tobias J. *Cancer and Its Management,* 3rd edn. Oxford: Blackwell Science, 1995.

4   Rudd GN. A survey of presenting symptoms in patients with recurrent head and neck cancers. Unpublished, 1996.

5   Koretz RL. Parenteral nutrition: is it oncologically logical? *J Clin Oncol* 1984; 2 (5): 534–539.

6   Larson DE, Burton DD, Schroeder KW, DiMagno EP. Percutaneous endoscopic gastrostomy. *Gastroenterology* 1987; 93: 48–52.

7   Mathus-Vliegen EMH. Feeding tubes and gastrostomy. In: Tytgat GNJ, Classen M, eds. *Practice of Therapeutic Endoscopy.* In press.

8   Saunders JR, Brown MS, Hirata RM, Jaques DA. Percutaneous endoscopic gastrostomy in patients with head and neck malignancies. *Am J Surgery* 1991; 162: 381–383.

9   Fresenius Ltd (UK). Freka®-PEG. Standard gastric set instruction booklet. Art. no. 7901051. Runcorn: Fresenius Ltd.

10 Leicester Royal Infirmary. *Tracheostomy—ENT Ward Guidelines.* Leicester: Leicester Royal Infirmary.

11 Shiley-Europe. *Tracheostomy Care.* Shiley instruction booklet. Staines: Shiley-Europe.

12 Rapport Y, Kreitler S, Chaitchik S, Algor R, Weissler K. Psychosocial problems in head and neck cancer patients and their change with time since diagnosis. *Annals Oncol* 1993; 4: 69–73.

13 McEleney M. The psychological effects of head and neck surgery. *J Wound Care* 1993; 2 (4): 205–208.

14 Kelly R. Nursing patients with oral cancer. *Nursing Standard* 1994; 8 (32): 25–29.

15 Burgess L. Facing the reality of head and neck cancer. *Nursing Standard* 1994; 8 (32): 30–34.

16: Palliative Care for Children

ANN GOLDMAN

Introduction

The death of a child is recognized as one of the greatest tragedies that can happen to a family. The family's grief and distress are intense and long lasting, and now that death in childhood is so uncommon, parents also experience considerable isolation. Today parents' expectations and plans barely even acknowledge the possibility of a child dying, and society as a whole has become unfamiliar and uncomfortable with the situation, and the ways to offer support. This includes medical and nursing staff too, who are affected both emotionally and often also by their lack of experience and confidence.

This chapter can only offer an overview of paediatric palliative care. It will identify the children for whom palliative care is appropriate, discuss some of their needs, particularly when they are different from an adults', and consider how services can be provided for them. Its aim is to provide an insight into the problems of the sick child and their family, and to encourage those caring for them to work together and with the family to provide as good a quality of life as possible.

Children needing palliative care

The nature of children needing palliative care differs significantly from that of adults in a similar situation. The number of deaths which can be anticipated and where palliative care can be planned is very much smaller, although the exact epidemiology is uncertain. Current estimates of prevalence suggest that in a health district of 250 000 people, with a child population of 50 000, five children are likely to die of a life-limiting condition in any one year: two from cancer, one from heart disease; and two from other conditions. In the same district there will also be around 50 children suffering from a variety of chronic life-threatening illnesses at any time, of whom about half will actively need palliative care [1].

Table 16.1 Main life-limiting conditions in childhood.

Malignant diseases
Degenerative disorders
Metabolic
Neurodegenerative
Cystic fibrosis
Muscular dystrophy
Organ failures
Heart
Liver
Kidney
Severe multiple disability
HIV/AIDS

The range of life-limiting conditions which affect children is wide (Table 16.1). Palliative care needs to be considered for all of these, not just cancer. Most of the illnesses are specific to paediatrics and many are very rare; some are familial and some have a protracted course, four broad groups can be identified [1]:
• Conditions where curative treatment may be possible but may fail. Palliative care is needed in times of prognostic uncertainty or when cure becomes impossible. Cancer is an example.
• Conditions where there are long periods of intensive treatment aimed at prolonging life, but premature death is still likely. Cystic fibrosis, muscular dystrophy, and HIV fit this pattern.
• Progressive conditions where treatment is entirely palliative and may extend over many years. Mucopolysaccharidoses and neurodegenerative diseases such as Batten's disease are examples.
• Conditions of severe neurological disability, such as severe cerebral palsy. These are not progressive, but result in susceptibility to complications and premature death.

Providing services for the family

Paediatric palliative care is very much a developing speciality, still defining and researching both the clinical care the children need and the best way to provide services. At present, the best way to provide for the needs of each child and family must be considered individually, in the context of the illness and of what is available locally.

Most family doctors will only see a few children with life-limiting illnesses in a lifetime's practice, and each of these is likely to have a different, probably rare, and possibly complex illness. Often a large network of health care professionals from many disciplines is involved in the care of any one child. These factors can make it difficult for the family doctor to gain experience and confidence in paediatric palliative care, and to define his or her role in the care of a child, particularly as that role may evolve and change as the child's illness progresses.

When a child is diagnosed with a life-threatening illness, the family rapidly learns a great deal about the disease and its management. If it is uncommon and especially if intensive treatments are needed, care may seem to focus around in-patient or out-patient hospital management. Families may build up very close relationships and develop confidence in the hospital staff. The primary health care team can easily feel superfluous and marginalized, and this can be misinterpreted by the family as lack of interest and concern. Misunderstanding can also occur with the contrasting situation of a child being cared for with long-term illness, who is almost entirely nursed at home by the family with very little or no hospital input. Here the primary health care team may feel overwhelmed by the task, and unsupported and put upon by the hospital services.

Since most children and families prefer to spend as much time as possible at home—and for those with prolonged illness this may be many years—the active involvement of the primary health care team is vital. Establishing one member from the team of professionals involved in the network of care as the key worker for each family can facilitate good communication and co-ordination of professional care. This ensures that all the family's needs are being met, without overlap or gaps developing. In most situations the professional who fulfils this role most effectively is a nurse.

Several models of paediatric palliative care exist at present, and are related to the type of illness the child has. The best established is for cancer, where the child's care is likely to be shared between a children's cancer centre some distance from where they live, their local paediatric department, and care at home. Paediatric oncology outreach nurse specialists are usually hospital based but travel out into the community. They offer expertise and experience in symptom management, psychosocial support, and liaise with the local paediatric community nurses and primary health care teams.

The children with other life-limiting diseases, especially those with a prolonged course where care is mainly home-based, have less well-structured provisions for care. Some families have support at home from generic paediatric community nurses, linked to the local hospital and able to act as key workers, but these are still only available in half the country. Some districts have developed multidisciplinary teams built up from local staff (e.g. paediatricians, nurses, social workers, therapists, and psychologists) who devote part of their time to working together as a palliative care team, but unfortunately these are still uncommon. In many cases arrangements have to be developed on an individual basis and there is a risk that families may be either neglected or the focus of inappropriate or uncoordinated help.

A number of children's hospices contribute to the facilities available. In 1996 there were 11 opened and 11 more in various stages of development [2]. These are all charitable organizations and have developed in response to a perceived need by families, offering a markedly different service from adult hospices [3]. They provide small comfortable 'home-from-home' facilities with accommodation and support for siblings and parents as well as the sick child. They are staffed by those experienced and qualified in the care of children, and have excellent facilities for play, education, and leisure for the children. The majority of children visiting the hospices have prolonged illnesses with considerable nursing needs for whom respite care is important. Relatively few children die at the hospices as most families choose to be at home. The hospices offer support through bereavement. Children with cancer are referred less commonly but those with a prolonged illness, such as brain tumours, or families with difficult social circumstances, may find the additional support valuable.

Palliative care needs

The principles of palliative care for children are similar to those for adults. The overall needs for children and their families have been summarized in the ACT Charter (Association for Children with life threatening or Terminal conditions and their families) (Fig. 16.1) [4].

Parents bear a heavy responsibility for nursing and personal care of their child, and most take on the burdens willingly. However, it is important to see parents in their role as part of the caring team whilst also acknowledging their need for support themselves. Siblings are especially vulnerable in the family and their needs must also be considered.

ACT Charter   for Children with Life-threatening Conditions and their Families

1 Every child shall be treated with dignity and respect and shall be afforded privacy whatever the child's physical or intellectual ability.

2 Parents shall be acknowledged as the primary carers and shall be centrally involved as partners in all care and decisions involving their child.

3 Every child shall be given the opportunity to participate in decisions affecting his or her care, according to age and understanding.

4 Every family shall be given the opportunity of a consultation with a paediatric specialist who has a particular knowledge of the child's condition.

5 Information shall be provided for the parents, and for the child and the siblings according to age and understanding. The needs of other relatives shall also be addressed.

6 An honest and open approach shall be the basis of all communication which shall be sensitive and appropriate to age and understanding.

7 The family home shall remain the centre of caring whenever possible. All other care shall be provided by paediatrically trained staff in a child-centred environment.

8 Every child shall have access to education. Efforts shall be made to enable the child to engage in other childhood activities.

9 Every family shall be entitled to a named key worker who will enable the family to build up and maintain an appropriate support system.

10 Every family shall have access to flexible respite care in their own home and in a home-from-home setting for the whole family, with appropriate paediatric nursing and technical support.

11 Every family shall have access to paediatric nursing support in the home when required.

12 Every family shall have access to expert sensitive advice in procuring practical aids and financial support.

13 Every family shall have access to domestic help at times of stress at home.

14 Bereavement support shall be offered to the whole family and be available for as long as required.

Association for Children with life threatening or Terminal conditions and their families
65 St Michael's Hill, Bristol, BS2 8DZ   Tel: 0117 922 1556   Registered Charity No. 1029659

Fig. 16.1 The Charter of the Association for Children with Life-threatening or Terminal conditions and their families (ACT).

Symptom management

THE CHILD'S AND PARENTS' ROLES IN MANAGEMENT DECISIONS

Parents fear the pain and other symptoms that their child may suffer and that they will not have the skills and confidence to relieve them. It is essential to provide them with detailed and honest information about the management of their child's current symptoms and any others which may be anticipated. Both they and the sick child need to take an active part in planning a practical and acceptable regimen of care, to exercise choice, and to retain their control and confidence.

As death approaches parents will need and value further information, including what signs might suggest that death is imminent and the possible modes of death. Professionals can sometimes be reluctant to undertake such frank discussion but knowing these details and having a clear plan of what to do as the situation changes can be key factors enabling families to cope successfully at home. Almost all families can be reassured that death will be peaceful, but if there are concerns about the possibility of sudden distressing symptoms such as convulsions, acute agitation, or bleeding, these should be discussed. It may be necessary to ensure that emergency drugs such as anticonvulsants, strong analgesics, and powerful sedatives are available in the house. Suitable doses and appropriate routes should be calculated ahead of time, so that the parents can give the drugs themselves or they are rapidly accessible for whichever professional is called.

Parents may wish, as most families do, to care for their child at home, but need to discuss other possibilities if that is not their choice. Those who are at home need access to advice and support 24 hours a day. The professionals involved need to plan this carefully so that those who are caring for the child locally, who may be in an unfamiliar situation, have back-up from others with experience in care of children and palliative care.

When a child has an uncommon illness it may be difficult for the local doctor or family to anticipate the problems and the symptoms which will develop as the disease progresses. As these relate closely to the diagnosis, specialist paediatricians and nursing staff with more experience of the particular illness should be able to advise. There are also disease-specific parent help groups for many rare illnesses which offer information. The organization Contact a Family is a useful starting point (see Useful Addresses, p. 377).

Children dying from cancer are likely to have a final illness lasting only a few months, although brain tumours tend to have a more protracted course. These children will almost certainly experience pain, depending on the sites and spread of the tumour. Other common problems include gastrointestinal symptoms such as nausea, vomiting, and constipation. Since bone marrow involvement is common in childhood tumours, anaemia and bleeding are often concerns. Dyspnoea, anxiety, agitation, and seizures may also occur.

In contrast, children with slower degenerative diseases suffer a different spectrum of problems, over a much longer period. Feeding difficulties, impaired intellect, convulsions, and communication and mobility problems are common. These increase as the illness progresses and respiratory difficulties and excess secretions may develop. Pain is usually less prominent, although muscle spasms may be troublesome.

As in adults, thorough assessment of any symptom is essential before developing a plan of management. This can be particularly challenging in children and has in the past contributed to the neglect and poor treatment of symptoms in children. Since the experience of pain and other symptoms is subjective, ideally the child should provide the information about their problems themselves. Their ability to do this will vary in relation to their level of understanding, experience, and communication skills. In preverbal children and those with severe developmental delay it can be particularly difficult.

Often, the use of a variety of approaches can help towards building up a more complete picture. For pain, a range of assessment tools, appropriate for different ages and developmental levels, have been developed but these are not available for other symptoms. These include colour tools, body charts, and faces scales [5]. They can be helpful when used alongside discussion with the child and the parents, and also careful observation both by the parents and staff. The contribution of psychological and social factors both for the child and family are often significant and are an important part of the assessment (Table 16.2).

When planning treatment the individual child's preferences need to be taken into account. Many find that taking a lot of medication is difficult, so complex regimens may not be possible. It is also important to find the most acceptable route for the child. The oral route is preferable;

Table 16.2 Factors to consider in assessing pain.

The pain itself
Child's opinion, parent and staff's observation
Sites—use body charts
Severity—pain tools, parent and staff observations
Timing—diaries
Nature—e.g. nerve pain
Precipitating and relieving factors
Coping skills of the child and family
Past experience of the child and family
Anxiety and emotional distress levels in the child and family
Meaning of the pain and underlying disease to the child and family

long-acting preparations are convenient and less intrusive. Children should be offered the choice between whole or crushed tablets or liquids. As a child's condition deteriorates the treatment plan often has to be simplified, routes of administration altered, and priority given to those drugs that contribute most to the child's comfort. Although rectal drugs are not popular in paediatrics they can have a role. Some children prefer them to using any needles, even subcutaneous, and they may be helpful in the final hours when the child's level of consciousness has deteriorated. If parenteral drugs are needed they are usually given subcutaneously, although if an intravenous line is already in place that can be used. Intramuscular drugs are painful and not necessary.

Doses of drugs for children are usually calculated according to their weight. Many of the drugs used in palliative care have not been recommended formally for use in children but a body of clinical experience has developed in the absence of many trials or extensive pharmacokinetic data [6,7]. In general neonates tend to need reduced doses relative to their size, whilst infants and young children may need comparatively higher doses and at shorter intervals than adults.

PAIN

After thorough assessment of pain a treatment regimen can be planned. This should consider the likely cause of the pain and whether this can be relieved by specific measures (e.g. radiotherapy for an isolated bony metastasis, antibiotics for a urinary tract infection). Then symptomatic relief can be addressed by combining pharmacological, psychological, and practical approaches. Analgesics often form the backbone to a plan but a combined approach is likely to be more successful.

The WHO ladder of analgesia (see p. 110) is equally relevant for children, with paracetamol, dihydrocodeine, and morphine sulphate forming the standard steps. Long-acting preparations are effective and particularly convenient. It is important to give families a short-acting preparation too, for breakthrough pain, and to explain their different roles carefully.

The myths perpetuating the undertreatment of pain in children have now been rejected. However, most doctors lack experience of using strong opioids in children, and this often results in unnecessary caution. Respiratory depression with strong opioids has not been a problem in children with severe pain. Indeed, recent studies of the pharmacokinetics of oral opioids and their metabolites suggest that in young children metabolism is more rapid than in adults and they may require relatively higher doses for analgesia. However, neonates and children under 6 months old require a lower starting dose of opioids because of their reduced metabolism and increased sensitivity.

Parents may be reluctant to have their children taking strong opioids. It is important to establish exactly what their concerns are. They may be anxious about the side-effects, but often it is related to their feelings that giving strong opioids represents an acknowledgement that their child is really going to die. Another common parental fear is that if opioids are started 'too early' there will be nothing left for later.

Likely side-effects include constipation, and so regular laxatives should be prescribed alongside the opioids. For some children relatively mild laxatives such as lactulose may be sufficient, but the majority will require a stimulant. Many children are initially quite sleepy; the parents should be warned about this, or they may fear that the child's disease has suddenly progressed and that death is imminent. Drowsiness usually resolves within a few days. Itching with opioids in the first few days is quite common and responds to antihistamines if it continues. Nausea and vomiting seem uncommon and routine antiemetics are not needed.

Non-steroidal anti-inflammatory drugs (NSAIDs) are often helpful for musculoskeletal pains, especially in children with non-malignant disease. Some caution is needed in children with cancer who have bone marrow infiltration because of the increased risk of bleeding. Neuropathic pain may be helped by antiepileptic and antidepressant drugs.

Headaches from central nervous system leukaemia respond well to intrathecal methotrexate. Headaches from raised intracranial pressure, associated with progressive brain tumours, are best managed with gradually increasing analgesics. Although steroids may seem helpful initially, the symptoms will inevitably recur as the tumour increases in size and a spiral of increasing steroid doses often develops. The side-effects of steroids in children almost always outweigh the benefits. There is rapid weight gain, dramatically changed appearance, and often marked mood swings. Both parents and the children themselves find these distressing.

FEEDING

An inability to feed and to nourish their child is very upsetting for parents and often makes them feel they are failing as parents. Also, sucking and eating are an essential part of all children's development, providing comfort, pleasure, and stimulation. Children with neurodegenerative diseases, and brain tumours in particular, often have problems with eating because of neurological damage. Others, such as those with cancers, will lose their appetite. Anticipation and careful discussion and planning of future care with the family is helpful, and can avoid having to make difficult decisions in a hurry. Nutritional goals aimed at restoring health often become secondary to comfort and enjoyment. Assisted feeding, via a nasogastric tube or gastrostomy, may be entirely correct for those with slowly progressive disease, but inappropriate for a child with a rapidly progressing tumour.

NAUSEA AND VOMITING

These are quite frequent problems in a variety of diseases. As in adults, antiemetics can be selected according to their site of action, and the presumed cause. Combining a number of drugs which act in different ways can help in resistant cases, as can the addition of a 5HT antagonist. Vomiting from raised intracranial pressure often responds well to cyclizine.

NEUROLOGICAL PROBLEMS

Watching a child have a seizure is extremely frightening for parents and they should always be warned and advised about management even if it is only a possibility. Children with neurodegenerative diseases often suffer with epilepsy as part of their ongoing disease and are taking long-term anticonvulsants, which can be adjusted when the pattern of seizures changes. For sudden acute onset of seizures a supply of rectal diazepam at home for the parents to use is extremely valuable. Subcutaneous midazolam can enable parents to continue to manage a child having severe repeated seizures at home.

Agitation and anxiety may reflect a child's need to talk about his or her fears and distress. In addition drugs such as benzodiazapines, haloperidol, and methotrimeprazine may provide relief, especially in the final stages of life.

RESPIRATORY SYMPTOMS

Dyspnoea, cough, and excess secretions can all cause distress to children and anxiety for their parents. If the underlying cause of the symptom can be relieved, even temporarily, this may be worthwhile, but if not, relief can be approached by combining drugs with practical and supportive approaches. Fear is often an important element in dyspnoea, and reassurance and management of anxiety may help to relieve symptoms. Simple practical measures such as finding the optimum position, using a fan, and relaxation exercises may all help.

The sensation of breathlessness can be relieved with opioid drugs, and small doses of sedatives such as diazepam are often helpful in relieving the associated anxiety. Children with gradually increasing hypoxaemia of chronic chest diseases may suffer from headaches, nausea, daytime drowsiness, and poor-quality sleep. Intermittent oxygen may help relieve these symptoms and can be given relatively easily at home. Children with dyspnoea in the later stages of malignant disease do not usually find oxygen helpful.

Excess secretions are often a problem for children with chronic neuro-degenerative diseases as their illnesses progresses and they are less able to cough and swallow. It may also occur for other terminally ill children as they approach death. Suction equipment is not usually helpful, but oral glycopyrronium bromide, or hyoscine hydrobromide, which can be given transdermally or subcutaneously, can reduce secretions.

ANAEMIA AND BLEEDING

The treatment of anaemia in the late stages of a child's life should be directed towards relief of symptoms rather than the level of haemoglobin, so regular blood counts are not needed. Parents should understand the purpose of transfusions and appreciate that as the illness progresses there is likely to come a point where transfusions no longer relieve symptoms and are therefore inappropriate, although early in the disease they may be valuable.

Florid bleeding, such as from haemoptysis or haematemesis, is extremely frightening for a child, distressing for the carers, and may leave the family with unforgettable painful memories. If this is a serious risk, such as in liver disease, then emergency drugs should be readily available and include an appropriate analgesic and sedative such as diamorphine and midazolam. Correct dosage should be calculated ahead of time and the drugs and syringes immediately accessible either at home or in hospital.

Many children with malignant diseases have widespread bone marrow infiltration and low platelets, but although petechiae and minor gum bleeding is common, serious bleeding is unusual. In general platelet transfusions are confined to bleeding that is severe or interferes with the quality of life, although children with an established history of bleeding throughout their illness may require regular platelet transfusions.

Support for the child and family

Support begins at the time of diagnosis and continues as the illness progresses,

Table 16.3 Predicting how well a family will cope.

Positive	Negative
Cohesive family	Over-involved family
Supportive family	Unconnected family
Flexible approach	Rigid approach
Open communication in family	Closed communication in family
Open communication with staff	Closed communication with staff
Good record with past stress	Poor record with past stress
	Previous parental psychopathology
	Concurrent stresses
	Single parent
	Parental strife
	Financial problems

through the child's death and into bereavement. All the family—the sick child, the parents, siblings, and the wider family—will be affected by the illness and may need help, both as a family unit and as individuals. A flexible approach, with time to listen and build up relationships, is important. A balance must also be sought in which the child's and family's problems are recognized but not overemphasized to the point that the family are disabled and their own resources diminished.

Although all families will suffer emotional distress the majority possess considerable strength and resilience and do find ways to continue to function effectively from day to day. A number of factors have been identified which can help predict a family's capacity to cope, and this knowledge can be helpful in identifying families who may be at extra risk and need particular support (Table 16.3). It is important also to be aware of any language difficulties or different cultural approaches to illness and death.

AT DIAGNOSIS

The time of diagnosis of a life-threatening illness is one of great turmoil for the family. Their grief begins at this time. The way in which the diagnosis is given has a powerful impact and forms the foundation for communication in the future. The family's expectations and pattern of life are disrupted and, especially if frequent hospital admissions are involved, many practical difficulties arise in day-to-day living so it can be easy for the parents and other children to feel overwhelmed, helpless, and out of control. Parents have a great need for information at this time and may value leaflets, contact with other parents in similar situations, and links with self-help groups (see Useful Addresses, pp. 377–381). The sick children face the trauma of being in hospital and the experience of unpleasant and frightening investigations and treatment. They may be particularly confused as explanations and understanding of what is happening may be delayed whilst parents themselves are just learning about the illness. Some parents may be reluctant to discuss the diagnosis with their children and need encouragement and help to do so.

AS THE DISEASE PROGRESSES

As the illness progresses the family have to live with the underlying conflict of maintaining some hope and semblance of day-to-day life in spite of persistent uncertainty. The parents may develop depression, anxiety, and sleep disturbance although they are often reluctant to speak of these problems unless asked specifically. Marital discord and loss of libido are also common. Parents often find difficulty in handling the children, particularly in maintaining discipline and boundaries for the sick child, and in balancing their time and emotions between the sick child and well siblings. If frequent hospital admissions are involved there are practical problems of travel, separation, and finance. If the child has heavy nursing needs, with physical disability and developmental delay, the burdens of care can be considerable. Parents may have very little time to themselves or time to devote to well brothers and sisters, and the opportunity for some respite care for the sick child, either at home or away from home, becomes essential.

The sick child may continue to experience regular hospital visits and unpleasant treatment and have gradually increasing symptoms and disability. Trying to maintain as normal a life as possible, maintaining friendships, education, and outside activities within the confines of the illness is a continual but important struggle. As the illness progresses extra support and special facilities and education may need to be introduced.

Most families employ some avoidance and denial as part of their coping strategy, including avoiding discussion and reminders of the illness, and this is normal. It helps protect them from extremes of emotion, allows them to live with the illness and function normally day to day, and to understand and recognize the situation gradually.

THE FINAL STAGES

Eventually it becomes clearer that not only is death inevitable but that the time of death is becoming quite close. This may be apparent from gradual deterioration in a long progressive illness or more abruptly such as after a relapse in cancer. The emotional impact at this time may be dramatic for parents, particularly for those who have held a very positive and 'fighting' approach throughout treatment. For others it is just a confirmation of what they have dreaded and known was inevitable all along. Sometimes there is a sense of relief that the uncertainty and suffering will soon be over, alongside the distress and sadness.

As well as information and discussion about the child's care parents need an opportunity to explore their own feelings and express their emotions. Parents may be able to talk to each other openly and offer each other support at this time, but more often they will cope in different ways and find that the whole experience is so physically and emotionally exhausting that they have little strength left to offer support either to each other or to their other children. Both the parents and well siblings often value the opportunity to talk to someone who is one step removed.

Many parents have never seen anyone die and will value the opportunity of talking about what may happen at the moment of death. They also appreciate information about the practical details of what to do after a person has died. Most will have been anticipating the funeral in their mind and are relieved to be able to acknowledge this and make some plans before the child has died.

An important issue at this time for parents is what to discuss with the child who is sick and with their other children. It is clear that children understand and learn about their illness and its implications whether the parents and the professionals encourage it or not. However, open discussion with children, particularly when death is a real possibility, can be very difficult to establish in practice.

Communicating with children must take into consideration their level of understanding about illness and the concept of death [6,7]. It also will be influenced by the child's previous experiences, the family's style of communication, and their own personal defences. Some approaches to helping families towards a more open and honest pattern of communication include:

- shifting the emphasis from 'telling' to 'listening';
- helping them identify the child's indirect cues as well as obvious questions;
- discovering the child's fears and fantasies;
- maintaining the child's trust through honesty;
- building up the whole picture gradually;
- explaining that communication need not rely on talking—drawings, stories, and play may be more effective and easier for children.

THE BEREAVED FAMILY

The grief suffered after the loss of a child has been described as the most painful, enduring, and difficult to survive, and it is associated with a high risk of pathological grief. Parents lose not only the child they have loved but their hopes for the future and their confidence in themselves as parents. It puts an additional stress on the marriage and alters the whole family structure. The brothers and sisters who are grieving often feel isolated and neglected as their parents can spare little time or emotion for them.

Ideally the professionals who know the family well and have been involved with them throughout the sick child's life should continue to be available through their bereavement. Grief is likely to continue over many years, and its depth and persistence is often underestimated. Parents value continuing contact with professionals who have known their child and the opportunity to talk about the child and their grief when others in the community expect them to 'have come to terms with it'. This support, initially more frequent and gradually decreasing, helps facilitate the normal tasks of mourning. Help can be offered for brothers and sisters, and information provided about appropriate literature, telephone helplines, and support organizations (see Useful Addresses, pp. 377–381). Most families will not need formal counselling but it is important to be able to recognize when there are signs of abnormal grief which may require referral for specialist help [8].

Conclusions

Helping to care for a child with a life-threatening illness, and for the family of such a child, is rarely easy. It presents many challenges both in the professional tasks which may be required and to our own emotional resources. However, even though the task may seem daunting, families greatly value professionals who have the courage to stay alongside them throughout their difficult journey, and there is personal satisfaction in being able to offer some help in an almost intolerable situation.

References

1 ACT/RCPCH. *A Guide to the Development of Children's Palliative Care Services.* Report of Joint Working Party of the Association for Children with life threatening or Terminal conditions and their families (ACT) and the Royal College of Paediatrics and Child Health (RCPCH). ACT/RCPCH, 1997.

2 ACT. *ACTPACK—Children's Hospices*. Bristol: Association for Children with life threatening or Terminal conditions and their families.

3 Dominica F. The role of the hospice for the dying child. *Br J Hospital Med* 1996; 38 (4): 334–343.

4 ACT. *ACT Charter*. Bristol: Association for Children with life threatening or Terminal conditions and their families.

5 Mathews JR, McGrath PJ, Pigeon H. Assessment and measurement of pain in children. In: Schechter N, Berde CB, Yaster M, eds. *Pain in Infants, Children and Adolescents*. Baltimore: Williams & Wilkins, 1993: 97–112.

6 Goldman A, ed. *Care of the Dying Child*. Oxford: Oxford University Press, 1994.

7 Davies B. Pediatric palliative care. In: Doyle D, Hanks G, Macdonald N, eds. *Oxford Textbook of Palliative Medicine*. Oxford: Oxford University Press, 1997: 1013–1096.

8 Hindmarch C. *On the Death of a Child*. Oxford: Radcliffe Medical Press, 1993.

17: Asthenia, Cachexia, and Anorexia

RICHARD WOOF

Introduction

Persistent weakness, tiredness, loss of appetite, and weight loss are all symptoms frequently experienced by patients with cancer and other life-threatening illnesses. They are encompassed by the terms asthenia, anorexia and cachexia.

Asthenia. Asthenia is characterized by the following:
• fatigue or easy tiring and reduced sustainability of performance;
• generalized weakness resulting in a reduced ability to initiate movement;
• mental fatigue characterized by poor concentration, impaired memory, and emotional lability.

Anorexia. Anorexia is the absence or loss of appetite for food.

Cachexia. Cachexia is a condition of profound weight loss and catabolic loss of muscle and adipose tissue. This is usually compounded by a chronic reduction in nutritional intake.

These conditions are often the first signs of a malignant process and are therefore important in diagnosis. In established disease, they are some of the most commonly experienced symptoms—occurring in approximately 50% of patients [1,2]—while also being relatively poorly controlled. The associated distress can be marked, especially in terms of body image and quality of life. In particular, cachexia is often associated with a shorter prognosis [3]. Although alleviating this suffering can be difficult, it is important for palliative measures to be actively considered when planning care.

Aetiology in cancer

In order to understand the aetiology of asthenia, cachexia, and anorexia, it is important to appreciate the following points.

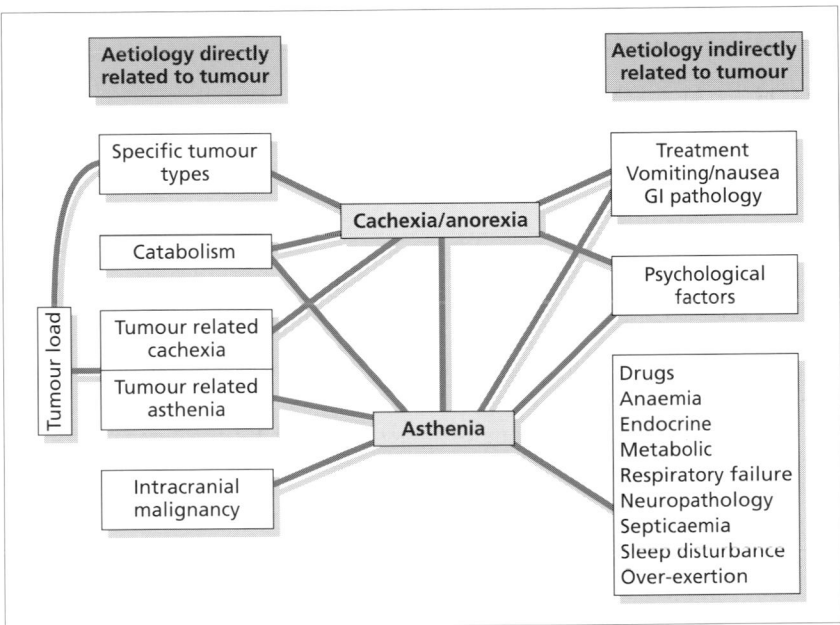

Fig. 17.1 The aetiology of asthenia and its relationship with cachexia.

- Asthenia, cachexia, and anorexia often coexist in individual patients.
- Cachexia and anorexia are major causes of asthenia.
- Asthenia, cachexia, and anorexia can have shared aetiology.
- Different aetiologies work synergistically to worsen symptoms.
- Multiple aetiologies often occur in individual patients.
- These symptoms can occur as a result of co-morbidity, unrelated to the terminal disease.

The close interrelationship between symptoms is illustrated in Fig. 17.1. Given that some of these causes may be reversible, it is clinically useful to have a clear understanding of the aetiology. This can be divided into two categories: (i) causes that are directly related to the effects of the tumour; and (ii) causes that occur as a consequence to complications and treatments of the malignant process.

Cachexia and anorexia directly caused by cancer

GASTROINTESTINAL TUMOURS

The physical presence of a tumour in the gastrointestinal tract will have a direct influence on the ingestion, digestion, and absorption of food.

TUMOUR-RELATED CACHEXIA

The catabolic metabolism found in some cancer patients is mediated by certain polypeptides known as cytokines. Their biological effects are varied, but include the following:
- increased basal metabolic rate;
- increased hepato-gluconeogenesis, using protein as substrate;
- increased glucose intolerance;
- altered lipid metabolism (e.g. increased lipolysis);
- anorexia.

The result of these processes is the breakdown of muscle and adipose tissue, leading to a clinical picture of cachexia.

Asthenia directly caused by cancer

TUMOUR-RELATED ASTHENIA

Chemical mediators are also thought to be influential in producing asthenia in isolation of cachexia and anorexia [4].

INTRACRANIAL MALIGNANCY

Asthenia is a sign of raised intracranial pressure.

Asthenia, cachexia, and anorexia indirectly caused by cancer

MEDICAL INTERVENTIONS

A wide variety of treatments can induce asthenia, cachexia, and anorexia, including chemotherapy, other drugs, radiotherapy, and surgery.

VOMITING AND NAUSEA

This subject is covered in greater detail elsewhere in this book (see Chapter 10). If nausea and vomiting are persistent, this will have nutritional consequences. Some of the causes of nausea and vomiting overlap with the aetiology for asthenia, cachexia, and anorexia.

GASTROINTESTINAL PATHOLOGY

A wide variety of complications of cancer can effect the gastrointestinal

(GI) tract to produce a combination of asthenia, cachexia, and anorexia. These include: constipation; gastroenteritis (e.g. *Clostridium difficile*); and oral complications (e.g. infections, stomatitis, dry mouth, taste alteration).

PSYCHOLOGICAL FACTORS

The complex interplay between mood, coping mechanisms, and learned food behaviour are potent aetiological factors. What is more, the psychological consequences of asthenia and anorexia can in return perpetuate the problem (see Fig. 17.2). This spiral of aetiology can also be influenced by the tiring effect of other unrelieved symptoms such as pain.

Distinguishing the biological manifestations of mood disturbance from organic disease can be difficult. However, it is important to make an accurate assessment of mood. Treatment for depression may be an important part of the overall management of the patient.

Some theorists have proposed that the symptoms of fatigue mimic those of advancing disease and so increase psychological distress. Consequently, some patients are upset by enquiries about their weight. Also carers can find a poor appetite in their loved one difficult to cope with. These points illustrate the importance of a sensitive approach by professionals when making assessments.

Indirect causes of asthenia

DRUGS

Drugs can produce fatigue, either by their sedative effects or as a result

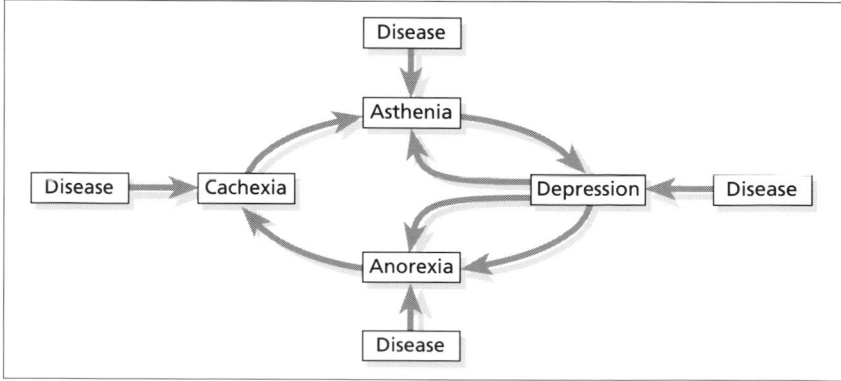

Fig. 17.2 The influence of mood in asthenia, cachexia, and fatigue.

of toxicity. In addition, changes in patients' weight and metabolism can aggravate these side-effects. Some of the common culprits include benzodiazepines, opioids, antidepressants, beta blockers, diuretics, anticonvulsants, and digoxin. Long-term steroids can produce fatigue due to proximal muscle weakness.

ANAEMIA

A combination of reduced haemopoiesis, nutritional deficiencies, and blood loss can all result in anaemia. Obviously, patients with primary haematological disease (e.g. leukaemia) or those having cytotoxic chemotherapy are particularly prone to anaemia.

METABOLIC CAUSES

Metabolic abnormalities of various types occur in terminally ill patients. These can be induced by a wide range of pathological processes and should be considered when assessing a patient with generalized weakness.
•   Malignancy: examples include hypercalcaemia (see Chapter 12), renal failure, hepatic failure, adrenal failure, and hypomagnesaemia.
•   Co-morbidity: diabetic control can be difficult in the terminally ill, especially if steroids are part of the therapeutic regime. Other examples of co-morbidity include thyroid diseases and inappropriate antidiuretic hormone (ADH) secretion.
•   Drug side-effects: the renal toxicity of certain drugs can cause troublesome disturbances of electrolytes.

RESPIRATORY FAILURE

Various pathological processes (e.g. pleural effusion, lung malignancy, co-morbidity) can result in respiratory failure. The resultant hypoxia and hypercapnia can contribute to asthenia.

NEUROLOGICAL CAUSES

Spinal cord compression. As outlined earlier in this book (see Chapter 12), this complication of malignancy is a palliative care emergency. In any patient who has 'gone off their legs', this diagnosis should always be considered as prompt treatment can prevent devastating paralysis.

Nerve compression. Due to a similar process of tumour pressure, more peripheral nerves can suffer loss of function (usually associated with pain). Although not as catastrophic as spinal cord compression, active treatment should be considered.

Paraneoplastic neurological symptoms. These conditions include peripheral neuropathy and polymyositis.

INFECTION

Terminally ill patients are especially vulnerable to infection and are more likely to be compromised by it. The symptoms of asthenia in these cases can be complicated by fever, confusion, and drowsiness. Asthenia experienced with infection may share chemical mediators with tumour-related cachexia and asthenia (i.e. cytokines).

SLEEP DISTURBANCE

There are many reasons why terminally ill patients should have a disturbed sleep pattern, not least uncontrolled coexisting symptoms. This simple explanation for asthenia should not be overlooked.

OVEREXERTION

The changing nature of an aggressive disease can make it particularly difficult for patients to adjust to their new levels of functioning. Indeed, to become less active could be interpreted by some as defeat. Maximizing quality of life requires achieving a balance between enjoying physical activity and the adverse effects of overexertion.

Asthenia, cachexia, and anorexia in non-cancerous conditions

Many disease processes can result in asthenia and anorexia. In chronic life-threatening conditions, these symptoms can become persistent and are associated with cachexia. For instance, in chronic obstructive pulmonary disease (COPD), cachexia is associated with a poorer prognosis [5]. Cardiac cachexia (cachexia associated with heart failure) is becoming increasingly recognized. It has an adverse influence on patients in terms of complications and clinical outcomes. The mechanisms behind this process are multifactorial, but include the effects of cytokines. Anorexia, cahexia and asthenia are common in patients with AIDS, not least to their susceptibility to infection and malignancy (see Chapter 13) [6]. Bowel complications of AIDS (e.g. villous atrophy, enterocyte dysfunction), produce malabsorption. Weight loss in AIDS tends to follow a fluctuating course, reflecting episodes of acute illness (infection) followed by periods of recovery. This is in contrast to the more progressive linear decline seen in cancer. Therefore, patients with AIDS have the potential for improvement in nutritional status, with active management.

Patients suffering from asthenia, cachexia, or anorexia associated with these and other illnesses deserve the same palliative treatment as patients suffering from cancer.

Assessment

As with symptom control in the rest of palliative care, a detailed holistic evaluation is important. Providing information to patients and their carers is vital for all aspects of the assessment and requires the use of skilful communication.

Management

Palliation often requires a variety of approaches to improve symptoms. Patients will benefit from their involvement in decision-making and goal-setting. Management can be divided into those measures aiming to relieve symptoms and those directed at treating the cause. Care plans should include constant review and reassessment.

General management: relieve the symptoms

SPECIFIC DRUGS

The following drugs can alleviate symptoms empirically. They should initially be used on a trial basis, with treatment being continued if benefit is confirmed.

Steroids. Dexamethasone 2–4 mg (or equivalent dose of alternative steroid), is useful for increasing appetite and energy [7]. The side-effects of these drugs can limit their use; they include: diabetes, psychological effects, immunosuppression, fluid retention, and proximal muscle weakness.

Progestogens. Megestrol acetate 160 mg daily [8] (increased to 800 mg if required), and medroxyprogesterone acetate 480–960 mg daily, can improve appetite and weight. These drugs are usually well tolerated but can cause mild oedema, impotence, and vaginal bloodloss.

Other drugs

Some authors have advocated the use of amphetamines and hydrazine sulphate, although evidence of their effectiveness is unclear and they are used rarely in the UK.

Complementary therapies

Complementary therapies may be beneficial to some patients (see Chapter 21).

MEDICAL TREATMENT OF COEXISTING SYMPTOMS

Active treatment of coexisting symptoms will contribute to well-being and alleviate asthenia.

NUTRITIONAL ADVICE

Nutritional support has benefits for patients, not only in terms of quality of life, but also for physical outcomes (e.g. increased tolerance to chemotherapy). However, studies have failed to show any convincing evidence for improved prognosis in cancer patients [9]. Equally, some patients can find dietary regimes arduous. Therefore, professionals have to provide advice that balances these pros and cons, taking into account patient well-being and the concerns of family and friends. Patients with AIDS-induced cachexia may benefit more from nutritional supplements as they recover from acute infections.

Nutrition can be deplete in many aspects; however, the main deficiency is in the form of energy. Dieticians are helpful in providing additional advice on nutritional needs of patients and are a source of information on dietary supplementation. At a more basic level, the following advice can be helpful.
- Make food interesting (plan meals).
- Eat a little and often.
- Use foods the patients like (discover their preferences and serve these more often).
- Prepare food that does not need a lot of chewing.
- Encourage fluids.

Table 17.1 Examples of commercially produced nutritional supplements.

Glucose supplements	Complete supplements (on prescription)	Complete supplements (over the counter)
Maxijul Fortical	Ensure Ensure plus Fresubin Fortisip	Build up Complan

- Use a small plate (this gives the impression of finishing a complete meal).
- Eat when hungry (have food at the ready).
- Lessen any emotional tension that may surround meal times.
- Suggest the use of aperitifs.

For some patients, commercially produced supplements are helpful (Table 17.1). Unfortunately they are not universally palatable and patients should be encouraged to experiment with different varieties and flavours (e.g. vanilla, chocolate, fruit, neutral, etc.). They are prescribable in the UK and are therefore free to most patients. They can come in powder or liquid forms.

IMMOBILITY

Deteriorating mobility is a consequence of asthenia and can result in pressure sores, incontinence, muscular stiffness, accidents, and reduced quality of life. If these problems are to be avoided, then poor mobility needs to be managed actively. This can be accomplished by employing a variety of measures.

- Walking aids (e.g. sticks, wheelchairs).
- Occupational therapy (e.g. rails, shower stool, raised chair cushions).
- Pressure area care (see Chapter 18).
- Physiotherapy to promote mobility and relieve muscular stiffness.
- Continence advice (e.g. commode, catheterization).
- Foot care to aid walking (e.g. chiropody).
- 'Monkey pole' to help patients move in bed.
- Reduction of hazards at home (e.g. attend to loose carpeting, remove house 'clutter').
- Nursing care at home (e.g. Marie Curie nurse).
- Lifting training for carers.
- Advice on rest periods and levels of activity.

The family and carers are important elements in mobility management.

Meals. Food is a basic need that evokes strong emotions in patients and their loved ones. Beliefs such as 'they are starving to death' and a natural desire to help can produce marked anxiety. Sensitive explanation of nutritional requirements and careful consideration of patients' needs can alleviate any tension concerning food.

Inactivity. Advancing weakness results in deteriorating levels of functioning that can impinge on previously enjoyed physical activities. This loss tends to be progressive and can lead to boredom or indeed depression. This should be recognized by professionals and thought be given to ways of helping. Hospices are particularly attuned to this need and can help arrange supported activities.

Mood disorder. This chapter has repeatedly emphasized the importance of mood disorder (e.g. depression and anxiety) on asthenia and anorexia. Assessments should always consider the emotional needs of patients. Effective communication and psychological support are important components of care. In the more profoundly affected patients, more structured counselling or drug treatment may be beneficial.

SPECIFIC MANAGEMENT: TREAT THE CAUSE

Looking at the aetiological factors involved in asthenia (see Fig. 17.1), it is apparent that active treatment of some of these causes may result in an improvement of symptoms. However, it is important to consider interventions carefully and discuss them with patients. For instance, before confirming anaemia by a full blood count, the patient has to be sure that they would be happy to go through with a transfusion and that they understand the chances of benefit. In many cases it is difficult to be sure of the best course of action. In practice this often results in a trial of treatment (transfusion in this case), whereby benefits are objectively evaluated so that decisions about ongoing management are informed by these facts. Decisions like this can only safely be made from the patient's perspective. These cost-benefit dilemmas form part of the management choices given below.
- Consider reducing or stopping causative drugs.
- Treat nausea and vomiting aggressively.
- Encourage the expression of anxieties or concerns.
- Actively treat clinical states of depression and anxiety.
- Consider blood transfusion in anaemia.

- Medical reversal of endocrine or metabolic complications, when appropriate and possible.
- Trial of oxygen therapy in hypoxia.
- High-dose steroids and specialist referral in suspected cord compression.
- Antibiotic treatment for infections, when appropriate.
- Reassert normal sleep pattern with non-pharmacological and drug treatments.
- Clearance of constipation.
- Mouth care.
- Consider vitamin B_{12} supplements in AIDS-related *Cryptococcus* infection of the bowel.

These specific measures often form part of a management plan which includes more general help. This multidimensional approach is more likely to alleviate symptoms.

Intravenous rehydration and artificial feeding: their role in palliative care

In caring for patients with poor oral intake, questions can arise about artificial hydration and feeding. In respecting the choices of patients it is difficult to give any firm direction on the role of these interventions in palliative care. However, there are specific circumstances when the appropriateness of these measures is clear.

ENTERAL FEEDING (see also Chapter 15)

In patients who have a 'reasonable' expectation of medium- or long-term survival/quality of life, enteral feeding has advantages that should be offered to such patients. These patients will tend to suffer from pathology of the head, neck, and upper gastrointestinal (GI) tract, or neuromuscular problems (e.g. MND). Specialist assistance is required for this, as simple nasogastric tubes are unacceptable in most cases.

INTRAVENOUS/SUBCUTANEOUS REHYDRATION

The debate about the value of intravenous hydration continues [10]. Various arguments are proposed. Some believe that intravenous fluids are an intrusion for patients and that the minimal symptoms of dehydration that do occur can be relieved equally effectively by mouth care. Others feel that unrelieved dehydration results in confusion, thirst, and reduced quality of life, all of which can be helped by intravenous or subcutaneous fluids. In the UK the former argument tends to hold sway in hospices, whereas hospitals have been known to hydrate terminally ill patients as part of the routine in the acute setting. Until research clarifies this debate and consensus is achieved, decisions about whether or not to hydrate artificially should only be taken after careful consideration of all the facts— especially in terms of the pros and cons for individual patients.

TOTAL PARENTERAL NUTRITION (TPN)

Because of the contraindications, complications, and uncertain value of TPN in palliative care, it has little place in the management of terminally ill patients. However, it may be beneficial preoperatively or before bone marrow transplant.

Summary

Asthenia, cachexia, and anorexia are a complex set of symptoms that frequently affect terminally ill patients with advanced disease. Although relieving these symptoms can be challenging, it may be possible, with careful assessment and management, to improve the quality of life of these patients.

References

1 Curtis EB, Krech R, Walsh TD. Common symptoms in patients with advanced cancer. *J Palliat Care* 1991; 7: 25–29.
2 Dunlop GM. A study of the relative frequency and importance of gastrointestinal symptoms and weakness in patients with far advanced cancer: student paper. *Palliat Med* 1989; 4: 37–43.
3 Dewys WD, Begg D, Lavin PT *et al*. Prognostic effect of weight loss prior to chemotherapy in cancer patients. *Am J Med* 1980; 69: 491–496.
4 Theolodgides A. Asthenins and cachectins in cancer. *Am J Med* 1986; 81: 696–698.
5 Chailleux E, Fauroux B, Binet F, Dautzenbery B, Polu J. Predictors of survival on patients receiving domiciliary oxygen therapy or mechanical ventilation. *Chest* 1996; 109: 741–749.
6 Grunfield C. What causes wasting in AIDS? *New Engl J Med* 1995; 333: 123–124.
7 Regnard C, Mannix K. Weakness and fatigue in advanced cancer. *Palliat Med* 1992; 6: 253–256.
8 Loprinzi CL, Ellison NM, Schaid DJ. Phase three evaluation of four dosages of megestrol acetate as therapy for patients with cancer anorexia and/or cachexia. *J Clin Oncol* 1993; 11: 762–767.
9 Shaw C. Nutritional aspects of advanced cancer. *Palliat Med* 1992; 6: 105–110.
10 MacDonald N, Fainsinger R. Indications and ethical considerations in the hydration of patients with advanced cancer. In: Bruera E, Higginson I, eds. *Cachexia-Anorexia in Cancer Patients*. Oxford: Oxford University Press, 1996: 94–109.

18: Pressure Area Care and the Management of Fungating Wounds

MARY WALDING

Introduction

Individuals in need of palliative care are already facing major readjustments due to diagnosis and prognosis. To develop skin wounds for whatever reason is a further challenge to their well-being. Illness and debility can disrupt the normal repair of skin and may contribute to further dermal breakdown. Distress may be caused by the physical or psychological effect on an individual, and it is impossible to separate the two in clinical care. Table 18.1 provides a summary of potential problems for a patient. The key to care is individual assessment and an awareness that a wound may dominate someone's life.

It is difficult to ignore such an obvious reminder of one's illness, and developing a wound may precipitate grieving for what a patient is losing. Denial is often associated with coping with this loss, and individuals may occasionally present with advanced fungating tumours that have previously been ignored. Treatment should respect the physical and psychological consequences and should always be what is acceptable to the individual. The ideal is to provide appropriate care that respects the patient's wishes and causes minimal disruption to their lifestyle.

Pressure sores

Pressure sores are also sometimes known as decubitus ulcers, pressure ulcers, or bed sores. No term accurately describes the pathology involved and for clarity of purpose this text will use the term 'pressure sore'. Pressure sores are a problem in the general hospital population, with an incidence of 3–14% [1], but are of greater concern in palliative care where studies have highlighted rates of 15–43% [2]. This is due to the multiple factors involved in the maintenance and healing of normal skin that are compromised in the individual who is seriously ill.

Table 18.1 Possible impact of skin damage on patients who are dying.

Physical	Psychological
Pain	Anxiety
Fatigue	Depression
Odour	Grief
Immobility	Feeling that the wound dominates their life
Lifestyle restrictions	Fear

Aetiology

A pressure sore arises as a result of pressure, friction, and shearing. They rarely occur in those who are healthy because an individual will react to discomfort and alter position. Exceptions may occur in accident situations where an individual may suffer a friction or shearing injury.

Propensity to develop pressure sores is related to problems with:

• the nutritional needs of the skin;
• damage to the integrity of the epidermis;
• inability to recognize or react to skin discomfort;
• impairment of the skin's ability to regenerate.

THE NUTRITIONAL NEEDS OF THE SKIN

Healthy skin requires nutrients and oxygen, which are provided via a good blood supply. This may be impeded by: poor dietary intake; hypoxia; pressure which compresses the capillaries; peripheral vascular disease, and diabetes. Blood supply also varies depending on the tissue type; for example, adipose tissue has a relatively poor blood supply and obese individuals will be at greater risk of pressure sore development because of this and the compression factor of their weight on vulnerable pressure points (see p. 286).

DAMAGE TO THE INTEGRITY OF THE EPIDERMIS

The epidermis may be damaged by the pressure, shearing, and friction forces discussed above. It may also be damaged by chemical means, either agents produced by the body, such as sweat, urine, and faeces, or ones applied to the skin. Cleansing products can often be harsh on vulnerable skin and the mode of application may cause shearing if care is not taken. Massage, in particular, can cause shearing between tissue layers if performed by an inexpert practitioner.

INABILITY TO RECOGNIZE OR REACT TO SKIN DISCOMFORT

Normally, discomfort or soreness caused by positioning will provoke an individual to move, thus preventing any damage to the skin. However, those with sensory or motor impairment may be unable to perform this preventative act, i.e. patients with neurological damage or major mobility problems.

IMPAIRMENT OF THE SKIN'S ABILITY TO REGENERATE

Some drugs and dermatological conditions may result in friable skin that is damaged easily. This is a particular problem with steroids as they also impair healing. Radiotherapy may also cause the skin to be vulnerable, and the entry and exit sites should be observed regularly for radiotherapy damage and indication of pressure problems (these are often difficult to differentiate between, so risk factors for pressure areas should also be assessed).

Vulnerable pressure points

Areas of the skin most likely to develop a pressure sore are those which tend to be in contact with support surfaces:
- buttocks and sacrum (sitting and lying);
- hips (lying on side);
- heels (lying or sitting in bed);
- elbows (lying on side);
- ears (lying on side);
- shoulders (lying on side);
- knees (lying on side).

Risk assessment

Assessment tools have been developed to enable health care professionals to identify those most at risk of pressure sores. As with all checklists, their value is primarily as *aides-mémoire* and as guides for allocation of resources, rather than as comprehensive indicators. Most assessment tools will differentiate between low-, medium-, and high-risk categories.

Reducing risk

Measures that can be employed to reduce the risk of pressure sores will depend on the needs and circumstances of the individual patient, but may include:

- nutritional support (consider involving the dietician);
- a mobility assessment by a physiotherapist;
- pain control (as this may improve mobility);
- skin hygiene;
- assessment and treatment of any incontinence problems (this may require a specialist referral);
- assessment of need for pressure-relieving support surfaces;
- regular observation of vulnerable pressure points;
- review of medication.

Mattresses and cushions

Areas vulnerable to pressure sore development are those which are in contact with a support surface. One of the ways of reducing the risk of developing pressure sores is to move the patient regularly. However, there is no evidence as to how often this should take place; traditionally nursing has taught that an immobile patient should be turned every two hours, but there is no evidence to support this. It has been noted that an individual will automatically shift their position every 20 minutes if able, but it is unrealistic to disrupt a patient this regularly.

A standard hospital mattress offers no pressure-relieving properties, neither is there evidence to suggest that soft mattress overlays (for example Spenco) are useful in preventing pressure sores. However, pressure-relieving support surfaces are available both in mattress and cushion form. It is equally important to consider the support surface when sitting as when in bed.

Categories of support surfaces

Support surfaces may be categorized as follows.

Profiled foam

There is some evidence of limited effectiveness with these aids, but they are not the ideal support surfaces for immobile patients. These are available as replacement mattresses, or as mattress overlays. Examples include: Cyclone; Transfoam; and Pro-pad.

Static air-filled

These can usually be adjusted so that the amount of air present in the mattress is appropriate for the individual. There are some air-filled mattresses available which are made of 'breathable' fabric and air is pumped through at a constant rate. They often have the benefit of temperature controls and low-friction fabric. Water mattresses work on the same principle, but have the disadvantage of weight and subsequent immobility. Examples include: Ro-ho; First-step.

Alternating air pressure

These consist of a system of cushions which are inflated and deflated in a preset alternating pattern, the cycle lasting several minutes. A wavelike motion may occasionally be felt. Examples include: Nimbus; Pegasus.

'Flotation' systems

These 'suspend' the individual on a cushion of air, creating negligible interface pressure. They tend to be large, expensive, and cumbersome, but are effective if an individual is bed-bound and immobile. The systems tend to be either cushion-based or bead-based. Whilst the individual will require assistance to move on bead-based beds, the advantage is great if a patient has a wound that produces a lot of exudate, or if incontinence is a problem, as fluids will sink to the bottom of the bed and be removed later without infection risks. Maintenance costs and storage problems mean that most units will hire these when needed. Examples include: Clinitron air flotation bed; Mediscus air flotation bed.

Assessment criteria

The price and sophistication of these mattresses varies widely and the most expensive is not necessarily the best. Each choice should be individual for the patient, taking into account their needs, abilities, and expectations. It is helpful to use a risk assessment tool (mentioned earlier) in order to prioritize need, for example:
• low risk score: profiled foam mattress;
• medium risk score: static air-filled mattress;
• high risk score: alternating-pressure air mattress.
The 'flotation' mattress may be reserved for exceptional circumstances

where the patient's comfort needs suggest that the properties of such a mattress may be helpful.

Treatment of pressure sores

The aim of wound care is to minimize patient distress and discomfort, and where possible promote healing. This can only be achieved through a holistic approach that considers the psychological and social issues discussed earlier alongside the physical problems.

Pain

Pain is often a problem associated with these sores and it should be addressed regardless of proposed treatment options—the individual may require a review of analgesia. Patients will often require prn. analgesia given about half an hour in advance of a dressing procedure. This may be an extra opiate dose or some paracetamol. Some patients who experience extreme pain and anxiety may find the use of Entonox gives relief.

Promotion of healing

It should not be assumed that pressure sores will not improve; they have been seen to heal even in individuals who were within weeks of death [2]. Care may be given to improve the risk factors, and wounds can be dressed appropriately in order to maintain a moist environment suitable for healing to occur.

Table 18.2 suggests dressings that are suitable for certain wound criteria. The recommendations may also be useful for wounds that are similar in nature, but not seen as pressure sores.

It is worth noting the advice that wounds be cleansed with an irrigation of warmed isotonic (0.9%) sodium chloride [3].

Infection

Wounds are often colonized by a variety of bacteria, but this only constitutes an infection if there is evidence to suggest that the body's own defence systems cannot cope with the bacterial load—for example there is redness, increased exudate, malodorous exudate, pain, or pyrexia [3]. The decision to swab a wound in order to identify appropriate antibiotic therapy should only be taken if the patient's prognosis indicates this or if the effects of the infection are difficult for the patient.

Table 18.2 Suggested dressings for pressure sores.

Appearance	Treatment
Intact skin; discoloured, erythema	Relieve pressure. Consider using a film dressing for protection unless the area requiring protection is the sacrum. Here a hydrocolloid is less easily displaced than a film dressing.
Damaged epidermis; slight damage to dermis	Hydrocolloid dressing. Leave *in situ* for 5–7 days if possible. If bleeding occurs, use an alginate dressing and a film dressing. Change daily.
Full thickness, skin loss	Fill cavity with a hydrocolloid gel or paste and cover with a hydrocolloid dressing.
Slough or necrotic tissue	Autolysis may be facilitated by maintaining a moist wound environment. Use a hydrocolloid or hydrogel. Enzymatic debriding agents may occasionally be useful.
Highly exuding wounds	Use hydrophilic foam sheets or cavity dressings. Use extra padding and film dressings to contain exudate. Wound drainage bags are also available.
Dressing examples	
Film dressings	Opsite, Bioclusive, Tegaderm
Hydrocolloid foam	Granuflex, Comfeel
Hydrocolloid paste	Granuflex
Hydrogel	Intrasite gel
Alginates	Kaltostat, Sorbsan
Enzymatic debrider	Varidase
Hydrophilic foam	Allevyn, Lyofoam

Fungating wounds

A fungating wound is a condition of proliferation and ulceration which arises when malignant tumour cells infiltrate and erode through the skin [4]. They develop most commonly from the following cancers: breast; head and neck; skin; and vulva.

The spread tends to be through tissues that offer the least resistance—between tissue planes, along blood and lymph vessels, and in perineural spaces [5]. Abnormalities in tissue growth in fungating tumours lead to areas of tissue hypoxia and consequent infection of the non-viable tissue. It is this that results in the characteristic malodour and exudate of fungating wounds.

Treatment

It may be possible to control tumour growth in order to prevent further problems associated with an invasive tumour. The options include:
* radiotherapy;
* surgery;
* chemotherapy;
* neutron therapy;

Table 18.3 Summary of treatment of fungating wounds.

Aim	Action
Control tumour growth	Consider radiotherapy, surgery, chemotherapy, neutron therapy, low-powered laser therapy, hormonal treatment.
Control malodour	Use occlusive dressings and charcoal pads. Consider the use of antibiotic therapy. Consider de-sloughing the wound. Use an air freshening unit and pleasant aromas; Consider the use of aromatherapy.
Control pain	Review analgesia, consider the need for co-analgesics.
Control exudate	Use highly absorbent dressings and padding. Occlude wound if possible. Consider the use of wound drainage (or ileostomy) bags. Consider the use of radiotherapy.
Control bleeding*	Consider radiotherapy. Consider using adrenaline 1 : 1000 soaks. Use padding and haemostatic dressings. Consider the use of silver sulphadizine or sucralfate paste. Is there a risk of tumour infiltrating a vessel? If so, consider potential patient and family needs.

* *See also* Chapter 12.

- low-powered laser therapy;
- hormone manipulation.

However, tumours do not always respond to palliative treatment and in these situations it is necessary to 'manage' the wound to minimize its impact upon the patient. Treatment options in this situation are summarized in Table 18.3.

DRESSINGS FOR FUNGATING WOUNDS

Fungating wounds are not going to heal, so conventional treatments to aid wound healing are less important than the priority of controlling odour and exudate. However, this is difficult to achieve, with many wounds requiring frequent dressing changes every day in order to control symptoms. These wounds are also complicated by their rapidly changing nature, therefore dressing plans will need to be flexible.

Useful dressings are: hydrophyilic foam, (e.g. Lyofoam, Allevyn; these are available as sheets or as cavity dressings);alginates (e.g. Sorbsan, Kaltostat); and semipermeable film dressing (e.g. Bioclusive, Opsite), which will help contain the odour and exudate.

Large amounts of padding with absorbent materials are sometimes helpful, as is the use of wound drainage or colostomy bags if the wound can be contained and the bags will adhere. It is also helpful to use medical adhesive (and remove with a suitable solvent).

There have been reported cases of moulded latex, similar to that used to create items for sets in the film industry, being used to make an occlusive barrier, through which the exudate may be drained with the use of a wound drain. This treatment depends on the availability of appropriate expertise.

There is much empirical discussion about various unorthodox treatments for fungating wounds—yoghurt, icing sugar, honey, sugar paste to name a few [6]. There is no research evidence to support the use of these, or that they are able to achieve anything that conventional dressings cannot.

TREATMENT OF MALODOUR

The malodour associated with fungating wounds can cause great distress as the individual feels permanently unclean and may isolate themselves for fear of offending others. It may also cause nausea and associated problems with appetite. Whilst the problem may be helped greatly through the use of occlusive dressings, other strategies may also need to be used, including the use of charcoal dressings, which will neutralize odour.

The odour is commonly caused by the anaerobic bacteria that will inhabit hypoxic and necrotic tissue. A successful treatment option is the use of metronidazole 200 mg orally t.d.s. However, the incidence of nausea associated with this drug often reduces compliance and it may be more effective to apply the antibiotic topically in the form of a gel. The disadvantage of this is cost, and the fact that this mode of application may be of little use when there are large quantities of exudate. It has been reported that clindamycin (300 mg q.d.s.) may be more effective than metronidazole [5].

De-sloughing the wound, i.e. removing the devitalized tissue, is also worth considering [7] although this should be done with extreme caution as de-sloughing may uncover further problems such as bleeding in a fungating wound.

It is often helpful to provide an air-conditioning unit for individuals with fungating wounds, or consider the use of air fresheners or aromatherapy oils—whatever they may find helpful.

TREATMENT OF BLEEDING

Fungating wounds tend to be vascular. The padding that is often necessary to contain exudate also has a useful protective function. If there is localized capillary bleeding then one of the following may be used (see also Chapter 12):

- alginate dressings (these have some haemostatic properties);
- topical adrenaline 1:1000, applied to a dressing pad;
- silver sulphadizine (should be avoided during radiotherapy as it can disperse the rays);
- sucralfate paste (crush a 1 g tablet and mix with KY jelly to an appropriate consistency);
- it is also worth considering the prophylactic use of tranexamic acid 1 g t.d.s. (see Chapter 12).

Fungating wounds can occasionally cause the rupture of a major blood vessel. The team caring for the individual should be aware of this and consideration given to the need to inform the patient and their family. It is sensible to follow precautions similar to a situation where a haemorrhage may be considered likely: to have a dark or red blanket to hand; to have gloves and pads; and to ensure there is adequate p.r.n. sedation and analgesia prescribed.

TREATMENT OF PAIN

Fungating wounds are often associated with pain that is difficult to control. Partly this is due to the effect of the tumour distorting nerve tissue, and there may be a role for the use of tricyclic antidepressants or corticosteroids for neuropathic pain (see Chapter 9). A lot of the pain may be due to and potentiated by the impact of the tumour and the experience for an individual. It may be necessary and helpful to involve the wider multidisciplinary team, including the complementary therapists. This is not to deny that the patient may indeed require large doses of opiates, plus the use of adjuvant drugs such as the non-steroidal anti-inflammatory drugs.

Conclusion

The management of both pressure sores and fungating wounds is one of the challenges of palliative care. Control of other symptoms is now often so effective that wounds may be seen as the most obvious indicator of a patient's disease. However, this chapter has suggested ways in which pressure sores may be prevented and how both these and fungating wounds may be treated in order to minimize their detrimental impact on the patient. The use of creative, patient-centred, multidisciplinary management can maximize our effectiveness as health care professionals in this area.

References

1 Reid J, Morison M. Towards a consensus: classification of pressure sores. *J Wound Care* 1994; 3 (3): 157–160.
2 Walding M, Andrews C. Preventing and managing pressure sores in palliative care. *Prof Nurse* 1995; 11 (1): 33–38.
3 Thomas S. *Wound Management and Dressings*. London: The Pharmaceutical Press, 1990.
4 Mortimer P. Skin problems in palliative care: medical aspects. In: Doyle D, Hanks G, Macdonald N, eds. *Oxford Textbook of Palliative Medicine*, 2nd edn. Oxford: Oxford Medical Publications, 1997.
5 Grocott P. The palliative management of fungating malignant wounds. *J Wound Care* 1995; 4 (5): 240–242.
6 Fairburn K. A challenge that requires further research. *Prof Nurse* 1994; 9 (4): 272–277.
7 Enck R. The management of large fungating tumours. *Am J Hospice Palliat Care* 1990; 7 (3): 11–12.

Further reading

Ivetic O, Lyne P. Fungating and ulcerating malignant lesions: a review of the literature. *J Adv Nursing* 1990; 15 (1): 83–88.

Mortimer P. Skin problems in palliative care: medical aspects. In: Doyle D, Hanks G, Macdonald N, eds. *Oxford Textbook of Palliative Medicine*, 2nd edn. Oxford: Oxford Medical Publications, 1997.

Ribbe MW, Van Marum RJ. Decubitus: pathophysiology, clinical symptoms and susceptibility. *J Tissue Viability* 1993; 3 (2): 42–47.

Surgical Materials Testing Laboratory. *A Prescriber's Guide to Dressings and Wound Management Materials*. Cardiff: VFM Unit, 1996.

Twycross R. *Symptom Management in Advanced Cancer*. Oxford: Radcliffe Medical Press, 1995.

Walding M, Andrew C. *The Prevention and Management of Pressure Sores at Sir Michael Sobell House*. Oxford: Sobell Publications, 1996.

19: Management of Lymphoedema

DENISE HARDY

Introduction

Lymphoedema is a progressive condition which results from insufficiency or failure of the lymphatic system, with or without coexisting venous insufficiency [1]. It results in the accumulation of protein-rich fluid in subcutaneous tissues. It is fortunately uncommon, but it can cause considerable distress. If left untreated it can become a crippling handicap to patients who are perhaps already weakened by advanced cancer. A heavy, oedematous limb has serious physical and psychological effects and may impair mobility, independence, and quality of life.

Early assessment and management should be implemented in order to minimize debility. For those in the UK who are uncertain about local services, the *Directory of Lymphoedema Services* is a useful reference point. It identifies specialist centres, referral details, and types of treatments available [2].

Aetiology

Lymphoedema occurs when there is a disturbance of the equilibrium between the transport capacity of the lymphatic system and the load of lymph to be cleared [3]. This may be due to: impaired lymphatic drainage; increased lymphatic load; or gravitational effects.

Impaired lymphatic drainage

Lymph node irradiation or excision obstructs lymphatic drainage routes and may result in the remaining vessels becoming overloaded. Patients at particular risk of developing lymphoedema are therefore those with breast, genital, or pelvic tumours who may have undergone surgery and/or irradiation to a major group of lymph nodes.

Lymphoedema may also result from congenital abnormalities of the lymphatics.

Increased lymphatic load

Increased lymphatic load can result from venous insufficiency or acute tissue inflammation. Initially the lymphatic system will respond by increasing lymph flow, but if the increase in load continues, drainage fails as the vessels become overloaded.

Gravitational effect

Dependent or gravitational oedema arises because of a lack of propulsion to blood and lymph flow in a limb. Patients who have neurological damage or who are immobile for other reasons are at high risk.

Other contributory factors

The following factors can also contribute to the formation of oedema [1]:
*   hypoproteinaemia;
*   heart failure;
*   fluid-retaining drugs (e.g. NSAIDs, steroids, some hormone therapies).

Characteristics of lymphoedema

In the early stages lymphoedema is soft, pitting, and reduces with elevation. The onset of swelling may be gradual or sudden, depending on the aetiology. Exacerbation of the swelling may occur following an infection of the limb.

Protein accumulation in the tissues results in fibrosis and thickening of subcutaneous tissues. Pitting of the skin becomes increasingly difficult and the limb swells.

Typical changes of chronic lymphoedema are [4]:
*   enhanced skin folds;
*   hyperkeratosis (warty, scaly skin changes);
*   lymphangiomata (blisters on the skin surface);
*   papillomatosis (a 'cobblestone' change to the surface of the skin).

Assessment of a patient with lymphoedema

Assessment of a patient with lymphoedema includes consideration of all possible aetiologies (see above), the physical effects on the patient, (including functional impairment), and the psychological and social effects on the patient and their carers.

History and examination

A thorough history can provide important information on the cause of the swelling. For example, swelling that develops immediately following surgery, radiotherapy, cellulitis, or thrombosis is probably due to acute inflammation and will subside once the inflammation has resolved. Some cancer treatments (e.g. radiotherapy or surgery to the groin or axilla) can result in swelling at any time from 6 weeks to 20 years after the event.

The examination of a swollen limb involves identifying the signs and extent of lymphoedema, together with determining the possible aetiologies and evidence of complications of the lymphoedema.

Determining the extent of the swelling is an important factor in choosing the appropriate treatment. Truncal swelling is identified by pinching folds of skin on both sides of the body: oedematous tissue is more difficult to pick up and will feel thicker on the affected side. In addition, patients may complain of swelling in and behind the axilla and may comment about marks left by undergarments on the affected side. A positive Stemmer sign is an indicator of lymphoedema in the leg (i.e. thickened skin folds of the toes which prevent pinching of the skin) [5].

A series of careful measurements will need to be taken for fitting of compression hosiery (see pp. 303–304). This should usually be done by a specialist practitioner.

SKIN CONDITION

The changes of chronic lymphoedema should be noted and the skin checked for dryness, fungal infections, cellulitis, and lymphorrhoea (leakage of lymph).

Acute cellulitis is particularly important to recognize and treat. It is not only a troublesome complication of lymphoedema, but can result in even more swelling.

BLOOD CIRCULATION

Signs of venous hypertension in limbs should be noted (i.e. distension of veins/cyanosis of limb), since venous obstruction or incompetence can influence the outcome of lymphoedema treatment. Should a deep vein thrombosis form in an already oedematous leg, compression treatment with hosiery or bandaging is usually postponed until 8 weeks after anticoagulant therapy has started [6]. This does not apply, however, to upper limbs where compression is often commenced in combination with anticoagulants. It is thought that veins in the arm have a small calibre and any emboli will not produce significant morbidity [1,3].

Arterial insufficiency is an absolute contraindication for the use of compression. Assessment by Doppler studies may be important before compression is applied.

NEUROLOGICAL FUNCTION

Many patients may complain of numbness or discomfort following surgery or radiotherapy. It is important to differentiate this from neurological deficit due to tumour infiltration, disease progression, or perineural oedema since this can cause progressive or complete loss of limb function and severe neuropathic pain.

Functional assessment is essential since a swollen limb often reduces function and mobility, affects posture and balance, and makes the limb uncomfortable to use. The resultant reduced function will perpetuate swelling, stiffness, and discomfort, and the patient may benefit from referral to an occupational therapist and/or physiotherapist.

PAIN

Lymphoedema does not cause acute pain. Most patients complain of tightness and aching due to the skin stretching over the swollen limb, and for some the weight of the limb can put a considerable strain on supporting joints and muscles causing aching and discomfort. When pain is more severe, it is important to consider the possibility of other complications and disease progression.

Patients' perceptions

Perceptions of body image are often affected by a swollen limb and can result in much psychological distress. It is crucial therefore to gain insight into an individual patient's experiences so that the therapist and patient may join in partnership to make decisions about future management.

Management

Management should begin early if good results are to be achieved. It is important to involve the patient as much as possible in setting realistic goals for treatment and in optimizing adherence to treatment.

Treatment aims include:
- preventing further development of lymphoedema;
- reducing swelling;
- alleviating associated symptoms;
- maximizing improvement and long-term control.

Management employs a combination of skin care, external support or compression, manual/simple lymph drainage, and exercise.

Intensive or reduction phase

Intensive treatment usually lasts 2–4 weeks and will require specialist help. The indications for intensive treatment are highlighted in Table 19.1. For cancer patients who do not have locally recurrent disease and whose life expectancy is more than a few weeks, reduction and control of the swelling is appropriate.

SKIN CARE

Care of the skin is a fundamental part of any management programme for patients with lymphoedema (see Table 19.2). Impaired local immunity (by removal of lymph nodes) and the presence of static protein-rich lymph in the swollen limb makes the patient prone to infection, which in turn can lead to further fibrosis and scarring of lymphatics. Keeping the skin intact and supple will reduce the risk of infection. Equally, reduction in the limb size will lessen the risk of infection by reducing the amount of static lymph.

EXTERNAL COMPRESSION

External compression in the intensive phase is achieved by the daily application of multilayer, graduated compression bandages. Compression

Table 19.1 Indications for the intensive phase of treatment [6].

Long-standing or severe lymphoedema
Awkwardly shaped limb
Deep skin folds
Damaged or fragile skin
Lymphorrhoea
Swollen digits

Table 19.2 Management of skin problems.

Dry flaky skin	Daily wash with soap substitutes. Daily application of bland moisturizing products, e.g. aqueous cream.
Hyperkeratosis	Moisturizing ointment to lift hard skin. Diprosalic ointment for small areas. Hydrocolloid dressings with steroid ointment for larger areas.
Contact dermatitis	Avoid irritant substance. Wash with bland emollients. Topical steroid ointments.
Fungal infections	Strict daily hygiene. Topical antifungal cream/powder. Keep area cool and dry. Long term treatment, if required with half strength Whitfields ointment.
Acute inflammatory episodes (cellulitis)	Penicillin V 500 mg q.d.s. 2 weeks (or erythromycin if patient is allergic to penicillin). Analgesia to relieve pain and fever. Rest and support of limb. Avoid compression in acute phase.
Lymphorrhoea	Non-adherent sterile dressing to leaking area. Application of compression bandages for 24–48 h, changing as necessary.

of the limb raises interstitial pressure, reduces lymph formation, and provides a firm outer casing for the limb muscles to work against.

Low stretch bandages (providing a low resting pressure and a high working pressure) are applied by a specially trained therapist whose experience ensures that the bandage provides even pressure around the limb. In awkwardly shaped limbs this can be achieved using soft foam or padding to smooth out the skin folds and promote a suitably smooth profile prior to bandage application. Graduation of bandage pressure ensures fluid is encouraged towards the trunk; this is achieved by bandage tension and overlap (the pressure being greatest distally). Bandages are replaced on a daily basis to ensure maintenance of adequate pressure. The improvement of the limb shape then enables the fitment of containment hosiery (see 'Maintenance phase' below).

EXERCISE

Exercise is important to promote the drainage of lymph and discourage pooling in the limbs. The most significant effects of exercise are highlighted in Table 19.3. Referral to a physiotherapist should be made if there is evidence of functional deficit or poor range of movement of a joint. The use of slings should be discouraged unless to relieve pain.

MANUAL LYMPHATIC DRAINAGE

Manual lymphatic drainage (MLD) is a very gentle form of massage used to encourage the flow of lymph from congested oedematous areas of the body to areas where it can drain normally [5]. If performed correctly, skin surface massage encourages the drainage of lymph. It is particularly useful for facial and truncal lymphoedema where external support or compression is not appropriate. Unless congestion is removed from the root of the limb, reduction in the limb itself will not be achieved.

A simplified form of this massage, simple lymph drainage (SLD), must be taught to patients and carers to ensure continued improvement (see Table 19.4).

Maintenance phase

Once effective reduction of the swelling has been achieved, the maintenance phase of treatment is implemented. The aim is to control lymphoedema using a combination of exercises, simple lymph drainage, and strong

Table 19.3 The value of exercise.

Increases lymphatic drainage by stimulating the muscle pump
Maintains and/or improves joint mobility
Improves posture and facilitates functional activities
Points to remember
Hosiery should always be worn during exercise
Movements should be slow, rhythmical and well controlled
Discourage over-exertion (this increase vasodilation lymph production)

Table 19.4 Simple lymphatic drainage—practical guidelines.

Simple lymphatic drainage (SLD) is based upon the principles of manual lymphatic drainage (MLD).

It is used within a lymphoedema treatment programme, particularly in the maintenance phase, and is designed to be taught to patients and their families.

Simplified hand movements stimulate contraction of the skin lymphatics. This 'milking' action improves superficial lymphatic drainage.

Movements are very slow, gentle and rhythmical with just enough pressure to move the skin over the underlying tissue.

SLD starts in the neck and unaffected lymphatics before working on the affected area. This ensures movement of fluid towards functioning lymphatics.

SLD is concentrated in the neck and truncal area, although the limb itself may be treated if required.

Daily treatments are required over a period of several months.

Creams and oils are not used during the SLD.

compression hosiery. Routine measures for continuing care are outlined in Table 19.5.

Hosiery is an important element in the maintenance phase of lymphoedema management. Any improvement gained through intensive

Table 19.5 Daily skin and general health care.

Protect the limb against trauma. Avoid sunburn.
Avoid injections/blood sampling in the affected limb.
Keep the limb spotlessly clean using soapless cleanser.
Moisturize the skin daily to avoid dryness.
Report signs of infection immediately—have antibiotics at hand.
Do not carry heavy bags/shopping with the swollen arm.
Avoid standing for long periods if the leg is swollen.
Use the swollen limb normally—avoid strenuous exercise.
Wear loose clothing to prevent further restriction.
Keep weight within normal limits—a normal, healthy balanced diet. Do not restrict fluids. Limit salt intake.
Do not ignore a slight increase in swelling size—contact the therapist as soon as possible.

Table 19.6 Containment hosiery—general information.

It must be evenly distributed and graduated, providing the most pressure at the hand/foot.
It must be firm fitting and comfortable.
It must never be too tight or painful.
Never fold over the top of the garment.
Wear all day—remove at night.
Avoid fitting following bathing or after moisturizing.
Must be worn during exercise and after manual lymph drainage.
Must be the correct size.

bandaging, exercise, or manual lymph drainage is lost if containment hosiery is omitted. There is a wide range of hosiery available, with varying compression classes. These range from class 1 (20–30mmHg at the ankle) to class 3 (40–50mmHg at the ankle). It is important to note that the European-manufactured hosiery has stronger compression than the equivalent class of British-manufactured hosiery. Lymphoedema usually requires class 3 hosiery. Guidelines for use of compression hosiery are given in Table 19.6.

Palliative phase

Reduction of swelling is, unfortunately, unrealistic for patients with locally recurrent advanced cancer, particularly when the trunk is congested. In these circumstances treatment of the limb will only result in an increase of oedema centrally. The palliative phase of lymphoedema management uses selected treatments, to address an individual's need and improve the quality of their life. Regular monitoring is required to adjust treatment to meet changing needs as the disease progresses.

Swelling often increases as tumour infiltrates into the skin and further compromises lymphatic drainage. Tissues can become very tense, hard, and indurated, and the skin is often discoloured and inflamed in appearance. Skin breakdown, ulceration, and lymphorrhoea are common. Swelling often extends beyond the root of the limb into the trunk and may involve the neck, head, or genitals.

Application of external support (in the form of gentle support bandaging, shaped Tubigrip, or containment hosiery) will counteract feelings of pressure within the limb. Patient comfort will dictate the pressure used.

Although diuretics play no role in pure lymphoedema, a venous element to the swelling may well respond to diuretic therapy. When lymphatic/

venous obstruction occurs due to recurrent tumour, a combination of high-dose steroid (dexamethasone 4–12 mg daily) and diuretics is worth considering to reduce peritumour oedema and pain.

Patients who are weak and debilitated and those with neurological dysfunction, such as spinal cord compression, are particularly at risk of dependent oedema. Gentle, regular, active or passive exercise will enhance lymph flow as well as preventing joint and muscle stiffness. Manual lymph drainage will help to ease truncal swelling and relieve tension in the affected limb.

Dependent oedema responds well to pressure and if there is no limb distortion, appropriate compression hosiery may be fitted as part of a plan alongside exercise and skin care. Pneumatic compression pumps (Flowtron, Centromed) may also be used provided the oedema does not extend into the trunk. These are particularly useful for softening longstanding fibrosis and reducing oedema. Appropriate compression hosiery should always be fitted afterwards.

Injury to tissues, infection, and discomfort are common features of this condition, and attention to them may make a difference between the patient preserving what little mobility remains, or becoming bed bound [1].

Conclusions

There is no doubt that the earlier lymphoedema treatment is introduced, the more successful it is, and that many of the distressing physical and psychological problems associated with this condition may be prevented. It is therefore essential that early signs of oedema are actively sought and that intervention instigated as soon as possible. Ideally this should include the early referral to a local lymphoedema specialist.

References

1 Badger C. Lymphoedema. In: Penson J, Fisher R, eds. *Palliative Care For People With Cancer,* 2nd edn. London: Arnold, 1995: 88–90.
2 British Lymphology Society. *Directory of Lymphoedema Treatment Services,* 2nd edn. Caterham, Surrey: British Lymphology Society, 1996.
3 Badger C, Twycross R. *Management of Lymphoedema: Guidelines.* Oxford: Sir Michael Sobell House, 1988.
4 Veitch J. Skin problems in lymphoedema. *Wound Manage* 1993; 4 (2): 42–45.
5 Mortimer PS, Badger C, Hall JG. Lymphoedema. In: Doyle D, Hanks G, Macdonald N, eds. *Oxford Textbook of Palliative Medicine,* 2nd edn. Oxford: Oxford University Press, 1997: 407–415.

6 Badger C. Palliation or reduction? A guide to selecting treatment for oedema in advanced disease. *Palliat Matters* 1996; No. 6: 1,4.

Further reading

Farncombe M, Daniels G, Cross L. Lymphoedema: the seemingly forgotten complication. *J Pain Symptom Manage* 1994; 9 (4): 269–276.

Foldi E, Foldi M, Weissleder H. Conservative treatment of lymphoedema of the limbs. *Angiology* 1985; 36: 171–180.

Leverick JR. *An Introduction to Cardiovascular Physiology.* London: Butterworth, 1991.

Regnard C, Badger C, Mortimer P. *Lymphoedema: Advice on Treatment,* 2nd edn. Beaconsfield: Beaconsfield Publishers, 1991.

Thomas S. Bandages and bandaging. The science behind the art. *Care Sci Pract* 1990; 8 (2): 56–60.

Woods, M. Patients' perceptions of breast cancer related lymphoedema. *Euro J Cancer Care* 1993; 2: 125–128.

20: Terminal Care and Dying

RICHARD WOOF, YVONNE CARTER,
BOB HARRISON, CHRISTINA FAULL
AND BRIAN NYATANGA

Introduction

Patients who are entering the last phase of their illness and for whom life expectancy is especially short, have health needs which require particular expertise. Professionals need to draw on all their palliative care skills, in order for patients to achieve a transition towards death that fulfils the wishes of the patient and of those close to them. A combination of a rapidly changing clinical situation and considerable psychological demands, pose professional challenges that can only be met with competence, commitment, and human compassion. It is important to remember that the nature of the terminal phase and subsequent death has particular consequences for the bereaved (see Chapter 7). In addition enabling patients to die with dignity and in comfort is a very valuable skill, which can bring immense professional satisfaction.

This chapter is concerned with how to care for patients whose health has deteriorated to the point when death is imminent. It includes how to recognize the terminal phase and how to manage the physical, psychological, and social needs of patients and their carers.

When is a patient terminally ill?

Terminal care is an important part of palliative care, and usually refers to the management of patients during the last few days, weeks or months of life, from a point when it becomes clear that the patient is in a progressive state of decline [1].

Although useful, this definition highlights the difficulty of characterizing the terminal phase, as it depends on a clinical assessment of subtle physical signs in order to predict a prognosis. Professionals require clinical acumen to discern between inevitable decline secondary to the primary disease and deterioration caused by a reversible complication or co-morbidity. These difficult decisions need experience and should be shared with the team (see Chapter 2).

It is useful to observe for the following signs as indicators of irreversible decline. This process is often gradual, but progressive.
- Profound weakness.
- Gaunt appearance.
- Drowsiness.
- Disorientation.
- Diminished oral intake.
- Difficulty taking oral medication.
- Poor concentration.
- Skin colour changes.
- Temperature change at extremities.

Principles of management

To provide quality terminal care, it is useful to be guided by the following principles. Although true for palliative care in general, these particular principles are applied more rigorously and intensely at this stage.

Consider the patient plus their family and friends as the unit of care, and encourage participation from all of these people. Perform a systematic assessment (see Box 20.1), and communicate the findings to the patient and their family/friends. Provide information and give support at all stages.

Relieve the patient's physical symptoms promptly. Consider the multifactorial nature of many symptoms, and remember the psychosocial component (e.g. fear) of certain symptoms. Avoid unnecessary medical intrusion—'First do no harm'. Stop all unnecessary drugs, while providing follow-up, continuity, and 24-hour emergency cover. Plan thoroughly for future problems, in what is likely to be a rapidly changing clinical picture.

Use a team approach, and listen to all suggestions and views. Involve all necessary resources for extra support at an early stage. Patients should be enabled to die in a place of their choosing. Their spiritual, as well as physical and psychosocial needs should be considered. Make every effort to reduce the morbidity due to bereavement among family and friends.

In summary: *think carefully, treat ethically, and review regularly.*

How to assess the needs of a terminally ill patient

Ideally, needs should be defined by the patient and be managed in terms of quality of life. However, in terminal care, it is not always feasible to

---

Box 20.1 Physical assessment checklist: what to look for

- Pain
- Shortness of breath
- Nausea/vomiting
- Agitation/restlessness/confusion
- Myoclonus and epilepsy
- Noisy breathing
- Urinary incontinence or retention
- Constipation
- Pressure areas/skin care
- Dry/sore mouth
- Difficulties swallowing
- Reversible complications/co-morbidity

---

make exhaustive assessments as communication with the patient may be difficult and accounts from carers can be inaccurate.

Professionals therefore have to share greater responsibility when making difficult decisions in situations where uncertainty exists. The wise practitioner is able to use professional experience combined with knowledge of the patient (previous symptoms, concerns, wishes), to perform a sensitive, problem-focused assessment. Box 20.1 outlines the components of a systematic assessment.

Treatment of common symptoms in terminal care

The management of many of the symptoms listed in Box 20.1 is covered elsewhere in this book and will therefore be only briefly mentioned here. This chapter will concentrate on those symptoms that are more specific to the terminal phase.

GENERAL NURSING CARE

The dependency of terminally ill patients demands a multidisciplinary approach, the basis of which is quality nursing care. Problems should be anticipated and actively prevented. It is important to try to involve family and loved ones in the nursing care of the patient. This can be particularly reassuring.

Basic nursing care includes the following:
- careful positioning of the patient;
- pressure area care;

- mouth care;
- bladder and bowel care;
- eye care.

Without the attention to detail that this entails, symptom control will be difficult.

PAIN CONTROL (see also Chapter 9)

Given that pain can change rapidly in the terminal phase, it is important to review patients repeatedly. Indeed, it is said that patients may often develop a new pain in the last 48 hours of life [2]. Do not assume that a non-communicative/semiconscious patient will not perceive pain. It is useful to ask repeatedly 'is the patient in pain?'.

SHORTNESS OF BREATH (see also Chapter 11)

Shortness of breath is a common symptom in the terminal phase [3]. It can result from direct involvement of the lungs from the primary disease (malignant or non-malignant) or following a secondary complication (e.g. anxiety, anaemia, infection, asthenia). It can be distressing to relatives. Be prepared to use non-drug (fans, open window, etc.) as well as drug treatments.

NAUSEA AND VOMITING (see Chapter 10)

The frailty of terminally ill patients puts them at risk of suffering from nausea and vomiting. This risk is increased as they are subject to the complications of rapidly advancing disease, polypharmacy, and anxiety.

CONFUSION

Confusion is common in patients with advanced illness, particularly in older people and those with chronic cognitive impairment (e.g. dementia, brain tumour). It occurs in up to 75% of patients in the last days of their illness. It is usually fluctuating in severity and characterized by:

- drowsiness;
- poor concentration;
- disorientation;
- poor short-term memory;
- inappropriate behaviour.

When it is severe, misperceptions, delusions, and hallucinations may also occur.

Most patients are very frightened. Many retain some insight and fear that they are going mad. It is very distressing to carers. It is perhaps the most difficult symptom to manage at home.

The management of confusion should be based on certain principles. Firstly, treat reversible causes (see Table 20.1). It is often challenging to balance the desire to investigate and discern a cause, with the need to protect patients from intrusive tests. Secondly, manage the patient in a suitable, quiet environment. Thirdly, make the patient safe. This may involve considering sedation if patients become agitated. Finally, acknowledge the distress and fears of the patient and carers and give clear explanations and reassurances where possible.

Table 20.1 Potentially reversible causes of confusion in patients with advanced disease.

Biochemical	Hypercalcaemia
	Hyponatraemia
	Uraemia
	Hyper- and hypoglycaemia
Infection	Urine
	Chest
Drugs	opioids
	benzodiazepines
	antidepressants
	anticonvulsants
	cimetidine
	steroids
	anticholinergics
Deficiency	thiamine
	alcohol
	benzodiazepine
	opioid
	adrenal steroid
Hypoxia	
Hypotension	
Extreme anxiety	
Severe pain	
Constipation	
GI bleed in patient with liver failure	

SEVERE RESTLESSNESS AND AGITATION

Terminal restlessness can be defined as increased purposeless movement in a patient who is near death [4]. Agitation can be understood as mental distress with or without disorientation.

Severe agitation, anguish, or aggression with risk to self or others is fortunately rare. It generally builds up over days to weeks although it may be acutely worsened or precipitated by a change of environment (e.g. admission). There are often some warning signs; these include: emotional unease or anguish, fluctuating disorientation, and psychotic features, particularly visual hallucinations and paranoid ideas.

Aetiology

Table 20.2 outlines the many causes of restlessness and agitation. Multiple aetiologies may coexist within any one patient. In elderly patients, pre-existing cognitive impairment (dementia) can predispose patients to suffer restlessness and agitation. Many of the causes listed in Table 20.2 also produce acute confusion.

Management

In spite of the limitations of assessment (see above, p. 309), it is important to consider the cause of the agitation and restlessness. In some cases simple measures can alleviate the cause and result in effective symptom control.
Basic care includes the following measures.
• Reassure the patient and make their environment comfortable (e.g. explanation, spiritual help, music, massage, good lighting).
• Reassure the family and friends.
• Ensure patient safety (e.g. prevent accidents). Most patients are frail and at risk of falling. Sedative drugs may cause hypotension and so increase this risk.
• Provide privacy.
• Assume a confident empathic approach.
Beyond this basic care, the team should consider the medical management of the patient.

Specific management: treat the cause. Some treatment options are covered in greater detail elsewhere in this book (e.g. pain, internal bleeding, shortness of breath). There are, however, some simple measures which can effect prompt relief from specific aetiologies.

Table 20.2 Causes of terminal restlessness and agitation.

Physical causes	Mental/emotional causes (terminal anguish)	Drugs	Biochemical causes
• Uncontrolled pain	• Anxiety	• Opioics	• Liver failure
• Full bladder	• Denial of advancing	• Psychotropics	• Renal failure
• Full rectum	disease	• Benzodiazepines	• Hypercalcaemia
• Immobility	• Fear of dying	• Hyoscine	• Hyponatraemia
• Dyspnoea	• Fear of losing control	• Steroids	• Hypoglycaemia
• Internal bleeding	• Unfinished business	• Digoxin	
• Cerebral	• Distress at leaving	• Anticonvulsants	
metastases	family	• Dopamine agonists	
• Infection	• Spiritual distress	• Withdrawal of drugs,	
• Hypotension	• Frustration with	e.g. opioids, alcohol	
• Nausea	predicament		

A full bladder is easy to determine, and catheterization is often an acceptable solution. A loaded rectum can be a cause of restlessness. Appropriate bowel care can result in calm (e.g. suppository, enema, manual evacuation) (see Chapter 10).

Immobility leads to bed-bound patients suffering joint stiffness, bed sores, and frustration. Nursing measures (e.g. pressure-relieving mattress, appropriate bedding, regular turning, and careful positioning) and suitable pain relief are all important.

Stop all unnecessary drugs, especially those with potentially toxic side-effects (steroids can be stopped abruptly in the terminal phase [5]). The use of antibiotics for infection can be viewed in terms of palliation. The decision to start such treatment has to be made in terms of quality of life. Administer oxygen therapy if the patient is hypoxic.

Non-specific management: control the symptoms (Table 20.3). In many cases it is inappropriate or not possible to treat the underlying cause, and

Table 20.3 Suggested therapeutic options for agitation and restlessness.

Sedative drug	Routes	Loading dose	Usual dose range over 24 hours	Comments
Midazolam	i.v., s.c., i.m.	2–10 mg	5–60 mg	Drug of choice for anxiety/anguish
Methotrimeprazine	i.v., s.c., i.m., oral	12.5–50 mg	12.5–150 mg	Also anti-emetic
Haloperidol	i.v., s.c., i.m., oral	1.5–10 mg	1.5–30 mg	Use lower dosages in elderly. May only need once daily administration. Also anti-emetic
Chlorpromazine	i.m., p.r., oral	25–50 mg	50–200 mg	Alternative
Diazepam	oral, p.r.	2–10 mg	6–30 mg	Rectal drug can be useful. Avoid with psychotic symptoms as the disinhibition can worsen symptoms

sedation with drugs is the mainstay of treatment. In an emergency situation a loading dose is often required, followed by regular maintenance, titrated according to response. Although large drug dosages are occasionally required, sedation should be kept to the minimum. In situations where repeated dosages have been necessary to induce calm, patients may sleep for long periods as a result of the cumulative effect of the drugs. Occasionally a combination of antipsychotic and benzodiazepines is more helpful than increasing doses of either alone.

MYOCLONUS AND EPILEPSY

Terminally ill patients can occasionally suffer myoclonic jerks (brief, shocklike activity in one or more muscle groups). These can be due to biochemical abnormalities, metabolic disturbance, or drugs (particularly opioids). They are considered as pre-epileptiform. The stopping or reduction in dose of causative drugs (e.g. strong opioids, anticholinergics) should be considered.

In the context of the terminal phase, the control of epilepsy includes first-aid measures and the emergency use of drugs until control is achieved. Subsequent prevention of fits relies on the continued use of previously prescribed drugs whenever possible, supplemented by regular use of sedating drugs (see Table 20.4).

NOISY 'BUBBLY' BREATHING

Noisy 'bubbly' breathing, often referred to as the 'death rattle', occurs because of the inability of the patient to cough up or swallow secretions from the oropharynx and trachea. Although often not troubling to the patient, it may cause considerable distress to relatives and carers.

Drug management

Anticholinergic drugs can help by reducing pharyngeal secretions (Table 20.5).

Non-drug management

Various techniques can assist in providing relief for patients with noisy breathing.
• Careful patient positioning (e.g. sitting up, recovery position).
• Gentle physiotherapy.

Table 20.4 Drugs to control myoclonus and epilepsy.

Drug	Route	Myoclonus		Epilepsy	
		Emergency	Prevention	Emergency	Prevention
Diazepam Diazemuls	p.r., oral i.v.	5–10 mg repeated every hour	10–20 mg at night	5–10 mg repeated every 5 minutes	20 mg at night
Midazolam	s.c., i.v., i.m.	2.5–5 mg repeated every hour	10–30 mg over 24 hours	2.5–15 mg repeated every 5 minutes	10–30 mg over 24 hours
Phenobarbitone (alternative in difficult cases)	i.v., s.c.		400–800 mg subcutaneously over 24 hours	100 mg i.v. over 2 minutes, or 200 mg s.c. every 15 minutes	400–800 mg s.c. over 24 hours
Clonazepam (particularly useful in myoclonus)	oral, s.c.		1–8 mg orally (0.5–5 mg s.c.) over 24 hours		

Table 20.5 Drugs to control noisy 'bubbly' breathing.

Drug	Route of administration	Regular dose	Maintenance dose
Hyoscine hydrobromide	s.l./s.c./i.v./i.m. Transdermal patch	200–400 μg every 2–4 hours	1.6–2.4 μg s.c. over 24 hours. (Transdermal patch: 1.5 mg every 3rd day)
Hyoscine butylbromide	oral/s.c./i.v.	10–20 mg every 4–6 hours	40–120 mg over 24 hours
Glycopyrronium	s.c.	0.2 mg 4 hourly	0.8 mg over 24 hours

- Nebulized normal (0.9%) saline 5 ml.
- Gentle oropharyngeal suction.
- Mouth care.
- Reassurance to family and friends.

URINARY INCONTINENCE AND RETENTION

Urinary incontinence is a common problem in the terminal phase, not least due to patient immobility. If ignored it can result in distress and agitation. Practical solutions are needed to overcome the problem: nursing assistance, pads, provision of commode, penile sheath, and catheterization. The incontinence adviser can be a help in complicated cases.

Retention of urine may occur for various reasons, including: prostatic outflow obstruction, drug therapy, or constipation. This can be extremely uncomfortable and warrant catheterization. Clearing any constipation and stopping aggravating drugs (especially anticholinergics) is advisable.

CONSTIPATION (see also Chapter 10)

A combination of drugs, immobility, dehydration, and disease process make constipation a particular problem in the terminal phase. As previously noted, it can distress patients to the point of agitation and restlessness. The use of laxatives is important and although patients may be frail, enema and suppositories may help.

PRESSURE AREA CARE/SKIN CARE (see also Chapter 18)

Terminally ill patients are particularly vulnerable to pressure sores. The team should anticipate this and prevent problems by using pressure-relieving aids and mattresses.

DRY/SORE MOUTH (see also Chapter 15)

Every assessment of a terminally ill patient should include the mouth. With careful use of medication and simple nursing measures, troublesome symptoms can be overcome.

DIFFICULTIES IN SWALLOWING (see also Chapter 10)

As patients become weak, they slowly lose their ability to swallow freely. Oral medication becomes harder to cope with and this should be seen as another opportunity to rationalize treatment. In the terminal phase it is generally inappropriate to commence artificial feeding or hydration (see Chapter 17).

Distressing acute terminal events

It is fortunate that distressing acute terminal events are rare. In addition, for many cancer patients they can be anticipated and the patient, the carers, and the professionals can plan ahead to minimize distress. Studies on patients dying from non-malignant chronic illness are not available. Table 20.6 shows the frequency of very distressing terminal events in hospice in-patients.

Table 20.6 Frequency of very distressing events in hospice in-patients (data from [2]).

Symptom	Frequency (% of patients)
Haemorrhage/haemoptysis	2
Respiratory distress	2
Restlessness	1.5
Pain	1

When such terminal events are managed badly, patient and carer distress may be magnified, bereavement may be more difficult and abnormal, and the team may feel failure and dissatisfaction. When managed well, the burden of suffering for patients and their carers may be greatly eased and many bereavement problems will be prevented. Great satisfaction may be gained by the team who work together to achieve this.

The principles of management of massive haemorrhage, respiratory distress, or other acute terminal incidents are similar irrespective of the type of event or the cause. Prevention may be possible if warning or herald signs are noted. Anticipation and planning, and preparation of carers and patients are essential. Families can often cope better with the event itself, and in bereavement, if they are sure that they can contact at any time a professional who knows the patient. Availability of care 24 hours a day, 7 days a week is invaluable in support of patients at home.

Such events are frightening and distressing for *everyone*—patients, carers, and professionals. Since most such events cause death within minutes the most important aspect of care is to stay with the patient. The urge to do something or get help should be resisted if this requires leaving the patient alone.

The main aims of drug treatment are:
• to reduce fear;
• to reduce pain;
• to reduce the level of awareness of the patient.
The oral administration of drugs is inappropriate since absorption will be too slow for efficacy. Box 20.2 lists drugs used in the management of distressing acute terminal events.

Ketamine should be used with great caution. It may be useful since it has a rapid onset of action, is both analgesic and anaesthetic, and does not require the preparation time of controlled drugs. It has a short-lived effect, however, and causes very unpleasant emergent effects, particularly if administered without a benzodiazepine. It is available only on a named patient basis in the community and probably will only be used by specialists.

Planning ahead

PATIENTS AT RISK

Patients at greater, and predictable risk of distressing terminal events fall into four groups.
• Patients with fungating tumours involving soft tissue around major blood vessels.

Box 20.2 Drugs used in the management of distressing acute terminal events

Benzodiazepine
- Diazepam 10–20 mg p.r.
- Diazemuls 5–20 mg i.v.
- Midazolam 5–10 mg i.m./i.v.

Opioid
- Diamorphine 2 × equivalent 4-hourly dose
- 10 mg i.m./i.v. if opioid naive

Other possible drugs
- Ketamine 20–100 mg i.m./i.v.*

---

* Caution: see text.

- Patients with pelvic tumour associated with fistulae involving the vagina and/or rectum.
- Patients with tracheostomal recurrent tumour.
- Patients with anterior, superior mediastinal or tracheal tumours.

DISCUSSION WITH CARERS, THE PROFESSIONALS, AND THE PATIENT

When there is a serious risk of such a terminal event many carers find it much less distressing to be forewarned despite the difficulty and distress of such a discussion. Occasionally, however, this knowledge and uncertainty is very disturbing to a carer (although they may still be better prepared to cope if such an event does happen). The discussion must be handled therefore with great sensitivity and followed-up with repeated support and review of the situation. Such a discussion should have three principal aims. First, to give an opportunity for the carer to voice their own suspicions and fears and discuss them in realistic terms. Second, to help the carer plan what they might do so that they can feel less helpless and fearful. Third, to ensure that the carer understands the optimum sources of professional support and how to contact them; for example, *not* to call 999, but instead to have the telephone numbers of the GP and emergency hospice/palliative care team beside the telephone.

Discussion of the possibility of a distressing terminal event with the patient is sometimes helpful. If a patient asks or is reported to be (or appears to be) worrying about such an event, facilitating discussion may allow a more realistic scenario to be portrayed with the opportunity to reassure the patient and the carer that suffering would be transitory and unconsciousness develop quickly, and to develop a plan of care together. It is also an opportunity to reassure many patients that such events are, in fact, very rare.

It is worth noting that many patients and carers worry about such catastrophic events when they are highly unlikely to occur in their particular circumstances. It is often helpful to ask if this is a significant fear in order to reassure the patient and carer that it *will not* happen. For example, the authors have met several patients who thought that their enlarging liver would eventually burst through their abdomen. Explaining that this would not happen brought tremendous relief.

There should also be discussion among the members of the professional team to:
- establish a clear plan of management and delegation of responsibilities;
- ensure all aspects of the plan are carried out;
- allow support and evaluation within the team should a distressing terminal event occur.

AVAILABILITY OF DRUGS IN THE HOME

When there is a possibility of an acute, distressing terminal event it is useful to ensure that the necessary drugs (see Box 20.3) are readily available. A specific 'emergency box' within the home is a helpful way of planning this.

MASSIVE HAEMORRHAGE

In addition to the general measures already outlined, it is useful to have to hand green, red or dark-coloured towels or blankets to reduce the visual and psychological impact of massive blood loss. Pressure on the bleeding site with a pillow or large pad may help (but may be very painful because of the tumour).

HAEMOPTYSIS

In patients with cancer massive haemoptysis usually occurs in those with a bronchogenic primary or as a consequence of a systemic coagulation dysfunction or fungal pneumonia in profoundly neutropenic patients. Patients with lung metastases and tracheolaryngeal primary tumours very rarely have massive haemoptysis.

There is often a warning of increasing, fresh haemoptysis.

CAROTID BLOW-OUT (see Chapter 12)

Carotid blow-out is more likely to occur in patients with recurrent tumour in a site previously treated with both surgery and radiotherapy. Death occurs within 2–3 minutes. There is often a herald bleed.

PELVIC BLEEDING

Tumours of the cervix, uterus, and rectum may erode into major pelvic blood vessels. This is often preceded by the formation of vesico-vaginal, recto-vaginal, or vesico-rectal fistulae, and with increasing loss of fresh blood.

Vaginal packing may be useful in some patients.

Many patients with pelvic tumours will have experienced venous obstruction and some may have been treated with warfarin. This is obviously an extra risk factor for massive haemorrhage.

GASTROINTESTINAL BLEEDING

Massive haematemesis is more usually due to peptic ulceration or oesophageal varices than tumour erosion into a major vessel. Patients with advanced cancer are often taking non-steroidal anti-inflammatory drugs (NSAIDs) and many are also taking steroids. They are therefore greatly at risk of peptic ulceration and there should be a proactive approach to watch for and treat characteristic warning signs in order to prevent catastrophic bleeding. Patients with, or with high likelihood of, oesophageal varices are generally well identified and appropriate planning can be made well in advance.

Psychosocial needs

Needs of patients

When assessing patient need, it is important to remember that some psychosocial problems may first present as poor control of physical symptoms (e.g. total pain, terminal agitation, sick with fear). Some of the common problems experienced are outlined in Box 20.3.

Also, factors such as personalities, relationships, and coping mechanisms are important to consider. Giving patients time and encouraging them to express their feelings is particularly important. However, patients must not be forced to engage with carers; some will not appreciate unrequested

---

Box 20.3 Psychosocial needs: what to look for

- Fear, e.g. the diagnosis, mode of death, drug side-effects
- Guilt, e.g. becoming a burden, past life experiences
- Anger, e.g. loss of dignity, missed opportunities, loss of independence
- Uncertainty, e.g. spiritual questions, prognosis, the future of the family
- Depression (as a consequence to the above)

'counselling'. Patients should also be allowed the option of denial as a legitimate coping mechanism.

In responding to patient concerns and providing emotional support, it is helpful to use the following guidelines.
- Where does the patient want to die and can this be guaranteed?
- Involve the patient as long as possible in decision-making.
- Answer patients' questions honestly. Give them time. Explanations may need to be repeated on several occasions.
- Patient confidentiality should be assured.
- Allay any fears about dying (uncontrolled symptoms, prolonged process, being alone, lack of warning).
- Space and privacy should be provided if the patient wishes.
- Consider the patient's spiritual needs. Respect cultural and religious differences.
- Reassure patients that their family will be offered bereavement support.
- Do not let the medical process obstruct the expression of affection between loved ones.
- Make careful enquiries about the patient's will and 'affairs'.

Needs of family/friends

The team members are often focused on the patient, giving family and friends little opportunity to express concerns. Often, all that is required is a recognition of the family's position and an expression of understanding. However, in certain circumstances it is important to explore difficulties at a greater depth. This assessment should cover physical (e.g. fatigue), psychological (e.g. depression), and social (e.g. finances) needs.

The family and/or friends should have access to professionals, both for information and to meet their own health needs. Information should be given, whenever patient confidentiality allows, even if this feels somewhat repetitious to the professional. Explain to the family or friends what they should do in an emergency, and confirm the 24-hour availability of professional care. The strain on the family and carers should be acknowledged and support offered as appropriate. It may be helpful for team members to determine the family's previous experience of death.

Families and carers often need to feel helpful and to know that their contribution is valued. This may include physical care (e.g. bathing). Families and friends should not be made to feel like intruders in the care of their loved one. They must be given every opportunity to stay with the patient, and visiting arrangements should be flexible. Reassure family members who find it too difficult to be at the bedside that the patient will not be left alone. Explain that even if comatose the patient may be aware of the family's presence. They may still be heard by the patient.

Dying in different settings

Patients can be looked after in various settings; each has inherent advantages and disadvantages (see Table 20.7). Although most people would prefer to die at home, unfortunately this is not achieved in many cases.

The importance of religion in dying

For those patients who possess a strong religious conviction as part of their spirituality, rituals around death are very important. Professionals should be respectful of this and act with sensitivity to these requirements.

This section aims to give a brief outline of some of the traditional practices of the main religions found in the UK. It is beyond this book to give a detailed account of all beliefs and rituals. What follows is a superficial overview, introducing professionals to what they may encounter in their care of certain patients (Table 20.8). Indeed, anticipating the religious needs of patients can be especially appreciated by both patients and their families.

It is also important to remember that in a pluralistic society such as the UK, religious law can be interpreted in various ways. Consequently, religious practices may be applied differently and should never be assumed.

Procedures after death

Diagnosing death

It is usually the responsibility of a doctor to diagnose death; however, in some hospices, nursing staff can perform this task. This can be done in various ways, although in terminal care a confirmation of somatic death

is made by observing the following:
- fixed dilated pupils;
- no heart sounds;
- no respiratory effort;
- no pulse.

How to prepare bodies after death

Relatives should be allowed the choice to see and spend time with the deceased person, not only during the act of dying but also afterwards. Professionals should make this easy for the bereaved and prepare the body appropriately. Policies exist within institutions with regard to 'laying out'; these should be followed with sensitivity to the wishes of family and friends. In particular, different cultural or religious practices should be respected (see Table 20.8).

Wounds should be covered with waterproof dressings and those handling the body should be warned of any risk of infection. Catheters, infusion lines, and Hickman lines should be removed (unless the case is being referred to the coroner). Those with infectious diseases may need to be placed in body bags (see Chapter 13).

A list of funeral directors can be given to patients; indeed the general practitioner (GP) or district nurse may be in a position to contact a firm for the family. Undertakers are available 24 hours a day and can prepare the body. Although not always immediately necessary, the body is often taken from the patient's home to the company's chapel of rest. These private companies attempt to accommodate the wishes of the bereaved by providing a range of services, although at a cost to the bereaved.

Organ donation

Patients carrying a donor card, or whose family consent, may be able to donate various organs and tissues. Generally speaking, organs are retrieved from patients who have died from cerebral trauma, intercranial haemorrhage, anoxic brain damage following cardiopulmonary arrest, or primary brain tumours. Certain contraindications exist for donation in general (e.g. over age 70, sepsis [10]) and for particular organs (long-term steroids and bone donation). As yet there are no nationally agreed guidelines.

Tissue and organ donation is rarely considered and although terminally ill patients may not satisfy the criteria, this does not apply universally and families should be given an opportunity to provide consent, if they wish.

Table 20.7 Advantages and disadvantages of different settings on patient care.

Setting	Number of deaths [6]	Advantages	Disadvantages
Home	• 29% of cancer deaths • 22% of non-cancer deaths	• Often preferred by patients [7] • Familiar surroundings and a non-medical environment • Family life maintained • Patient in control (e.g. decisions, visitors, cultural/spiritual needs) • Home is generally a more peaceful environment • Familiar with medical staff (GP and District Nurse)	• Pain control may be inadequate [8] • Specialist palliative care services not always available for non-malignant disease • Professional help not as accessible • Patients may not be protected from unwelcome visitors • Burden of care giving falls upon the relatives and friends who may be unable or unwilling to cope • Disruption of family life • Financial consequences to care at home • Critically ill patients may need intensive support (e.g. daily or twice daily visit by GP)
Nursing/ residential home	• 7% of cancer deaths • 16% of non-cancer deaths	• Immediate access to nursing care (except in residential care) • The family is relieved of the burden of care • Familiar GP will have ongoing responsibility for medical care	• Financial implications for patients and families • Standards of care may be variable, being limited by resources. • Surroundings are unfamiliar • Families may experience guilt; 'don't put me in a home'

Hospital	• 50% of cancer deaths • 57% of non-cancer deaths	• Medical and nursing expertise is readily available • Burden of care is removed from the family • Patients and families may feel safe knowing that doctors and nurses are available	• Staff knowledge on symptom control may be limited • Families may feel there is a lack of specialist medical and nursing attention [9] • Patients may feel isolated on a busy unit • Nursing care may be limited by resources • Symptoms may be poorly controlled • Care is more orientated to cure. • Unfamiliarity with staff • Family may not be encouraged to participate in the care of the patient • Visiting hours may be restricted
Hospice	• 13% of cancer deaths • <1% of non-cancer deaths	• Immediate access to specialized staff, within a multidisciplinary team • Palliative care philosophy is widely applied (see Chapter 1) • Most have a higher staff ratio of qualified nurses • Generally less noisy, more peaceful environment than hospitals • Bereavement support is generally more available	• Hospices may be perceived as 'a place to die' • Unfamiliar surroundings. • Some hospices may be perceived as being too 'religious' • Many hospices may not meet the needs of patients from ethnic minority groups (although this could be true of other settings)

Table 20.8 Overview of rituals around death for main UK religions.

Religion	Death rituals	Disposal of the body
Christianity	• Traditionally a priest performs the last rites prior to death (prayers of forgiveness and sacrament if possible) • Individuals may wish to pray with the dying patient	• Body can be touched by non-Christians • Body is cleaned and covered by white sheet • Body can be buried or cremated • Funeral directors assist in much of this preparation • The religious component of bereavement occurs at the funeral service.
Islam	• Patient should face Mecca if possible • Mullah (religious leader) may whisper prayers in patient's ear	• Traditionally the body should not be touched by non-Muslims • Washing and preparing the body follows precise rules • Burial should occur within 24 hours or as soon as possible • Post-mortems and organ donation are resisted • Burial is the traditional means of disposal of the body
Hinduism	• Brahmin priests may perform rituals that allow forgiveness of sins • A thread may be left around the wrist to show that the patient has received a priest's blessing • Devout Hindus may wish to die on the floor, being close to mother earth	• Correct funeral rites are believed to be important for the future of the deceased's soul • Body is washed and put in normal clothes • Only men can perform funeral rites, preferably the eldest son • Cremation is used to dispose of the body • Bereavement involves 10 days of mourning, each day has a particular ceremony
Sikhism	• A reader from the temple will recite hymns, if the patient is too weak to do this personally • At death attendants may utter words of praise (Wonderful lord, Wonderful lord)	• The body is washed and placed in a shroud • Religious artefacts worn by patient will be left—'the 5 K's' (e.g. wooden comb, iron wrist band, short sword, undershorts, uncut hair)

Continued

Table 20.8 *Continued*

Religion	Death rituals	Disposal of the body
		• Traditionally Sikhs are cremated • Friends and family consider visiting the bereaved as a duty and may provide food
Judaism	• Psalms are recited and the patient should not be left alone • Pillows should not be removed from beneath the head (is believed to hasten death)	• The body should be left for 10 minutes after death • The body may be laid on the floor, with feet pointing to the door • Preparation of the body can be precise and is performed by Jews who specifically deal with the dead • Burial should occur within 24 hours of death • Bereavement is structured with religious ceremony
Buddhism	• The patient will wish to die with a 'clear mind' and may use chanting to achieve this. This influences the nature of the next incarnation • There may be a wish to avoid distractions, e.g. sedating drugs, over-crowding of room, intrusions etc. • Most Buddhists believe that consciousness remains in or near the body for 8–12 hours post death. This may mean that some Buddhists would prefer the body not to be touched during this period	• Ideally the body should not be moved or washed before the arrival of a Buddhist monk • Disposal of the body may be by burial, cremation or embalming, depending on the nationality of the deceased

Obviously it is important for professionals to be fully conversant with local policy and approach relatives with appropriate sensitivity. Additional advice is provided by local tissue transplant co-ordinators. They are able to speak to relatives and arrange tissue retrieval.

Death certificates (Medical Certificate of Cause of Death)

The death certificate (Fig. 20.1) must be issued by a registered medical practitioner. It cannot be issued in the following circumstances.
• Patient not attended in their last illness by a medical practitioner.
• The certifying doctor has not examined the body or seen the patient in the 14 days prior to the death.
• The cause of death is unknown or appears unnatural.
• The cause of death is associated with an anaesthetic, industrial disease, surgery, fracture, violence, or suicide.

In these cases the coroner must be informed and a post-mortem may subsequently be performed. If doubt exists, it is always worthwhile discussing the case with the coroner or the coroner's officer (police representative of the coroner).

The certificate must be completed accurately and with no omissions. The data are used to compile national statistics on mortality. Details on how to fill out death certificates are outlined at the front of the certificate book. The certificate is then taken to the Registrar of Births, Marriages and Deaths (usually by a relative), whereupon a Certificate for Disposal is issued; this needs to be given to the undertaker. If the body is to be cremated, a second form needs to be completed by two independent doctors (usually the certifying doctor and another doctor who is at least 5 years post-registration).

Post-mortem

A post-mortem may be a mandatory requirement (cases referred to the coroner). This is a legal requirement and cannot be refused. Post-mortems can also be requested in order to clarify medical detail of the death; these are known as hospital post-mortems. Relatives can refuse hospital post-mortems.

Summary

Care for patients who have reached the terminal phase of their illness poses many challenges to professionals. Good quality palliative care at this point often requires increased professional support of patients and their loved ones. Following a death there are certain practical requirements that need to be dealt with professionally and with sensitivity to the feelings of the bereaved.

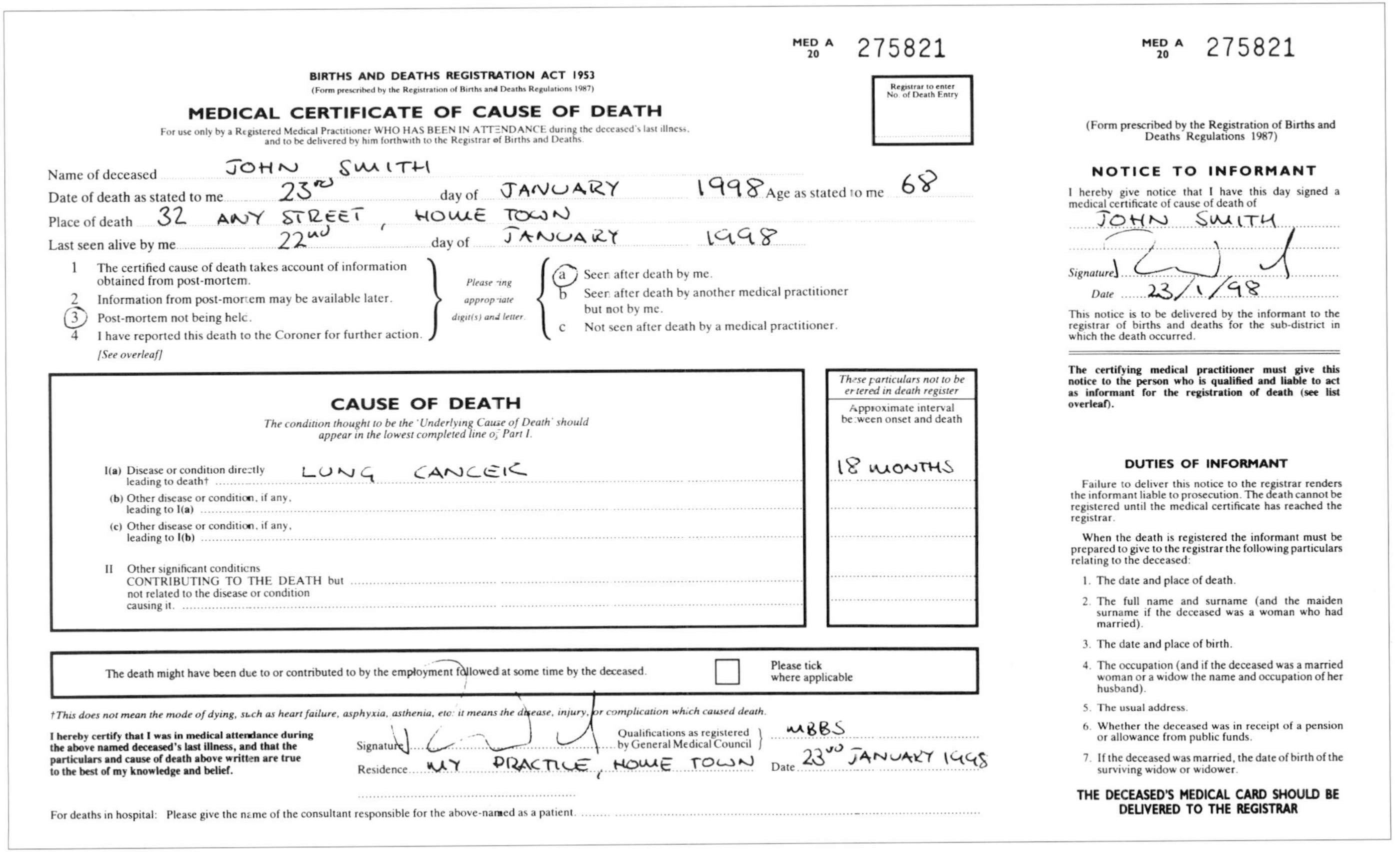

Fig. 20.1 The Medical Certificate of Cause of Death.

References

1 National Council for Hospice and Specialist Care Services. *Specialist Palliative Care: A Statement of Definitions*. Occasional Paper, No. 8, London: NCHSCS, 1995.

2 Lichter I, Hunt E. The last 48 hours of life. *J Palliat Care* 1990; 6: 7–15.

3 Boyd KJ. Short terminal admissions to a hospice. *Palliat Med* 1993; 7: 289–294.

4 Lovel T. Restlessness in end stage disease. *Palliat Care Today* 1994; 31: 12–13.

5 Working Party on Clinical Guidelines in Palliative Care. *Changing Gear—Guidelines for Managing the Last Days of Life in Adults*. London: National Council for Hospice and Specialist Palliative Care Services, 1997.

6 Addington Hall J, McCarthy M. Dying from cancer: results of a national population based investigation. *Palliat Med* 1995; 9: 295–305.

7 Townsend J, Frank AO, Fermont D *et al.* Terminal cancer care and patients' preference for place of death. *BMJ* 1990; 301: 415–417.

8 Cartwright A. Changes in life and care in the year before death 1967–1987. *J Publ Health Med* 1991; 13: 81–87.

9 MacCabee J. The effect of transfer from a palliative care unit to nursing homes— are patients' and relatives' needs met? *Palliat Med* 1994; 8: 211–214.

10 UK Transplant Co-ordinators' Association. *Organ Donation and Transplantation— Information for Doctors, Nurses and other Professionals*. London: HMSO, 1992.

21: Complementary Approaches to Palliative Care

CATHERINE ZOLLMAN AND
ELIZABETH THOMPSON

Introduction

The last 20 years have seen a dramatic increase in the use of complementary medicine (CM). Palliative care settings appear to be no exception to this observation. Of hospices responding to a survey in 1992, 70% offered massage and aromatherapy services [1]. In fact there are similarities between many complementary approaches and the care provided by a palliative care unit which make the combination potentially attractive. This chapter will explore these similarities and show how CM and orthodox palliative medicine might truly 'complement' each other.

Confusion surrounds the term 'complementary medicine' and other terms which are sometimes used interchangeably (Table 21.1). One possible definition of CM is:

Areas of medicine that are generally outside current accepted medical thought, scientific knowledge or university teaching [2].

However it is defined, CM describes a very heterogeneous group of approaches, some of which have features in common, while others have conflicting theories and practice. For the purposes of this chapter, we have not considered psychotherapy, cognitive/behavioural approaches, or counselling under our definition of CM.

The appropriateness of CM in holistic palliative care

Palliative care acknowledges that a patient's physical symptoms cannot be fully understood or helped without an appreciation of emotional, psychological, and social factors. Likewise, many CM practitioners claim to have a holistic perspective. The central tenets of anthroposophy, a philosophical and therapeutic system developed by Rudolf Steiner, are a good example of this approach (see Box 21.1).

Both palliative care and many CM disciplines take an 'individualized' approach, i.e. that what is of greatest importance is not the underlying diagnosis, but how it affects the individual patient and their quality of

Table 21.1 Assumptions about complementary medicine (CM).

Statement	Comments
Alternative	Implies used instead of orthodox treatment. In fact the majority of CM users appear not to have abandoned orthodox medicine.
Not provided by the NHS	CM is increasingly available on NHS. 39% of GP practices provide access to CM for NHS patients [3].
Unregulated	Osteopaths and chiropractors are now state registered and regulated. Other CM disciplines will probably soon follow.
Natural	Many conventional pharmacological products are derived from natural products e.g. plants and minerals. Conversely CM can involve unnatural practices.
Holistic	As in conventional medicine, there are practitioners who take a holistic approach to their patient and there are those who are more reductionist in outlook.
Unproven	There is a growing body of evidence that supports the claim that certain types of CM are effective in certain clinical conditions.
Irrational—no scientific basis	Basic science research is beginning to give an understanding of the mechanisms of some types of CM (e.g. acupuncture, hypnosis [4,5])
Harmless	There are reports of rare but serious adverse effects associated with some CM use [6].

life. Many CM treatments also contribute to a pleasurable sense of being cared for and thereby improve quality of life.

Existential questions and concerns form a regular feature of work with people with advanced disease. Some CM disciplines include a spiritual

> **Box 21.1 Central tenets of anthroposophy**
>
> • Each individual is unique
> • Scientific, artistic, and spiritual insights may need to be applied together to restore health
> • Life has meaning and purpose—the loss of this sense may lead to a deterioration in health
> • Illness may provide opportunities for positive change and a new balance in our lives

dimension and can recognize and address symptoms at this level. Many CM practitioners will explicitly acknowledge potential spiritual concerns.

Both palliative and complementary medicine, which are person-centred rather than disease-centred, have strategies that ensure it is never the case that 'there is nothing more to be done'; patients' symptoms can be improved, relationships healed, preparations for death embraced, etc. Realistic hope can sustain people.

As with the best of palliative care nursing, many CM approaches involve practitioners and patients in a degree of physical contact which legitimizes touch and human contact.

The benefit of any intervention, particularly in advanced illness must clearly outweigh any harm. Except for some notable exceptions (see later sections) CM approaches have very few harmful effects if used appropriately.

Most palliative care units have a 'low-tech' atmosphere where patients are helped to feel at home. Most CM approaches require a minimum of equipment and can be readily practised by the bedside, at home or in a day centre. Techniques can even be taught to relatives or patients themselves as well as volunteers and medical and nursing staff.

Potential problems with CM approaches in palliative care settings

Guilt and responsibility

One of the most important potential adverse effects of CM that has been observed is the generation of guilt. Many CM disciplines support the belief that the way people behave and look after their bodies influences their state of health. They also place great emphasis on the role of self-healing. These two axioms can develop into a two-edged sword. On the one hand they can promote greater independence and self-esteem by reversing the patient's traditional role of sitting back and letting the doctors do the work. On the other they can create a burden of responsibility and guilt in patients who come to believe that they are the cause of their own illness and that the reason they are not getting better is because they are not trying hard enough, eating well enough, or being good enough to people. CM practitioners, particularly those who are unused to working with patients with a terminal disease, must be very aware of these risks.

Increasing denial

CM can be used as a psychological or emotional support in the face of progressing disease or impending death. However, there is a fine line between this and a potential for increasing an unhelpful pattern of denial, which can risk delaying or even preventing appropriate adjustment and acceptance. This is not unique to CM: inappropriate use of conventional oncological treatments may have similar effects.

Masking important symptoms

Use of CM can mask or disguise the development of complications which require urgent conventional medical treatment (e.g. incipient cord compression). It may also mask disease progression for which further conventional symptomatic treatment is superior (e.g. radiotherapy to bony metastases). Regular medical reassessment of all patients with new or persistent symptoms is mandatory.

Antagonism and communication difficulties

There is often an element of faith in some of the principles of CM and disagreement about the effectiveness of various techniques. It is possible that those who do not share these beliefs (either family members or conventional medical carers) will feel antagonized by a patient's decision to seek CM treatments. This can lead to isolation and fragmentation of care, placing patients in the difficult position of having to choose between conflicting advice.

Financial

The financial implications of CM for both patient and health service purchasers need to be carefully considered. CM treatments are labour intensive but generally cost little in terms of medication or equipment. Cost-effectiveness is not established.

Supervision and responsibility

CM practitioners will often be working outside the conventional management structures of the NHS. Some may be working as volunteers. Job descriptions, limits to practice, review procedures, lines of clinical and management responsibility, and codes of conduct all need to be clearly and carefully defined.

Interprofessional issues

Many conventional health care professionals have undergone CM training but other CM practitioners will have trained outside the multiprofessional environment of an NHS hospital. The language they use and the way in which they conduct their practice may therefore be unfamiliar to medical, nursing, and other health care professionals. This can lead to misunderstandings and frustration. The presence of CM practitioners at multidisciplinary team meetings can be problematic initially, but with time, familiarity and mutual respect can develop.

Contraindications to specific therapies

Accepted contraindications to the use of the various therapies are listed below in the relevant sections. Except where specifically stated, these lists have been developed by CM practitioners and teachers through a mixture of experience, educated guesswork and commonsense. Research-based supporting evidence is not generally available.

Acupuncture

Acupuncture, the ancient Chinese art of healing using the insertion of fine needles to 'cure' or palliate symptoms, has origins dating back to at least 2500 BC. The *Yellow Emperor's Classic of Internal Medicine* [7] describes amongst other concepts, an elaborate system of diagnosis based on vital energy, or 'Qi', and meridians, which are a series of invisible lines joining acupuncture points together.

The patient is treated using thin needles inserted in a carefully chosen combination of specific acupuncture points. The needles are left *in situ* or stimulated by hand for up to 20 minutes. In addition, some needles are stimulated using electro-acupuncture equipment, using 'moxibustion' (a technique involving heat and herbs), or given painless stimulation using low-level laser therapy.

Over the last 30 years, solid evidence has accumulated on many of the basic mechanisms of action of acupuncture [4], including stimulation of multiple endogenous opioids, release of serotonin (which can influence mood), autonomic effects, alteration in blood supply, and increased production of corticosteroids. However, more basic scientific research is needed.

Many patients feel very relaxed and some feel slightly drowsy after their first acupuncture treatment. Some even feel somewhat euphoric. Patients can be treated lying down or sitting up. They often feel a combination of sensations such as heaviness, numbness, tingling, and soreness around the needles, a phenomenon called 'de Qi' (pronounced 'ter chi').

Indications for acupuncture

Acupuncture is used for a wide variety of problems and symptoms, and the WHO publish a list of common conditions helped by acupuncture [8].

Painful conditions

Painful conditions, such as those affecting muscles and bones, are especially amenable to treatment using acupuncture. Uncontrolled studies in patients with malignancy show that a reduction in consumption and side-effects of conventional analgesics is sometimes possible using acupuncture to treat bone pain, nerve pain, and pain due to soft tissue disease [9]. However, pain relief for malignant conditions is generally of shorter duration than for non-malignant conditions and tolerance to the effects of acupuncture may be more of a problem in the former. If disease progression occurs, duration of pain relief can decrease. Acupuncture can also be helpful for syndromes including postsurgical and postradiotherapy pain syndromes.

Breathlessness

In a series of 20 patients with disabling, advanced cancer-related breathlessness, use of acupuncture was associated with clinical improvements measured both subjectively and objectively [9].

Nausea and vomiting

Nausea and vomiting (including chemotherapy-induced symptoms) have been reduced by acupuncture and transcutaneous electrical nerve stimulation (TENS), and these effects appear to be reproducible. A systematic review of acupuncture antiemesis found that 11 out of 12 good-quality, randomized, placebo-controlled trials favoured acupuncture [10].

Stroke

Patients in a randomized controlled trial who were treated twice a week after a stroke, had earlier rehabilitation, better motor function, balance, and activities of daily living, shorter hospital stays, and improved quality of life compared with control patients [11].

Other conditions

Miscellaneous problems such as changes in bowel habit due to radiation, ulcers, bedsores, depression, itch, and hiccup may also be helped by acupuncture [9].

Safety, adverse effects, and recommended contraindications

Generally acupuncture has a low side-effect profile. Acupuncturists should have a thorough knowledge of anatomy and physiology and of the diagnostic process. Deep needling, where needles could cause internal damage, should be avoided. Disposable needles should be used to prevent the risk of infection to patients.

Acupuncture should not be used for patients with significantly impaired clotting. Needles should not be used in a lymphoedematous limb. Patients with an unstable spine should not have treatment over the spine. Patients fitted with pacemakers should not have electro-acupuncture.

Dietary interventions

Although 'healthy eating' advice is a mainstay of general health promotion and disease prevention strategies, the use of diet as a *treatment* for established disease (other than certain well-defined deficiency or intolerance syndromes) is rare in contemporary Western medicine.

Indications and evidence on dietary intervention

Dietary interventions may be used with a variety of aims. These include: enhancing general well-being; reducing cancer risk; improving immune function; speeding recovery from treatment; and improving prognosis. Table 21.2 illustrates the wide spectrum of possible dietary interventions.

Complete dietary regimes can be arduous, prolonged, and involve an upheaval of daily life. It is particularly important with terminally ill patients, to balance realistic chances of benefit with the likely adverse effects. Choosing and maintaining a strict anticancer dietary regime can be, for some, an important coping strategy.

The body of evidence on the effects of dietary intervention is growing, and the case for a link between various dietary factors and development of certain cancers in humans seems well established [12]. Research into whether dietary change *after* diagnosis can affect outcome is ongoing and reviewed elsewhere [13]. The main findings are summarized below.

Supplements have been shown to cause regression of precancerous lesions: for example, vitamin A and beta-carotene have reversed oral leukoplakia in tobacco chewers, and vitamins A, C, and E have reduced colonic crypt cell proliferation in patients with adenomatous polyps.

In addition to the accepted links between saturated fat intake and *development* of breast cancer, there appears to be a negative correlation between the percentage of total energy derived from fat and *disease-free survival* in patients with oestrogen receptor-positive breast tumours.

The Gerson clinic in New Mexico recently published a report of consecutive patients with malignant melanoma attending the centre for metabolic therapy [14]. Although the survival rates were impressive, the result of this uncontrolled study might be explained by selection bias and pre-existing differences between Gerson patients and 'average' melanoma patients. However, an unpublished study suggests that Gerson patients may have reduced requirements for morphine and non-steroidal anti-inflammatory drugs (NSAIDs) in late-stage disease, and a lower incidence of hypercalcaemia from bone metastases.

Possible tumour regressions have been reported in a small series of breast cancer patients treated with coenzyme Q10. This requires replication under more stringent conditions.

Table 21.2 Types of dietary intervention.

Type of intervention	Principles on which intervention is based	Details of intervention
Shift to a more healthy pattern of eating	Basic diet can be modified to improve health, e.g. UK government 'Health of the Nation' White Paper (1993) or US Committee on Diet, Nutrition and Cancer (1983)	*Increase* proportion of fresh fruit, vegetables and wholegrain cereals (esp. organic produce) *Decrease* total fat (esp. animal derived), smoked & cured foods
Ingestion of nutritional supplements (vitamins, minerals etc. normally found in the diet) 3 different philosophies.	1 Ingestion at RDA (recommended daily allowances) prevents deficiency due to inadequate dietary consumption.	For example, vitamin C, beta carotene, vitamin B complex, CoQ10, selenium, zinc, evening primrose oil and vitamin E
	2 Ingestion at doses higher than RDA used to compensate for increased nutritional need, e.g. pregnancy, lactation.	Supplements often available in liquid or powder preparations.
	3 Ingestion at mega-doses uses supplements as pharmacological agents to treat disease.	Can involve taking more than 18 tablets a day.
Complete dietary regimes	Dietary regimes used as complete treatments for disease, e.g. the metabolic therapy described by Dr Max Gerson in the 1950s; Livingstone–Wheeler regime; macrobiotic diet, etc.	*Gerson*—strict vegetarian diet; salt, alcohol and nicotine excluded; freshly pressed vegetable juices, coffee enemas, potassium supplements and enzymes.
		Livingstone–Wheeler— diet as above plus vaccine prepared from patient's own blood.

Considerable controversy surrounds the trials of high-dose vitamin C undertaken in the 1970s and 80s. The negative results of two well-conducted controlled clinical trials are still disputed on methodological grounds by proponents of this therapy.

Laetrile, an extract from apricot kernels, was shown to have no beneficial effects but considerable toxicity in a controlled clinical trial.

Specific adverse effects of dietary intervention

Reported adverse effects of dietary interventions are rare and problems are unusual when following reputable professional advice. Malnutrition from strict anticancer diets has been described anecdotally. The incidence of this problem is unknown; however, patients with cachexia are at particular risk. Hypervitaminosis A has been reported when high range therapeutic doses are prolonged, especially if liver function is disturbed. Vitamin A can be teratogenic. Orange skin pigmentation, which is harmless and reversible, occasionally occurs with high doses of beta-carotene.

Prolonged zinc supplementation can cause copper deficiency, and selenium toxicity has been reported at doses just above the therapeutic range.

Vitamin C is generally regarded as safe, although at huge doses, diarrhoea may limit bowel tolerance. Vitamin C is a urinary acidifier at doses of 4–8 g/day and therefore increases the toxicity of methotrexate if used concurrently. High doses of folic acid supplementation may antagonize the therapeutic effects of methotrexate. Evening primrose oil has been reported to exacerbate temporal lobe epilepsy.

A theoretical concern that antioxidants may interfere with cancer cell death during active anticancer treatment has yet to be addressed.

Healing

Spiritual healing is a process whereby a practitioner focuses intention to produce a change in another living system. Although viewed by many orthodox practitioners as one of the more 'fringe' of the complementary therapies, patients find healing acceptable and helpful with few, if any, side-effects. It is not necessary for patients or healers to hold any particular religious or spiritual belief.

Healing is practised under various names (therapeutic touch, non-manual touch therapy, psychic healing, etc.) but can be broadly classified into two differing approaches.
• *Laying on of hands*—where the healer's hands are placed gently on or near the body of the patient with a 'healing intention'. The process usually takes 15–20 minutes. Patients may experience warmth, tingling, or relaxation during or immediately after the procedure.
• *Distance healing*—where the patient and healer(s) may be physically

separated by large distances and where meditation, prayer, or other focused intent is used by the healer(s). The patient may not necessarily know that healing is taking place.

Both approaches may involve visualization techniques such as seeing patients surrounded in light, picturing them fit and well, or clearing images of disease from their bodies.

Evidence for the effectiveness of healing

Despite the lack of a clear mechanism of action, there is a body of evidence which suggests that healing can have statistically significant effects. That said, most of the work is from *in vitro* or animal experiments and much remains unpublished except in thesis form. There are no published trials of healing in a palliative care context. The evidence has been extensively reviewed and referenced elsewhere [15]. Two examples are given here.

In the first example, 393 patients admitted to a coronary care unit (CCU) were randomly allocated to receive intercessionary prayer (IP) from a group of Christians based outside the hospital or to receive no distant healing. Patients and assessors were blind to treatment allocation. Treatment group patients had significantly fewer complications (cardiac arrest, pneumonia, intubation, requirement for antibiotics or diuretics) during their CCU stay [16].

The second example concerns studies in psychiatric and hospitalized patients. These have demonstrated significant anxiolytic effects of healing when compared to sham or placebo procedures [17].

Adverse effects and safety issues

There are no published reports of adverse reactions to the procedure of healing itself, although there are anecdotal reports of patients stopping necessary medication after seeing faith healers. The Confederation of Healing Organizations (CHO), which represents healers in the UK, has published a Code of Conduct for members which advises them against making diagnoses and giving medical advice.

Provided that practitioners and patients are clear about the limitations of therapy, and there is regular reassessment by medically trained professionals, healing can be considered a very safe therapy. However, sensitivity concerning the religious beliefs and customs of the patient is necessary.

Herbalism

Herbalism, or phytotherapy, is the study and practice of using plant material for medicinal and health promotion purposes. Much of modern pharmacological prescribing has its roots in ancient herbal traditions. However, herbalists hold that isolation and extraction reduces efficacy and increases toxicity. They believe in a wider and more balanced pharmacology of plants, and therefore prefer to use organically grown, whole plant preparations.

For clarity we can divide the topic into its main branches: Chinese herbalism, Western herbalism, and specific herbal 'cures'.

Chinese herbalism

Chinese herbalists use a traditional system of diagnosis, observing the pulse and the tongue, to decide on an individual prescription, often containing a number of herbs. They may combine this with acupuncture treatment.

Western herbalism

A Western herbalist takes a case history, exploring physical, psychological, and emotional dimensions, which centres on looking for a pattern of disturbance or disease. Individualized prescriptions are determined by key symptoms thought to correspond to dysfunction in certain organs. Herbs are usually administered as tinctures or alcohol-water extracts, but elixirs, pills, ointments, pessaries, and suppositories are also used.

Specific herbal 'cures'

Some individual herbal preparations are purported to have anticancer effects or to enhance conventional cancer treatments by reducing toxicity or increasing efficacy. They can be used singly or as part of regimes, such as the Gerson therapy. Some commonly encountered remedies are listed below.
* Iscador, a preparation, of the mistletoe plant, is part of a wider medical approach known as anthroposophy, founded by Rudolf Steiner in 1920.
* 'Juzentaihoto' (JTT), a Chinese herbal preparation popular in Japan and the USA.
* 'Essiac' (burdock, sheep sorrel, turkey rhubarb, and slippery elm bark);
* *Astralagus membranaceus* or 'huang qi', from the root of the milk-vetch plant—claimed to have tonic and immunostimulant properties;

- 'Kombucha'—a mixture of bacteria and yeast grown in birch leaf tea;
- Hoxsey's herbs—a herbal mixture shown to have cytotoxic effects in animal test systems.

Evidence for effectiveness of herbal medicine

Iscador has been shown to have immunostimulatory properties and increase natural killer cell activity [18]. Reduction of radiotherapy induced T-cell suppression has been seen in mice, and a trial is being undertaken to replicate this in breast cancer patients.

Preliminary research from Japan claims that JTT can improve chemotherapy-associated myelosuppression and quality of life in advanced breast cancer patients [19]. JTT can aid biological recovery from radiation in mice, and has been associated with an increase in natural killer cell activity in postoperative patients with gastrointestinal cancers [20].

One laboratory-based study of *Astralagus membranaceus* with interleukin-2 showed a 10-fold potentiation of interleukin activity when the combination was used compared to interleukin alone [21]. Another study using a distilled fraction of the same herb showed a reversal of cyclophosphamide-induced immunosuppression in rats [22].

A meta-analysis of randomized clinical trials comparing *Hypericum* (St John's wort) with conventional antidepressants in mild depression showed similar efficacy with considerably lower toxicity for the herbal product [23].

There are no clinical trials which substantiate the claims made for Essiac, Kombucha, or Hoxsey's herbs.

Experienced herbalists anecdotally report success in treating nausea in the terminally ill patient when other conventional methods have failed.

Adverse effects

Although an extensive review of herbal safety published in the *Food and Drug Law Journal* in 1992 states that 'there is no substantial evidence that toxic reactions to herbal products are a major source of concern' [24], there have since been a few reports of severe idiosyncratic reactions such as acute hepatitis and irreversible rapidly progressive interstitial renal fibrosis following the ingestion of traditional Chinese herbs [6].

Side-effects of Iscador are similar to that of interferon, with high fevers, headaches, and muscle pains. Liver pain has been observed in patients with liver metastases.

Given the large number of people using herbal remedies, there are very few reports of serious adverse effects. However, reporting systems are largely informal, and available evidence is therefore unreliable. The National Poisons Unit and the University of Exeter are establishing databases of validated reports of adverse events attributed to herbal products.

Homoeopathy

Homoeopathy ('homoeo', similar, plus 'pathos' illness) is based on the 'law of similars'—the principle of treating like with like—meaning that symptoms of disease are treated with medicines capable of producing similar symptoms when given to healthy individuals.

The homoeopathic method was described in 1790 by the German physician, Samuel Hahnemann. During experiments to reduce adverse effects, he discovered that serial dilution made medicines less toxic but paradoxically more active—particularly when dilution was combined with vigorous shaking. This process is called 'potentization' and is considered to increase the therapeutic action of the remedy.

The homoeopath identifies patterns emerging from a holistic clinical history and matches these with features of known homoeopathic remedies to make an individual prescription. Remedies can be prescribed in tablet or liquid form and are easily administered in the terminal phase without interfering with other medications.

Indications for homoeopathy

In theory any patient could benefit from homoeopathy, though in practice it is applied in cases where conventional alternatives have proved ineffective. Homoeopathy is said to have most chance of helping where the patient is able to relate their story and where symptoms are vivid. It can be very useful where the patient is stuck in a particular emotional state, such as despair or fear. When the pattern of an individual patient fits that of a known remedy closely, homoeopaths claim a greater chance of success.

Homoeopathic preparations of conventional chemotherapeutic agents have been prescribed concurrently with chemotherapy to try to reduce toxicity. The theoretical concern that anticancer activity may also be reduced is currently being examined.

Evidence for the effectiveness of homoeopathy

Reproducible evidence from methodologically rigorous, triple-blind randomized placebo-controlled trials in patients with asthma and hay fever has demonstrated that homoeopathic preparations can have clinically significant effects which are superior to placebo [25]. All told, over 100 controlled clinical trials of homoeopathy have been systematically reviewed [26]. Although many were methodologically poor, over three-quarters of trials favoured homoeopathy. A meta-analysis of 89 trials in various clinical conditions showed homoeopathy to be consistently superior to placebo [27]. However, there are virtually no published data concerning its use in palliative care.

Case studies suggest that one remedy may not produce any response whereas another, which fits the symptom pattern more closely, may be followed by dramatic improvement in key symptoms as well as non-specific improvements in anxiety and psychological adjustment. In an uncontrolled study of 50 consecutive patients from the Royal London Homoeopathic Hospital cancer clinic who received a package of complementary care including homoeopathy, quality of life (as measured by the Rotterdam Symptom Check List) improved, while physical symptoms remained stable even though 74% had metastatic or recurrent disease on entering the study [28]. The study had a high drop-out rate, and results therefore need careful interpretation.

Adverse effects

There are no known toxic effects of homoeopathy. However, patients and homoeopaths describe a phenomenon known as aggravation—the development of new symptoms or a worsening of existing symptoms. This is said to be transient and to respond quickly to decreasing the frequency or stopping the remedy.

Massage, aromatherapy, and reflexology

The use of touch to relieve discomfort is probably one of the most instinctive and oldest therapies in existence.

Massage, which can be defined as therapeutic soft tissue manipulation, is a component of many traditional systems of medicine. Swedish massage is the form on which most current European techniques are based.

Aromatherapy is massage using essential oils—aromatic plant extracts prepared by distillation—which are said to have different properties (relaxing, invigorating, antiseptic, purifying, etc.). A combination of diluted essential oils will be selected to suit the preference and nature of the patient.

Reflexology is a technique whereby the feet are massaged in a way which is claimed to affect the functioning of the organs of the body. Specific areas of the feet (reflex zones) are said to correspond to individual organs, and massaging these areas can either give the therapist diagnostic information or lead to therapeutic change in the corresponding organ.

Massage techniques have been extensively employed in palliative care settings [1] and have been adapted for these circumstances, for example by using gentle massage strokes to avoid overtreating frail patients. Treatments can be given by independent massage therapists but increasingly trained nurses, physiotherapists, and occupational therapists are providing massage and aromatherapy. If essential oils are used, they must be diluted with a carrier oil (e.g. sweet almond oil) and can be used singly or in established combinations of 4–5 low-toxicity oils.

Indications and effects of massage therapies

Practitioners using massage in palliative care settings have reported psychological, emotional, and physical benefits for patients and staff. The research base is rigorously and extensively reviewed elsewhere [29]. Key points emerging are summarized below.

Psychological effects. A small number of well-conducted randomized controlled trials support the claim that massage is effective in relieving anxiety in institutional settings. Effects on depression are less clear.

Emotional effects. The pampering and pleasure received during a massage can be one of the few positive physical experiences for a patient with advanced disease—in the words of one patient: 'it was done so lovingly and gently. The whole experience has made me feel I was worth caring about' [30]. Practitioners also report an effect of massage in improving the body image of patients who have undergone mutilating surgery.

Massage may lead to emotional release although patients can be nurtured and supported without feeling they have to 'open up' and talk.

Physical effects. Massage is frequently used for pain relief, perhaps alleviating pain through reduction in anxiety and muscle tension, although there are almost no reliable research data on the subject. Lymphoedema is now widely treated using specialist massage and bandaging techniques.

There are also anecdotal reports describing improvements in sleep patterns, lethargy, fatigue, terminal agitation, and restlessness after massage.

Interpersonal significance. Massage gives staff and relatives a way of spending time and being with the dying patient.

Use among staff. Staff support systems sometimes include massage, and practitioners report that these sessions are used to 'unload' problems. As one member of staff puts it: 'Massage allows me to "take in" so that I can "give out"' [29].

Evidence comparing the different massage therapies

Randomized trials comparing aromatherapy massage with massage using carrier oil alone [30,31] have provided results which are difficult to interpret owing to a number of methodological flaws. There seems at least to be a suggestion that essential oils may augment the effects of massage in reducing anxiety and some physical symptoms.

Reflexology is one of the most sparsely researched of the complementary disciplines, and claims that it has greater efficacy than a simple foot massage are currently unsubstantiated.

Adverse effects and recommended contraindications

Providing massage is gentle and care is taken in moving and lifting patients, adverse effects are rare. As with other CM disciplines, contraindications reflect established practice rather than documented side-effects. No serious adverse events with aromatherapy have been documented.

Limbs affected by deep vein thrombosis should not be massaged, and extreme caution should be exercised when massaging close to bone metastases. Skin recovering from radiotherapy should generally be avoided. Patients with abnormal clotting or platelets should be massaged with great care.

The variety and concentration of aromatherapy oils is limited to avoid theoretical risks of overexposure or interaction with concurrent medication.

Although vigorous massage close to active tumour sites is generally avoided, there are no known reports of metastatic spread being promoted by massage.

Mind-body techniques: hypnosis, meditation, relaxation, and visualization

Mind-body medicine encompasses a wide range of therapeutic interventions which address psychological and emotional issues with the aim of altering physical symptoms and possibly disease processes.

Techniques encompassed by the term 'mind-body approaches' include counselling, psychotherapy, therapy involving hypnosis, cognitive-behavioural techniques, neurolinguistic programming (NLP), relaxation, yoga, visualization, and meditation.

Hypnosis

Hypnotic techniques increase a patient's suggestibility and responsiveness to psychological approaches by using an altered state of consciousness, or 'trance'. Hypnotic techniques can be used to augment any number of psychotherapeutic or psychological techniques, from hypno-analysis to cognitive behavioural techniques. Therapy incorporating hypnosis is only as good as the underlying therapy and therapist. However, a recent meta-analysis of trials comparing identical cognitive-behavioural interventions delivered alone or with hypnosis, showed a substantial enhancement in treatment outcome with adjunctive hypnosis [32].

Meditation

Meditation is a process by which the mind is stilled to facilitate a calm and pleasant experience of the present moment. It may also, but does not necessarily, have a spiritual dimension (Table 21.3).

Visualization and imagery

Imagined scenes, objects, places, or people are used in many mind-body techniques to enable a change in subjective experience. A favourite beach or beautiful garden are popular images.

Table 21.3 Categories of meditation techniques.

Concentrative meditation Involves focusing the mind on the breath, an image (real or imagined) or a sound (often repeated). Through this concentration the mind becomes more tranquil and aware.
Mindfulness meditation Attention is opened to whatever enters the mind without judgement or worries so that eventually the mind becomes more calm and clear.

Most of these techniques can be taught and applied in one-to-one sessions or facilitated groups by therapists or doctors and nurses with appropriate training. Using audio tapes and headphones, patients can practise the technique anywhere at home or in hospital and many learn to 'customize' the methods to suit themselves.

Indications and effects of mind-body techniques

HEALTH ENHANCEMENT

Relaxation and visualization techniques have been used to promote relaxation and a general feeling of well-being whilst undergoing stressful experiences such as chemotherapy or bone marrow aspiration.

RELIEVING OR PALLIATING SPECIFIC SYMPTOMS

Studies have indicated efficacy of mind-body techniques in certain situations. For example, the pain of oral mucositis was much reduced in patients undergoing bone marrow transplantation who had relaxation and imagery training [33]. Pain in patients with advanced cancer was reduced by deep-breathing, progressive muscle relaxation, and imagery training [34].

Several studies have demonstrated that anxiety and nausea related to chemotherapy respond well to mind-body approaches, especially in children and adolescents. Anticipatory nausea and vomiting have been helped by hypnosis [35].

PROGNOSTIC: ALTERING THE COURSE OF DISEASE

Very few studies have examined the effects of mind-body interventions on the progression of cancer. Results are contradictory and it is too early to draw definite conclusions in this controversial area.

Carl Simonton encouraged cancer patients to use images such as sharks eating cancer cells or armies of soldiers in battle, to enhance immune function, and augment the effect of conventional treatment. An uncontrolled study in 225 selected cancer patients reported survival figures 'as much as twice as long' as national averages [36]. However, the study had profound methodological flaws, such as non-representative sample and lack of any staging or prognostic data.

A well-publicized, but methodologically flawed, study on the Bristol Cancer Help Centre programme showed a significant survival disadvantage for intervention patients [37]. The results need cautious interpretation owing to the non-randomized nature of the study and the absence of any measures of compliance.

Spiegel and co-workers, while conducting a randomized study of a 12-month psychosocial group intervention to improve quality of life in patients with metastatic breast cancer, found a clinically and statistically significant survival advantage in intervention patients compared with controls [38].

Adverse effects and contraindications

Providing that any therapist who employs hypnotic techniques has the appropriate training and background experience, mind-body therapies are generally very safe. Therapists need to be aware of the psychological vulnerability of cancer patients and the limited time available for patients with terminal illness to deal with deep trauma or ingrained patterns of behaviour. Realistic goals of therapy need to be agreed and often techniques used symptomatically are more appropriate than an analytic approach.

The World Health Organization (WHO) cautions that hypnosis should not be used in patients with psychosis, organic psychiatric conditions, or antisocial personality disorders.

Documented adverse effects of sustained meditation include grand-mal seizures in established epileptics and acute psychosis in individuals with a history of schizophrenia.

Conclusions

This chapter has begun to explore the similarities between palliative care and complementary approaches, and to examine the relevance of individual complementary therapies to the palliative care setting. As practitioners individualize their patients' care they may be asked about therapies with which they are unfamiliar and inexperienced. Although there is no evidence that any of the complementary approaches can cure cancer, there is much that demonstrates their ability to improve symptoms and quality of life. Discussing the relevance of complementary medicine (CM) in individual cases openly and with an awareness of this evidence can facilitate a profound and therapeutic patient/carer relationship.

By integrating the best of orthodox and complementary care, it may be possible to meet more of the needs of palliative care patients. Continuing research, particularly in conventional settings, is necessary to establish the most appropriate strategy for future developments.

Acknowledgements

The authors would like to thank Dr Jacqueline Filshie of the Royal Marsden Hospital, Sutton, for her section on acupuncture, and to acknowledge the contributions and advice of Keith Robertson, Director of Education, Scottish School of Herbal Medicine, and Andrew Vickers and Rebecca Rees of the Research Council for Complementary Medicine (RCCM).

References

1 Wilkes E. *Complementary Therapy in Hospice and Palliative Care*. Sheffield: Trent Palliative Care Centre, 1992.
2 Ernst E, Henstschel C. Diagnostic method in complementary medicine. Which craft is witchcraft? *Int J Risk and Safety in Med* 1995; 7: 55–63.
3 Thomas K, Fall M, Parry G, Nicholl J. *National Survey of Access to Complementary Health Care via General Practice*. Sheffield: Medical Care Research Unit, 1995.
4 Pomeranz B, Stux G, eds. *Scientific Bases of Acupuncture*. Berlin, Heidelberg, New York: Springer Verlag, 1989.
5 Crawford HJ, Gruzelier JH. A midstream view of the neuropsychophysiology of hypnosis: recent research and future directions. In: Fromm E, Nash MR, eds. *Contemporary Hypnosis Research*. New York: Guilford Press, 1992: 227–266.
6 Vanherweghem JL, Depierreux M, Tielemans C *et al*. Rapidly progressive interstitial renal fibrosis in young women: association with slimming regimen including Chinese herbs. *Lancet* 1993; 341: 387–391.
7 Veith I. *The Yellow Emperor's Classic of Internal Medicine*. Berkeley: University of California Press, 1972.
8 Bannerman R. Acupuncture: the World Health Organisation view. *World Health* 27/28 December 1979; 24–29.
9 Thompson JW, Filshie J. Transcutaneous electrical nerve stimulation (TENS) and acupuncture. In: Doyle D, Hanks G, McDonald N, eds. *The Oxford Textbook of Palliative Medicine*, 2nd edn. Oxford: Oxford University Press, 1997: 421–437.
10 Vickers AJ. Can acupuncture have specific effects on health? A systematic literature review of acupuncture anti-emesis trials. *J Roy Soc Med* 1996; 89: 303–311.
11 Johansson K, Lindgren I, Widner H, Wiklund I, Johansson BB. Can sensory stimulation improve the functional outcome in stroke patients? *Neurology* 1993; 43: 2189–2192.
12 Doll R. *Causes of Cancer*. Oxford: Oxford University Press, 1981.
13 Goodman S. *Nutrition and Cancer: State-of-the-Art*. London: Green Library, 1995.
14 Gar Hildenbrand GL, Hildenbrand LC, Bradford K, Cavin SW. Five-year survival rates of melanoma patients treated by diet therapy after the manner of Gerson: a retrospective review. *Alternat Ther Health Med* 1995; 1 (4): 29–37.
15 Benor DJ. *Healing Research*, Vols 1–4. Munich, Oxford: Helix, 1993–95.
16 Byrd RC. Positive therapeutic effects of intercessory prayer in a coronary care unit population. *South Med J* 1988; 81 (7): 826–829.
17 Simington JA, Laing GP. Effects of therapeutic touch on anxiety in the institutionalised elderly. *Clin Nurs Res* 1993; 2 (4): 438–450.

18 Hajto T. Immunomodulatory effects of Iscador: A viscum album preparation. *Oncology* 1986; 43 (Suppl. 11): 51–65.

19 Adachi I. Role of supporting therapy of Juzentaihoto (JTT) in advanced breast cancer patients. *Jap J Cancer Chemother* 1989; 16 (4): 1538–1543.

20 Okamoto T. Clinical effects of Juzendaiho-to on immunologic and fatty metabolic states in post-operative patients with gastrointestinal cancer. *Jap J Cancer Chemother* 1989; 16 (4): 1533–1537.

21 Chu D, Sun Y, Lin JR. A fractionated extract of *Astralagus membranaceus* potentiates lymphokine-activated killer cell cytotoxicity generated by low-dose recombinant interleukin-2. *Chin J Mod Develop Trad Med* 1989; 9 (6): 325, 348–349.

22 Chu DT *et al*. Immune restoration of local xenogenic graft-vs.-host reaction in cancer patients *in vitro* and reversal of cyclophosphamide- induced immune suppression in the rat *in vivo* by fractionated membranaceus. *Chin J Mod Develop Trad Med*. 1989; (6): 326, 351–354.

23 Linde K, Ramirez G, Mulrow CD, Pauls A, Weidenhammer W, Melchart D. St John's wort for depression: an overview and meta-analysis of randomised clinical trials. *BMJ* 1996; 313: 253–258.

24 McCalels RS. Food ingredient safety evaluation. *J Food Drug Law* 1992; 47: 657–665.

25 Reilly D, Taylor M, Beattie NGM *et al*. Is evidence for homeopathy reproducible? *Lancet* 1994; 334: 1601–1606.

26 Kleijnen J, Knipschild P, Ter Riet G. Clinical trials of homoeopathy. *BMJ* 1991; 302: 316–323.

27 Linde K, Clausius N, Ramirez G. Are the clinical effects of homeopathy placebo effects? A meta-analysis of placeb-controlled trials. *Lancet* 1997; 350: 834–343.

28 Clover A, Last P, Fisher P, Wright S, Boyle H. Complementary cancer therapy: a pilot study of patients, therapies and quality of life. *Comp Ther Med* 1995; 3: 129–133.

29 Vickers A. *Massage and Aromatherapy: A Guide for Health Professionals*. London: Chapman & Hall, 1996.

30 Corner J, Cawley N, Hildebrand S. An evaluation of the use of massage and essential oils on the wellbeing of cancer patients. *Int J Palliative Nurs* 1995; 1 (2): 67–73.

31 Wilkinson S. Aromatherapy and massage in palliative care. *Int J Palliative Nurs* 1995; 1 (1): 21–30.

32 Kirsch I, Montgomery G, Saperstein G. Hypnosis as an adjunct to cognitive behavioural psychotherapy: a meta-analysis. *J Consult Clin Psycholol* 1995; 63: 214–220.

33 Syrjala KL, Donaldson GW, Davis MW, Kippes ME, Carr JE. Relaxation and imagery and cognitive-behavioural training reduce pain during cancer treatement: a controlled clinical trial. *Pain* 1995; 63 (2): 189–198.

34 Sloman R, Brown P, Aldana E, Chee E. The use of relaxation for the promotion of comfort and pain relief in persons with advanced cancer. *Contemporary Nurse* 1994; 3 (1): 6–12.

35 Redd WH, Andresen GV, Minagawa RY. Hypnotic control of anticipatory emesis in patients receiving cancer chemotherapy. *J Consult Clin Psychol* 1982; 50: 14–19.

36 Simonton OC, Matthews-Simonton S, Sparkes TF. Psychological intervention in the treatment of cancer. *Psychosomatics* 1980; 21 (3): 226–233.

37 Bagenal FS, Easton DS, Harris E, Chilvers CED, McElwain TJ. Survival of patients with breast cancer attending Bristol Cancer Help Centre. *Lancet* 1990; 336: 1186–1188.
38 Spiegel D, Bloom JR, Kraemer HC. Effects of psychosocial treatment on survival in patients with metastatic breast cancer. *Lancet* 1989; 298: 291–293.

Further reading

Lerner M. *Choices in Healing*. Cambridge, Mass.: MIT Press, 1994.
Lewith G, Kenyon J, Lewis P. *Complementary Medicine: An Integrated Approach*. Oxford General Practice Series. Oxford: Oxford Medical Press, 1996.
Sharma U. *Complementary Medicine Today: Practitioners and Patients*, rev. edn. London: Routledge, 1995.
Vickers A. *Massage and Aromatherapy: A Guide for Health Professionals*. London: Chapman & Hall, 1996.
Defining the Question: Research Issues in Complementary Medicine, Parts I & II. London: Research Council for Complementary Medicine, 1997.

The scope and nature of this book have meant that references have had to be kept to a minimum. A more extensive reference list of the evidence relating to complementary medicine in palliative care is available from Dr Catherine Zollman, Research Council for Complementary Medicine.

22: The Syringe Driver

JEREMY JOHNSON

Introduction

Syringe drivers are lightweight, portable infusion pumps, usually electrically or mechanically operated, capable of delivering precise doses of medication over a set period of time, most commonly 24 hours (Fig. 22.1).

In palliative care the role of the syringe driver has been firmly established by its ability to administer subcutaneous infusions of analgesics, either as single agents, or in combination with other compounds such as antiemetics, sedatives, or anticholinergic drugs [1–7].

The use of the syringe driver in palliative care

Apart from the obvious advantages syringe drivers are useful because they:
- are comfortable for ambulant patients;
- provide 'steady-state' plasma concentrations of drugs;
- avoid the necessity for repeated injections (this is important in frail, cachectic patients);
- sustain infusion over 24 hours or longer.

However, they do have some disadvantages. For example, they entail the need to anticipate the patient's requirements over the next 24 hours. Any alteration in symptoms may necessitate additional injections to supplement the infusion regimen (the boost button is not suitable for this: see below, p. 361 and Appendix (p. 372). Some patients find the syringe driver obtrusive and disconcerting, while it is regarded by some, professionals and lay persons, as a 'last rite'.

Delivery of drugs by the subcutaneous route may be vital in patients who cannot swallow or who are nauseated and vomiting, but in those who can take and absorb oral medication a subcutaneous infusion delivered by syringe driver is unlikely to improve symptom control and may be problematic and inconvenient to the patient, as well as costly.

Indications

The syringe driver may be indicated in the following situations:
- persistent nausea or vomiting;
- oral/pharyngeal lesions;
- difficulty swallowing;
- poor alimentary absorption;
- aversion to oral medication;
- intestinal obstruction;
- profound weakness/cachexia;
- comatose or moribund patient;
- patient choice.

Setting up a syringe driver for subcutaneous infusion
(see also Appendix)

PREPARING THE PATIENT AND CARERS

Prior to commencing an infusion, spend time with the patient and their carers explaining the nature and intention of the procedure. Many have reservations and some fear that the institution of a syringe driver equates with impending death. Invite questions, acknowledge anxieties, and reassure where appropriate.

EQUIPMENT

The following equipment should be assembled before setting up a syringe driver: a battery; a Luer-Lok syringe (usually 10 or 20 ml); an infusion-giving set with fine-gauge (23 or 25 G) butterfly needle; clear adhesive dressing (Opsite or Tegaderm); and a suitable diluent, i.e. sterile water for injection and a syringe driver.

PREPARING THE DRIVER

The Graseby syringe drivers (Fig. 22.1) are the most widely used (see the Appendix for details).

CHOICE OF SITE FOR THE BUTTERFLY NEEDLE

Suitable sites for placement of the butterfly needle include: the upper chest; outer upper arm; anterior abdomen; and thighs. The exact placement

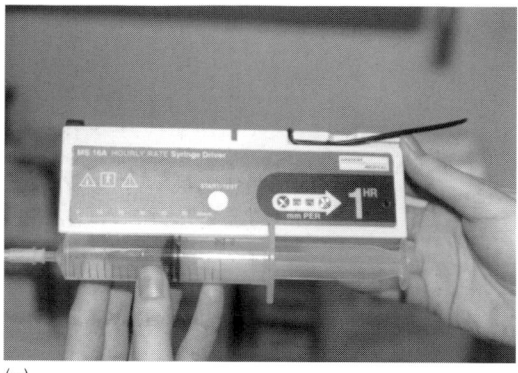

(a)

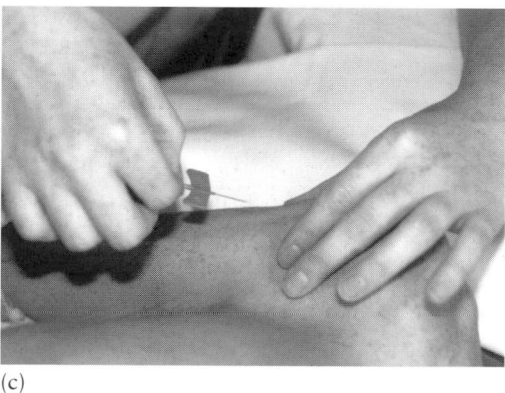

(b)

(c)

Fig. 22.1 Setting up a syringe driver. (a) Draw up medication and set rate of delivery. (b) Attach loaded syringe and clamp to driver. (c) & (d) Insert fine-gauge butterfly needle into skin. (e) Loop tubing and secure with transparent dressing. (f) Final set up.

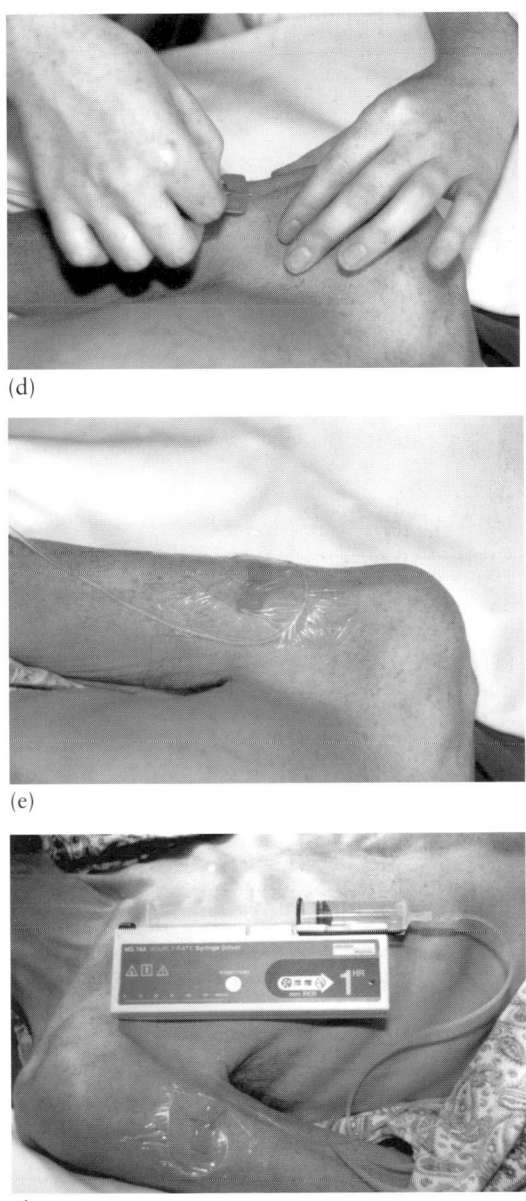

(d)

(e)

(f)

Fig. 22.1 *Continued*

may be influenced by the patient's preference, by the disease process, and by common sense.

Take care to avoid the deltoid area in bed-bound patients who require regular turning, and sites over bony prominences in cachectic patients. Also avoid broken skin, areas of inflammation, and oedematous/lymphadematous areas.

Regular checks

It is essential that the following checks are made regularly throughout the period of use:
- check for signs of irritation or inflammation at the injection site;
- check for evidence of leakage at the various connections;
- check that the driver is working (light flashing/intermittent motor noise);
- check that the set rate is correct;
- check for signs of crystallization or precipitation (cloudiness);
- check that the tubing is not kinked.

Changing the site of the infusion

Change the infusion site only when necessary, i.e. if it is painful, or appears to be inflamed or swollen. The frequency of this will depend on the combination of drugs used. Single-agent diamorphine infusions can last for several days, those with benzodiazepines and certain antiemetics may be alright for 2–3 days, whereas if cyclizine or a phenothiazine is used, daily changes may be necessary. The extension set and needle should generally be changed at each resiting.

Alteration of drug dose

If drug dosages need to be altered the syringe should be recharged rather than the infusion rate altered. Alteration of the rate will deliver *all* of the drugs at an increased or decreased rate. It will also alter the time of next recharge of the syringe, and may lead to times without infusion if district nurses are planning visits at the same time each day.

Changing the infusion rate can potentially lead to an overdosage (or underdosage) if the rate is not checked and reset at each syringe recharge. It also makes it more difficult to calculate the actual dose of each drug the patient is receiving daily.

Problems and their solutions

Should there be persistent problems with irritation at the injection site

consider the following options:
- reducing the concentration of drugs (i.e. larger volume);
- changing the drug—or consider an alternative route;
- mixing drugs with 0.9% saline (if miscible);
- using a Teflon (e.g. Jelco) cannula (but this can kink);
- adding hydrocortisone 100 mg or dexamethasone 1 mg to the infusion;
- adding 1500 units of hyaluronidase to the infusion. This is an enzyme that breaks down connective tissue locally and increases diffusion.

THE BOOST BUTTON (GRASEBY MS26)

Do *not* use the 'boost button' for top-up medication or breakthrough analgesia on a regular basis. Each boost advances the plunger 0.23 mm: this will shorten the total infusion time by about 7–8 minutes. The equivalent of a 4-hourly dose of analgesics would require approximately 30 clicks of the button! Furthermore all other drugs present in the infusion will also be given with each bolus. Instead additional medication may need to be given by injection or suppository.

Drugs used in syringe drivers

General recommendations

Table 22.1 lists the major drugs that may be infused using a syringe driver in palliative care. It is not, however, an exhaustive list, and other chapters should be consulted for drugs appropriate to specialist needs. The following recommendations offer guidelines for the selection, preparation, and usage of drugs with the syringe driver.
- The maximum recommended concentration for single-agent diamorphine is 250 mg/ml (though concentrations up to 400 mg/ml have been reported).
- Keep the number of drugs combined in a single syringe to a minimum (generally two or three).
- Water for injection is the preferred diluent for most drugs except non-steroidal anti-inflammatory drugs (NSAIDs), which mix better with 0.9% saline.
- Dilute diamorphine *prior to* mixing with other drugs.
- Do not use 0.9% saline to dilute cyclizine—there is a high risk of precipitation as insoluble cyclizine chloride.

Table 22.1 Drugs used in syringe drivers. This list is not exhaustive; it covers many of the drugs used in palliative care. See other chapters for specific indications and usage.

Medication	Trade name and ampoule size	Indication	Dose range per 24 hours	Comments
Analgesics				
Diamorphine hydrochloride [8]	Crystalline powder 5,10,30,100,500 mg Reconstitute with water	Pain Dyspnoea	Start: • One-third total daily dose of oral morphine • 10–20 mg in opioid naive patients • Increase as necessary by 30–50% increments • No maximum dose	• Opioid of choice for s.c. infusion • Highly soluble§ • Do not exceed 250 mg/ml • Loading dose (equivalent to 4 h) may be required initially s.c. • If converting from fentanyl TTS usually remove patch 6–12 hours prior to starting syringe driver
Methadone [9] [10] ‡	10 mg/ml 1, 2, 3.5, 5 ml	Diamorphine intolerance	One-fifth estimated daily dose of oral morphine	• Can have unacceptable adverse reactions at injection site • Wide variation in individual plasma concentration • Long half life—tendency to accumulate • Rectal route an alternative
Ketamine [11] [12]†	Ketalar 10 mg/ml/20 ml amp 50 mg/ml/10 ml amp 100 mg/ml/5 ml	Difficult cancer pain, especially of neuropathic origin	Start 100–150 mg/day Titrate against effect Increase to 300–700 mg/day	• Inhibits NMDA receptor • Psychomimetic side-effects (may need midazolam/haloperidol cover) • Contraindicated in raised intracranial pressure and fits • Caution in hypertension/cardiac problems

Drug	Preparation	Indication	Dose range	Notes
Fentanyl [13] ‡	Sublimaze 50 μg/ml 2 ml and 10 ml	Alternative, if significant side-effects with diamorphine	100–1000 μg (rarely 2000 μg)	• Available in the community on named patient basis only Advantage over TTS patch: • achieve pain control rapidly • delivery of high and low doses
Tramadol [14] ‡	Zydol 50 mg/ml 2 ml	Weak opioid (step 2)	60–600 mg	Reduce oral dose by 30% for s.c. equivalent
NSAIDs Diclofenac ‡	Voltarol 25 mg/3 ml	Bone pain Ureteric colic	75–150 mg	• Infusion sites often a problem • Do not mix with other drugs • Dilute with 0.9% sodium chloride
Ketorolac [15] ‡	Toradol 10 mg/ml 30 mg/ml	As above	30–60 mg	• Well tolerated • Caution in renal failure • Can be nephrotoxic • Short term use only (few days because of nephrotoxicity) • High incidence of upper GI bleeding • Dilute with 0.9% sodium chloride
Naproxen [16]	As above		550–600 mg	• Precipitates easily with morphine

Continued on p. 364

Table 22.1 *Continued*

Medication	Trade name and ampoule size	Indication	Dose range per 24 hours	Comments
Antiemetics				
Metoclopramide*	Maxolon and non-proprietary 5 mg/ml 2 and 20 ml	Impaired gastric emptying	30–120 mg (rarely 180 mg)	• D_2 antagonist • Non-sedating • Occupies large volume • Possibility of extrapyramidal/dystonic side effects or tardive dyskinesia with prolonged use and in younger women
Haloperidol*	Serenace and haldol 5 mg/ml 10 mg/ml 2 ml	Drug induced nausea Metabolic causes Antipsychotic	2.5–10 mg 10–30 mg	• Central D_2 antagonist • Mildly sedating • Maximum concentration: 2 mg/ml • Settles agitation and psychosis
Cyclizine*	Valoid 50 mg/ml	Intestinal obstruction Movement induced nausea	50–150 mg	• Antihistamine (H_1) and anticholinergic • Drowsiness can be a problem • Compatibility problems
Ondansetron ‡	Zofran 2 mg/ml 2 and 4 ml	Chemotherapy or radiotherapy induced vomiting (not usually s.c. route)	8–24 mg	• $5HT_3$ antagonist • Expensive

Granisetron ‡	Kytril 1 mg/1 ml 1 and 3 ml	Chemotherapy or radiotherapy induced vomiting (not usually s.c. route)	3–9 mg	• $5HT_3$ antagonist • Expensive
Sedative and antiemetic Methotrimeprazine [17] [18]*	Nozinan 25 mg/ml 1 ml	Nausea Confusion Restlessness Psychosis	12.5–50 mg 25–200 mg	• Effective antiemetic • Extremely useful for terminal agitation • Occasional skin reactions • If used as a single agent dilute with 0.9% sodium chloride
Sedative Midazolam [19] [20]	Hypnovel 2 mg/ml 5 ml 5 mg/ml 2 ml	Anxiety Terminal restlessness Dyspnoea Anticonvulsant Myoclonus	10–100 mg (common range 10–30 mg)	• Water soluble benzodiazepine • Bio-availability via s.c. route: 40% • Large inter-individual variability in steady-state plasma level
Clonazepam †	Rivotril 1 mg/1 ml	Anxiety Terminal restlessness Anticonvulsant Neuropathic pain	0.5–8 mg/24 hr	• Less water soluble than Midazolan • Irritant

Continued on p. 366

Table 22.1 *Continued*

Medication	Trade name and ampoule size	Indication	Dose range per 24 hours	Comments
Anticholinergic				
Hyoscine hydrobromide ‡	0.4 mg/ml 1 ml 0.6 mg/ml 1 ml	Terminal bronchial secretions and additional sedation	0.8–3.2 mg	• Dry mouth—extra attention with oral hygiene • May cause confusion
Hyoscine butylbromide [21] [22]†	Buscopan 20 mg/ml 1 ml	Severe colic Intestinal obstruction	20–120 mg	• May be as effective as the hydrobromide for bronchial secretions—and much cheaper
Steroids				
Dexamethasone†	Sodium phosphate 5 mg/ml Equivalent to 4 mg/ml Dexamethasone Decadron 4 mg/ml Equivalent to 4.17 ml of above	Raised intracranial pressure Reduction in peritumour oedema	5–20 mg 4–16 mg	• Compatibility difficulties (see Table 22.2) • Use separate syringe driver if necessary

Glycopyrronium Bromide	Robinul 0.2 mg/ml 1 and 3 ml	As above	0.4–1.2 mg	• less likely to cause confusion than Hyoscine Hydrobromide
Anticonvulsants				
Phenobarbitone‡	200 mg/ml 1 ml	Fits' in terminal distress	600–1600 mg	• Not water soluble • Use second syringe driver if necessary
Clonazepam†	See above			
Midazolam*	See above			
Miscellaneous				
Octreotide [23]†	Sandostatin 50µg 100µg/ml 1 ml 200µg/ml 5 ml 500µg/ml 1 ml	Reduces: GI secretions Volume of vomit in intestinal obstruction Volume of entero-colic fistula Watery diarrhoea, especially in HIV/AIDS	150–600µg	Expensive

* Frequently used; † Sometimes used; ‡ Rarely used; § Solubility of morphine salts: diamorphine HCl = 625 mg/ml, morphine acetate = 400 mg/ml, morphine tartrate = 100 mg/ml, morphine sulphate = 45 mg/ml. Contraindicated: the following are all too irritant to be used subcutaneously; diazepam, prochlorperazine and chlorpromazine.

Storing drugs or preparations in a refrigerator, or wearing a syringe driver outdoors in cold weather may reduce solubility of the active agents. Protect the syringe from light—many drugs are subject to photodegradation, so put the syringe in an opaque pouch, holster, or pocket.

If the contents of the syringe become cloudy or discoloured before or during infusion, the syringe should be discarded immediately. Should incompatibility problems persist and alternative drugs or routes are not available, then a second syringe driver may be required.

Unlicensed drugs

Many of the drugs commonly used in a palliative care setting are not specifically licensed for administration by s.c. infusion. This should not necessarily preclude their use in this form. The licensing of drugs relates to the marketing, and in many cases pharmaceutical companies may not have applied for a licence for the product to be used in this manner. The Medicines Act of 1968 allows considerable freedom for doctors to prescribe and use unlicensed drugs if they consider it appropriate. Drugs prescribed in this way may be dispensed by pharmacists and administered by nurses. It may be worth consulting with other colleagues prior to using an unusual drug or dose outside the usual range.

Mixing drugs in syringes

A survey of UK hospice practice found a diverse range of drugs and doses used in combination for subcutaneous infusion via a syringe driver [25]. An invariable component was diamorphine, usually administered with an antiemetic and/or sedative. However, 18 of the 28 drugs reported had been used infrequently and by fewer than 5% of the units. For the majority of these there is little evidence confirming efficacy by this route of delivery and no reliable data regarding compatibility or stability.

COMPATIBILITY

Consideration of the compatibility of drugs is vital to ensure efficacy of therapy. Interactions between drugs can be difficult to predict and may produce a number of effects, including a reduction in stability or changes in solubility resulting in precipitation or crystallization (Fig. 22.2). This may cause the infusion cannula to become blocked, the injection site to become inflamed, and the treatment to be ineffective.

Physical compatibility

Most drugs used in syringe drivers are water soluble and can be mixed. However, phenobarbitone (made up in propylene glycol) is immiscible with aqueous solutions and should *not* be used in the same syringe as other drugs.

Drugs such as phenytoin and diazepam made up in an oily solution are unsuitable for delivery by the subcutaneous route. If delivered intravenously they should not be mixed with water-soluble drugs.

Chemical incompatibility

The major factor leading to incompatibility is the relative concentration of each drug. Other factors include pH, storage conditions, temperature, and ionic strength.

STABILITY

Many salts in aqueous solution undergo degradation: for example diamorphine is hydrolysed to 6-mono-acetylmorphine and morphine. Using spectroscopy and high-performance liquid chromatography, several studies have examined the stability of diamorphine under a variety of conditions [26–31]. At concentrations of up to 20 mg/ml, diamorphine is stable for 15–18 days (i.e. less than 5–10% loss of potency). The addition of midazolam or hyoscine hydrobromide does not appear to significantly affect this.

Depending on relative concentrations, the addition of haloperidol, cyclizine, or metoclopramide may reduce the stability time considerably and also lead to loss of the antiemetic from the solution (Fig. 22.2) [24,28,29,32].

Table 22.2 indicates the compatibility and stability of two-drug mixtures for at least 24 hours [33]. Higher concentrations may lead to lower efficacy due to instability or precipitation of drugs.

The stable concentrations of some three drug combinations (respective maximum doses in a 10 ml infusion) are given below.

- Diamorphine up to 70 mg/ml + midazolam up to 4 mg/ml + hyoscine hydrobromide up to 0.17 mg/ml (700 mg diamorphine + 40 mg midazolam + 1.7 mg hyoscine hydrobromide).

Table 22.2 The compatibility of drugs combined in a syringe for s.c. infusion.

	Diamorphine	Metoclopramide	Haloperidol	Cyclizine	Methotrimeprazine	Midazolam	Hyoscine hydrobromide	Hyoscine butylbromide	Dexamethasone	Octreotide
Diamorphine		c‡ √√	c† √√	c* √√	√√ Stable at any concentration of either drug	√√ Stable at any concentration of either drug	√√ Stable at any concentration of either drug	√√ Stable at any concentration of either drug	c	√√
Metoclopramide	c‡ √√		n	p	n	√	√√	n	√√	
Haloperidol	√√ c†	n		√	n	√√	√	√	p	√√
Cyclizine	c* √√	p	√		√	c	√	√√	p	p
Methotrimeprazine	√√	n	n	√		√√	√	√	p	√√
Midazolam	√√	√	√√	c	√√		√	√	p	√√

Hyoscine hydrobromide	√√	√√	√	√	n	√√
Hyoscine butylbromide	√√	n	√	√	n	
Dexamethasone	c	√√	p	p	p	p
Octreotide	√√	√√	p	√√	√√	p

√√ compatible at therapeutic concentrations—some published evidence.

√ compatible at therapeutic concentrations—common usage but no published evidence.

c = caution at higher concentrations.

p = likely to precipitate

n = generally not a clinically useful combination (same group of drug or counteracting effects)

* Stable up to diamorphine up to 20 mg/ml + cyclizine up to 20 mg/ml (Figure 22.2). This implies that 150 mg of cyclizine (standard 24 h dose) will mix safely with up to 200 mg diamorphine in a 10 ml infusion). Higher concentrations of diamorphine are probably only stable with lower concentrations of cyclizine. Diamorphine any concentration + cyclizine up to 6.7 mg/ml (i.e. 67 mg of cyclizine in 10 ml infusion or 130 mg in a 20 ml infusion is stable with diamorphine at doses >200 mg in 10 ml or >400 mg in 20 ml).

† Stable up to diamorphine up to 10 mg/ml + haloperidol up to 1 mg/ml (i.e. diamorphine 100 mg is stable with up to 10 mg of haloperidol in a 10 ml infusion). Also stable up to diamorphine any concentration + haloperidol up to 0.75 mg/ml: (i.e. 7.5 mg of haloperidol is the maximum stable dose to use with >100 mg diamorphine in a 10 ml infusion).

‡ Stable up to diamorphine up to 25 mg/ml + metoclopramide up to 5 mg/ml (i.e. diamorphine 250 mg is stable with up to 50 mg of metoclopramide in a 10 ml infusion).

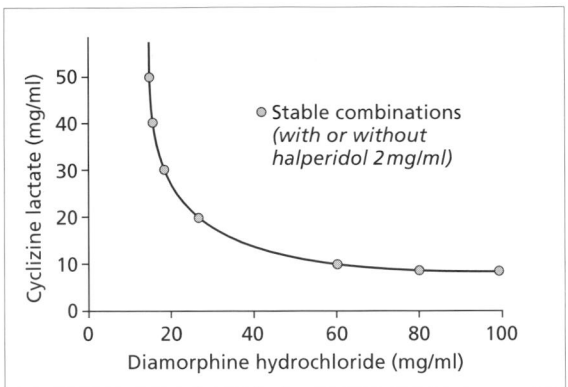

Fig. 22.2 A graph showing the stability and compatibility of diamorphine and cyclizine combinations in water for injections after storage for 24 hours at room temperature in plastic syringes. From [24] with permission.

• Diamorphine up to 70 mg/ml + midazolam up to 4 mg/ml + haloperidol up to 0.5 mg/ml (700 mg diamorphine + 40 mg midazolam + 5 mg haloperidol).
• Diamorphine up to 45 mg/ml + methotrimeprazine up to 7.5 mg/ml + hyoscine hydrobromide up to 1.2 mg/ml.

Concluding remarks

Overenthusiastic and indiscriminate use of the syringe driver should be avoided. Many drugs can be given effectively by other routes (e.g. sublingual, buccal, rectal, transdermal). Opioids administered via a syringe driver do not give 'better' analgesia than when given orally unless there is a problem with absorption or administration via the latter route. However, should a parenteral route be necessary, in most instances subcutaneous administration is preferable to the intravenous or intramuscular routes [34]. Once symptoms are controlled, it is often possible to reconvert medications to the oral formulations.

Appendix

Instructions for the use of Graseby model syringe drivers

As Graseby models are the most widely used they will be described here. Although the same principles apply it is essential that manufacturer's instructions are followed where other makes are employed:

1   Insert battery; alarm will sound for a few seconds.

2   Press start/boost button. Motor will run for a short while as safety circuits are checked.

3   Release start button.

4   Set the rate of delivery. Since the syringe bore varies with different manufacturers what is important is not the volume but the *length* of the infusion fluid.

(a) The rate of delivery is calculated as:

$$\frac{\text{length of infusion volume}}{\text{delivery time}}$$

For example, 48 mm in 24 hours.

(b) The MS 16 is set at mm/h (usually 0.2 mm per hour).

(c) The MS 26 is set at mm/day (usually 48 mm per 24 hour).

(d) For most makes of 10 ml syringes the volume of fluid for 48 mm is 9–10 ml.

(e) For the BD plastipak 10 ml syringe the volume ifs approximately 8 ml.

5   Draw up the medication into the syringe and dilute to the appropriate volume with sterile water for injection.

Note: in calculating the total volume, sufficient solution needs to be made up to allow for 'priming' the giving set, i.e. filling the whole line including all Luer connections. For most sets this 'dead space' accounts for an extra 0.5–1.0 ml (Baxter microvolume set: 0.5 ml, Graseby 100 cm: 0.75 ml).

6   Start driver by pressing start/boost button—light will flash every 20–25 seconds.

Note: driver can only be switched off by removing battery.

7   Protect mixture from light by using a holster or carry case.

References

1   Russell PSB. Analgesia in terminal malignant disease. *BMJ* 1979; I: 1561.

2   Dickinson RJ, Howard B, Campbell J. The relief of pain by subcutaneous infusion of diamorphine. In: Wilkes E, Lenz J, eds. *Advances in Morphine Therapy*. The 1983 International Symposium on Pain Control. Royal Society of Medicine International Symposium series, no. 64. London: Royal Society of Medicine, 1984: 105–110.

3   Oliver DJ. The use of the syringe driver in terminal care. *Br J Clin Pharmacol* 1985; 20: 515–516.

4   Coyle N, Mauskop A, Maggard J, Foley KM. Continuous subcutaneous infusions of opiates in cancer patients with pain. *Oncol Nurs For* 1986; 13: 53–57.

5   Beswick DT. Use of syringe driver in terminal care. *Pharm J* 1987; 239: 656–658.

6   Burera E, Brenneis C, Michaud M, Chadwick S, MacDonald RN. Continuous

subcutaneous infusion of narcotics using a portable disposable device in patients with advanced cancer. *Ca Treat Rep* 1987; 71: 635–637.

7   Bottomley DM, Hanks GW. Subcutaneous midazolam infusion in palliative care. *J Pain Symptom Manage* 1990; 5: 259–261.

8   Jones VA, Murphy A, Hanks GW. Solubility of diamorphine. *Pharm J* 1985; 235: 426.

9   Bruera E, Fainsinger R, Moore M *et al*. Clinical note: local toxicity with subcutaneous methadone. Experience of two centres. *Pain* 1991; 45: 141–143.

10 Fainsinger R, Schoeller T, Bruera E. Methadone in the management of cancer pain: a review. *Pain* 1993; 52: 137–147.

11 Luczak J, Dickenson AH, Kotlinska-Lemieszek A. The role of Ketamine, an NMDA receptor antagonist, in the management of pain. *Prog Palliat Care* 1995; 3: 127–134.

12 Mercadante S. Ketamine in cancer pain: an update. *Palliat Med* 1996; 10: 225–230.

13 Paix A, Coleman A, Lees J *et al*. Subcutaneous fentanyl and sufentanil infusion substitution for morphine intolerance in cancer pain management. *Pain* 1995; 63: 263–269.

14 Luczak J, Kotlinska A, Sopata M, Baczyk E, Porzucek I. Patient-controlled analgesia with Tramadol in palliative care. 7th World Congress on Pain, Paris, 1993.

15 Blackwell N, Bangham L, Hughes M, Melzack D, Trotman I. Subcutaneous Ketorolac—a new development in pain control. *Palliat Med* 1993; 7: 63–65.

16 Toscani F, Barosi K, Scazzina M *et al*. Sodium naproxen: continuous subcutaneous infusion in neoplastic pain control. *Palliat Med* 1989; 3: 207–211.

17 Oliver DJ. The use of Methotrimeprazine in terminal care. *Br J Clin Pract* 1985; 39: 339–340.

18 Baines M. Management of intestinal obstruction. *Baillière's Clinical Oncology* 1987; 1: 357–371.

19 Amesbury BDW, Dunphy KP. The use of subcutaneous Midazolam in the home care setting. *Palliat Med* 1989; 3: 299–301.

20 Bleasel MD, Peterson GM, Dunne PF. Plasma concentrations of Midazolam during continuous subcutaneous administration in palliative care. *Palliat Med* 1994; 8: 231–236.

21 De Conno F, Caraceni A, Zecca E, Spoldi E, Ventaridda V. Continuous subcutaneous infusion of hyoscine butylbromide reduced secretions in patients with gastrointestinal obstruction. *J Pain Symptom Manage* 1991; 6: 484–486.

22 Bausewein C, Twycross R. Comparative cost of hyoscine injections. *Palliat Med* 1995; 9: 256.

23 Riley J, Fallon MT. Octreotide in terminal malignant obstruction of the gastrointestinal tract. *Euro J Palliat Care* 1994; 1: 23–25.

24 Grassby PF, Hutchings L. Drug combinations in syringe drivers: the compatibility and stability of diamorphine with cyclizine and haloperidol. *Palliat Med* 1997; 11: 217–224.

25 Johnson I, Patterson S. Drugs used in combination in the syringe driver—a survey of hospice practice. *Palliat Med* 1992; 6: 125–130.

26 Allwood MC. Diamorphine mixed with antiemetic drugs in plastic syringes. *Br J Pharmaceutical Pract* 1984; 6: 88–90.

27 Collins AJ, Abethell JA, Holmes SG, Bain R. Stability of diamorphine hydrochloride

with haloperidol in prefilled syringes for subcutaneous infusion. *J Pharm Pharmacol* 1986; 38 (Suppl.): 51.

28 Regnard C, Pashley S, Westrope F. Anti-emetic/diamorphine compatibility in infusion pumps. *Br J Pharmaceutical Pract* 1986; 8: 218–220.

29 Allwood MC. The compatibility of high dose diamorphine with cyclizine or haloperidol in plastic syringes. *Int J Pharmacy Pract* 1991; 5: 120.

30 Allwood MC. The stability of diamorphine alone and in combination with anti-emetics in plastic syringes. *Palliat Med* 1991; 5: 330–333.

31 Allwood MC, Brown PC, Lee M. Stability of injections containing diamorphine and midazolam in plastic syringes. *Int J Pharmacy Pract* 1994; 3: 57–59.

32 Fawcett JP, Woods DJ, Munasiri B, Becket G. Compatibility of cyclizine lactate and haloperidol lactate. *Am J Hosp Pharm* 1994; 51: 2292.

33 Grassby PF. Personal communication, 1996.

34 Hanks GW, Conno Fde, Rpamonti C, Ventafridda V *et al*. Morphine in Cancer Pain: Modes of Administration. Expert Working Group of the European Association for Palliative Care. *BMJ* 1996; 312: 823–826.

Further reading

David J. A survey of the use of syringe drivers in Marie Curie Centres. *Euro J Cancer Care* 1992; 1: 23–28.

Dover SB. Syringe driver in terminal care. *BMJ* 1987; 294: 553–555.

Nicholson H. The success of the syringe driver. *Nursing Times* 9 July 1986: 49–51.

Oliver DJ. Syringe drivers in palliative care: A review. *Palliat Med* 1988; 2: 21–26.

Useful Addresses

Palliative care services information

Association of Community Health Councils
30 Drayton Park, London N5 1PB
Tel. 0171 6098405

British Lymphology Society
PO Box 1059, Caterham, Surrey

Hospice Information Service
St Christopher's Hospice, 51–59 Lawrie Park Road, Sydenham, London
SE26 6D2
Tel. 0181 7789252

Hospice Pharmacists' Association
Membership Secretary: Tel. 01727 858657 ext. 217
Professional Relations Officer (Mary Allen): Tel. 01442 252314

Mildmay Mission Hospital (AIDS Hospice)
Hackney Road, London E2 7NA
Tel. 0171 7392331

Milestone House (AIDS Hospice)
113 Oxgangs Road North, Edinburgh EH14 1EB
Tel. 0131 4416989

National Council for Hospice and Specialist Palliative Care Services
7th Floor, 1 Great Cumberland Place,
London, W1H 7AL
Tel. 0171 7231639

Association for Palliative Medicine of Great Britain and Ireland
11 Westwood Road, Southampton, SO17 1DL
Tel. 01703 672888

Research Council for Complementary Medicine
60 Great Ormond Street, London, WC1N 3JF
Tel. 0171 8338897

Patient/carer support groups

AIDS Ahead (for the deaf)
Unit 17, Macon Court, Herald Drive, Crewe, Cheshire CW1 1EA
Voice: 01270 250736 *or*
Text: 01270 250743

Alzheimer's Disease Society
Gordon House, 10 Greencoat Place, London SW1P 1PH
Tel. 0171 3060606

Association for Children with life threatening or Terminal conditions
and their families (ACT)
65 St Michael's Hill, Bristol BS2 8DZ

BACUP (cancer information and support)
3 Bath Place, Rivington Street, London EC2A 3JR
Tel. 0171 6132121

Blackliners
Eurolink Centre, 49 Effra Road, London SW2 1BZ
Tel. 0171 7387468

Body Positive (HIV support)
51B Philbeach Gardens, London SW5 9EB
Tel. 0171 3735237

Cancer Care Society
21 Zetland Road, Redland, Bristol BS6 7AH
Tel. 0117 9427419

Cancer Link (directory of cancer support and self-help)
17 Britannia Street, London WC1X 9JN
Tel. 0171 8332451

Carers' National Association
20–25 Glasshouse Yard, London EC1A 4JS
Tel. 0171 4908818

'Changing Faces' (support for people with head and neck cancers)
1 & 2 Junction Mews, London W2 1PN
Tel. 0171 7064232

Child Death Helpline (a confidential helpline for anyone affected by the death of a child)
Tel. 0800 282986

Contact a family (support for families caring for children with disabilities and special needs)
170 Tottenham Court Road, London W1P 0HA
Tel. 0171 3833555

Disabled Living Centre Information Service
Disabled Living Foundation (DLF), 380–384 Harrow Road, London W9 2HU
Tel. 0171 2896111

Huntington's Disease Association
108 Battersea High Street, London SW11 3HP
Tel. 0171 2237000

Let's Face It (support for people with head and neck cancers)
14 Fallowfield, Yateley, Surrey GU17 7LW
Tel. 0181 9312827 (London office)

London Lighthouse (AIDS hospice: information and support)
111–117 Lancaster Road, London W11 1QT
Tel. 0171 7921200

MacFarlane Trust (haemophilia)
PO Box 627, London SW1H 0QH
Tel. 0171 2330342

Mainliners
38–40 Kennington Park Road, London SE11 4RS
Tel. 0171 5825434

Motor Neurone Disease Association
David Niven House, 10–15 Notre Dame Mews, Northampton NN1 2PR
Tel. 01604 250505
MNDA Helpline: Tel. 0345 626262

Multiple Sclerosis Society
25 Effie Road, Fulham, London sw6 1ee
Tel. 0171 6107171

National Association of Citizen's Advice Bureaux
115–123 Pentonville Road, London n1 9lz
Tel. 0171 8332181 and in local directories

Naz Project (Asian HIV/AIDS)
Palingswick House, 241 King Street, London w6 9lp
Tel. 0181 7411879

Parkinson's Disease Society
215 Vauxhall Bridge Road, London sw1v 1ej
Tel. 0171 9318080

Positive Partners and Positively Children
The Annexe, Jan Rebane Centre, 12–14 Thornston Street,
London sw9 obl
Tel. 0171 7387333

Terrence Higgins Trust
52–54 Grays Inn Road, London wc1x 8ju
Tel. 0171 8310330

Home Office Drugs Branch
Room 230, 50 Queen Anne's Gate
London sw19 9at
Tel. 0171 2733000

Index

cytomegalovirus (CMV) infections 205,
   208, 213
   gastrointestinal 215
   peripheral neuropathy 221
   retinitis 217

dantrolene sodium 128, 231
day-care units 25, 28
deafferentation pain 104
death
   anxiety 74–5
   certificate 208, 330–31
   denial 89
   diagnosis 320
   with dignity 68
   fear of 74–5, 89, 93, 237
   at home 48
   lack of experience of 88–9
   leading causes 45
   numbers in local population 44, 45
   procedures after 320–7
   religious practices 320, 328–9
   in society 74–6
death rattle 315–17
decubitus ulcers *see* pressure sores
degenerative disorders, in children 257,
   261–2
dehydration
   in dying patients 70–1
   in hypercalcaemia 188
demulcents 160
denial 95, 284
   complementary therapy increasing 336
   death 89
dentures 155
depression
   asthenia/cachexia and 275
   in breathlessness 163
   on hearing bad news 93
   missed diagnosis 68
   in motor neurone disease 237
dermatitis
   contact, in lymphoedema 301
   seborrhoeic 218
despair 93
developing countries 5
dextromethorphan 160 1, 170
dextromoramide 112, 120
dextropropoxyphene 112
diabetes mellitus 188, 276
diamorphine 111, 113, 116
   after fentanyl patch discontinuation
      119–20
   in breathlessness 170, 173
   in drug users 209, 210–11
   fentanyl patch size and 118
   in gastrointestinal obstruction 143
   relative potency 112
   in severe pain 132

spinal 130
subcutaneous infusion 361, 362
   compatibility with other drugs 368–9,
      370
   stability in mixtures 369–72
   in terminal phase 238, 328
diarrhoea 198
   in AIDS 214–16
Diazemuls 316, 320
diazepam
   in breathlessness 172, 233
   in motor neurone disease 236
   in severe pain 132
   in stridor 253
   in terminal phase 314, 316, 320
diclofenac 124, 363
diet
   in gastrointestinal obstruction 144–5
   healthy 339–40, 341
   supplements 279–80, 340, 341
   see also feeding; nutrition
dietary interventions 339–42
   adverse effects 342
   indications and evidence 340–2
dietary regimes, complete 340, 341
dietician 22
diflunisal 124
dihydrocodeine 111, 112, 170
disability, in motor neurone disease 229,
   234–5
discharge planning 35–6
district nurse 18
diuretics, in lymphoedema 304–5
doctors 16
   barriers to communication 89–90
   communication between 96–7
   in community care 17–18
   palliative medicine 17, 26
   see also general practitioners
docusate, sodium 143, 147, 150
domiciliary specialist medical opinion
   17–18
domperidone 139, 153
dorsal root ganglion block 129
Dosett weekly pill dispenser 40, 41
dothiepin 126
double effect principle 69
dressings
   for fungating wounds 292
   for pressure sores 289, 290
drugs
   in asthenia and cachexia 278–9
   controlled *see* controlled drugs
   diarrhoea-inducing 216
   emergency
      acute terminal events 320
      availability in home 35–7, 261, 321
   fatigue due to 275–6
   inducing nausea 138